医学论文英文摘要写作

A Guide to Writing English Abstract for Medical Research Paper

第 3 版

李朝品　王先寅　编著

科学出版社

北京

内 容 简 介

本书是一部医学论文英文摘要写作指南，共十一章。第一章为概论，总体介绍了摘要写作的意义、分类及基本要求；第二章至第七章详细讲解了医学论文英文摘要写作的核心要素，包括内容和语言措辞等；第八章系统地概述了摘要写作中的数值表达；第九章讲解了语法修辞。此外，根据我国作者在英文摘要写作方面的习惯，第十章特别介绍了摘要翻译的原则和方法。第十一章为英文摘要写作中常见错误分析，从词法、句法到篇章逻辑结构，分析了作者在写作中的常见失误。本书附录包含致谢和投稿信的撰写方式，论文文后参考文献著录标准和格式，以及典型期刊摘要结构及版式，可为读者提供更直观的参考模板。

本书可作为医学院校本科生和研究生的教学用书，也可供广大医务工作者、医学科研人员撰写医学论文英文摘要时参考，同时可为医学院校专业英语教师提供教学设计思路及第一手备课资料。

图书在版编目（CIP）数据

医学论文英文摘要写作 / 李朝品，王先寅编著. —3 版. —北京：科学出版社，2021.3
ISBN 978-7-03-068157-7

Ⅰ. ①医… Ⅱ. ①李… ②王… Ⅲ. ①医学-英语-论文-写作 Ⅳ. ①R

中国版本图书馆 CIP 数据核字（2021）第 034534 号

责任编辑：杨小玲 董 婕 高峥荣/责任校对：杨 赛
责任印制：赵 博/封面设计：陈 敬

科学出版社 出版
北京东黄城根北街 16 号
邮政编码：100717
http://www.sciencep.com
天津市新科印刷有限公司 印刷
科学出版社发行 各地新华书店经销
*
2004 年 2 月第 一 版 由人民卫生出版社出版
2021 年 3 月第 三 版 开本：787×1092 1/16
2021 年 3 月第一次印刷 印张：27
字数：633 000
定价：88.00 元
（如有印装质量问题，我社负责调换）

前　　言

随着科技全球化，国际间学术交流日益频繁，对专业技术人员英语水平要求也越来越高。为实现高效、快捷、广泛的医学研究成果共享与交流，美国国立医学图书馆创建的基于 MEDLINE 为来源的检索数据库 PubMed，为广大读者提供了信息获取平台。PubMed 收录的文献数据核心为医学及与医学相关领域的健康科学研究成果，我国出版的中文期刊中华系列医学杂志上所刊载的医学论文英文摘要均被收录于该数据库。

改革开放数十载，虽然我国在英语教学手段和方法方面尝试了一系列改革举措和创新，并取得了长足进步，但是，广大医学生和医疗卫生工作者因语言环境所限，对医学专业英语掌握仍然不够，尤其是写作能力。医学英语作为专业用途英语（English for specific purposes，ESP），无论从语义、语用及文体特征方面均有别于通用英语（general English）。因此，只有掌握 ESP 的特点，才可写出得体的英文摘要，从而实现医学科研成果精准而无障碍的交流。为帮助广大医学生、医疗卫生工作者及医学科研人员提升医学论文英文摘要写作能力，我们曾于 2004 年首次编写出版了《医学论文英文摘要写作》。本书的雏形是我们给医学本科生、研究生讲授专业英语的教学资料，后期在教学过程中不断完善而成，在此基础上，本书于 2009 年再版。

《医学论文英文摘要写作》是一部针对医学论文英文摘要写作的指南用书，由多年从事专业英语教学及医学教育的专家学者共同努力撰写而成。所引实例资料：一是取材于国内外部分主流医学期刊，为读者提供真实的原始语言素材；二是作者历年在教学、编校审稿过程中所收集的案头资料，这些语言资料既是精华荟萃，又是经验积累。编写的内容博取众家之长，全面、系统地概述了医学论文英文摘要写作的所有要素，同时还介绍了英文摘要写作中的语言修辞及中文摘要翻译方法等内容。常见错误分析，以及分散于各章节有关摘要的写作重点、难点分析讲解，可帮助读者克服母语负迁移所带来的影响。

《医学论文英文摘要写作》自 2004 年问世以来，一直深受广大读者的认可与青睐。然而，越是众赐厚爱，越让我们倍感不安，作为一部指导英文摘要写作的专著，既不能写成百科全书式，也不能写成万花筒式。百科全书虽可包罗万象，但势必增加读者的负担，甚至导致读者无所适从，而万花筒看起来较美，但五颜六色也会造成视觉疲劳。因此，十几年来，我们一直在反思、斟酌，通过教学调研、同行讨论，以期进一步完善，终于形成了第 3 版。

全书由十一章及四个附录构成，全面介绍了医学论文英文摘要写作的要素。第一章为概论，总体介绍了英文摘要写作的意义、分类及基本要求。第二章至第七章详细讲解了医学论文英文摘要写作的核心要素，包括内容和语言措辞等。第八章系统地概述了英文摘要写作中的数值表达。第九章讲解了语法修辞。根据我国作者在英文摘要写作方面的习惯，第十章特别介绍了摘要翻译的原则和方法。第十一章为英文摘要写作中常见错误分析，从词法、句法到篇章逻辑结构，分析了我国作者在写作中的常见失误。附录包含了致谢和投稿信撰写方式、论文文后参考文献著录标准和格式及典型期刊摘要结构及版式，可为读者提供更直观、更快捷的参考模板。

本书以近几十年来应用语言学领域研究成果为基础，从语义、语用，对比语言学角度系统讲解了医学论文英文摘要写作，其主要特色如下。

第一，准确实用。书中所选实证资料取材于国内外部分主流医学期刊，采用英汉/汉英对照编排，读者不仅能从中体验到真实的原始语言素材，而且可以通过中英对照，体悟汉语和英语语言在专业表达上的异同；以模仿语言习得为学习过程，从而高效地提高自己的写作能力。

第二，全面新颖。虽然市场上有类似的著作，但个性化特征明显，未能详尽阐述英文摘要写作中的相关重点、难点，而本书编写以教学实践与审稿中总结的经验和教训为基础，博采众家之长，内容更为系统、全面。

第三，针对性强。本书主体尽管是针对医学论文英文摘要写作的专著，但不限于此。全书不仅详尽分析了英文摘要写作中的所有要素，而且介绍了英文摘要翻译方法和常见错误分析、关键词的选取、语法修辞、英语基本句型及其扩展等，这些内容均可为作者提供借鉴资料。

第四，受众群体更广泛。本书可作为教学用书，供医学院校本科生、研究生学习之用，可为从事医学专业英语教学的教师提供教学备课资料；也可供医疗卫生工作者、医学科研人员撰写医学论文英文摘要时参考。

本书引用了大量的文献资料，尤其是我们长期在教学过程中收集的资料，但因时间过久，无法确认出处，只能在此深表感谢与歉意。我们期盼完美，但本书势必存在瑕疵。正所谓"旁观者清"，但愿不要因为我们在某些问题方面的一家之言而给读者带来误导。同时，我们也希望得到同行专家、学者的赐教。另外，有两方面问题需要说明，一是，本书为语言学习用书，书中某些例证资料的时效与专业研究进展是不同的两件事，即我们需要掌握的是语言，而非医学研究进展；二是，一些引自国内中文期刊的例证，有中英文不对应现象，以及个别统计学数据瑕疵，为尊重原刊，本书引用时不做任何处理，希望读者阅读时重点关注英语语言素材本身，书中所附中文翻译主要用于辅助理解。本书编者学识有限，书中难免存在瑕疵，敬请读者给予批评指正。

李朝品

2020 年 5 月

第 2 版前言

岁月不居。屈指数来，《医学论文英文摘要写作》首版已五载有余。如今，大小书店却难觅其踪，由此看来，本书还是得到了广大读者的认可，这也让编者倍感欣慰和一丝鼓励。欣喜之余，不免也有些惆怅。用什么来回馈广大读者的厚爱？唯有使原著进一步完善。两年前，我们着手材料收集工作，为此次修订再版做了充分准备。

随着科技全球化，国际学术交流日益频繁，社会对专业技术人员的外语水平要求也越来越高。改革开放数十载，我国在外语教学手段和方法方面尝试了一系列的改革和创新并取得了长足的进步，但广大的外语学习者，尤其主修医学科学的学习者由于受到种种客观条件限制，对医学专业英语的掌握还十分薄弱。因此，很难满足他们的工作、学习和学术交流的需要。同时，为了与国外同行进行信息交流，我国国内主办的各类医学学术期刊均要求写出英文摘要。虽然有为数不多的涉及此类写作的专著，遗憾的是，这些著作基本上是单纯讲述写作格式及一般表达，未能全面分析医学英语的特点。

医学英语为医务人员、各临床部门在临床应用、科研及教学、医学基础及医学服务等实践中所使用的专门语言（English for specific purposes）。无论从语义、语用及文体特征，医学英语均有别于通用英语（general English）。因为专用英语有其自身的特点：①满足特定行业的需要，在某些学科内使用；②涉及的内容特殊，即专门化的内容。例如"老年患者"，从语用及伦理角度看，宜用"elderly patients"而禁忌"old patients"。又如"疾病"，与之对应的英语表达有"disease；illness；sickness；condition；trouble；affection；ailment；complaint；indisposition；disorder；malady；lesion"，根据语义学理论，词汇可以在一个共同概念的支配下结合在一起，而两个或几个不同的词项具有相同（或相近）的成分定义，就成为同义词。据此，当我们需要表述这一概念时，该如何选择？对于医学写作中的语态使用问题，通常众说纷纭。在语言实践中，又该如何取舍？诸如此类的问题无时无刻不困扰着我们学习者和作者。本书对此做了深入分析与释疑。

鉴于《医学论文英文摘要写作》已经出版数载，我们不仅在使用中发现了某些不足，同时也收到了广大热心读者的中肯建议。此次修订仍然沿用首版的十个章节，但突出了以下几个方面：①更换了首版中大量例证，在注意内、外刊兼顾的原则前提下，大量例证直接取材于在国际医学领域具有极高影响力的外刊，英语为其母语的英、美作者，目的是为读者提供更地道的（authentic）的原始语料素材；②吸收了近十几年来应用语言学在医学英语方面的最新研究成果，如语义学、语用学、等效翻译理论等，以便那些深受母语（汉语）思维习惯干扰的读者体察英、汉语言在表达上的差异；③针对我国作者在写作中常犯的语言措辞不当之错，为了避免与其他专著重复，删除了首版第八章"医学论文中动词语态与时态"，同时，借助于作者自建的医学英语语料库以及在长期审稿工作中所积累的资料，增写了"英文摘要写作中常见错误分析"；④各章节后增加了相应的练习，为读者提供了更多的语言实践机会；⑤以常见的结构式摘要为主，兼顾其他类型，如"资料性摘要"等。总之，此次修订不仅做了大篇幅的资料更新，而且内容更为翔实，覆盖面更广。

　　千虑必有一失。叩盼各位专家学者及广大热心读者不吝赐教，以期日后更为完善，为我国医学研究进一步参与到国际交流而尽绵薄之力。

李朝品

2003 年 6 月于芜湖

第 1 版前言

时代的列车已驶入 21 世纪，医学科学也进入到一个高速发展的新时期，医学界每天都有大量论著问世，学术论著的交流和传播对医学科学的发展起着重要的促进作用。要跻身医学科学的国际学术交流，写好医学论文，尤其是写好医学论文英文摘要是非常重要的环节。为了使学生在学习过程中，能对医学论文写作的基础知识有所了解，我们在教学过程中开设了医学写作的辅修课程，受到了学生的欢迎，也积累了一些资料，形成了课堂教学的教案。鉴于国内有关如何撰写医学论文英文摘要的教材尚少，现将《医学论文英文摘要写作》的教案进行整理充实，印刷出版，以期对撰写医学论文英文摘要能有所帮助。

本书着眼于医学专业论文英文摘要的写作，简明扼要地介绍了医学论文英文摘要的标题、作者与单位的书写、内容、结构、数值表达法、动词的时态和语态、语法修辞、常用句型及例句等。因由教案整理而来，本书适用于医学院校本科生、研究生、青年教师、临床医师、护师等学习之用和撰写医学论文英文摘要时参考，也适合于专业英语教师开设医学写作辅修课程教学参考等。

本书的素材主要来源于在医学写作上具有权威性的文献和专著，例句和例文主要摘引自部分国外医学期刊和中华医学系列期刊；有关院校的同行和学生也为本书提出不少建设性意见和建议，正是由于他们的关心和支持，使得该教案能得以形成，在此对大家的关心和支持表示衷心感谢！

由于作者水平有限，本书欠妥之处在所难免，欢迎读者批评指正，以利完善、修订。

李朝品

2003 年 6 月于淮南

目　　录

前言

第 2 版前言

第 1 版前言

第一章　概论 …………………………………………………………………………… 1

一、医学论文英文摘要的撰写意义 ………………………………………… 1

二、英文摘要分类 ……………………………………………………………… 2

三、结构式英文摘要写作内容及格式 …………………………………… 7

四、练习 …………………………………………………………………………… 19

第二章　医学论文英文标题写作 ……………………………………………… 21

一、英文标题组成 ……………………………………………………………… 22

二、英文标题句式 ……………………………………………………………… 26

三、英、汉标题比较 …………………………………………………………… 35

四、英文标题中冠词省略及常见名词与介词搭配 ………………… 50

五、英文标题概念表达常用句式结构 ………………………………… 62

六、练习 …………………………………………………………………………… 67

第三章　医学论文英文署名与工作单位 …………………………………… 70

一、署名 …………………………………………………………………………… 70

二、工作单位及属地 …………………………………………………………… 74

三、练习 …………………………………………………………………………… 89

第四章　医学论文英文摘要"Objective"写作 ………………………… 91

一、非动词不定式引导的"Objective" …………………………………… 91

二、动词不定式引导的"Objective" ……………………………………… 95

三、"Objective"句中动词形式的选择 …………………………… 108

四、练习 …………………………………………………………… 109

第五章 医学论文英文摘要"Methods"写作 …………………………… 111

一、"Methods"写作中应包含的内容 ……………………………… 112

二、"Methods"写作中的表达方法 ………………………………… 119

三、主要研究手段的表述 …………………………………………… 125

四、研究方案的表述 ………………………………………………… 127

五、"Methods"写作中的常用动词及词组 ……………………… 130

六、"Methods"句中动词形式的确定 …………………………… 140

七、"Methods"写作中常用"方法、手段" ……………………… 142

八、练习 …………………………………………………………… 145

第六章 医学论文英文摘要"Results"写作 ……………………………… 148

一、"Results"总体写作要求 ……………………………………… 148

二、"Results"写作中的常用词及短语 ………………………… 152

三、"Results"写作中的难点和重点 …………………………… 174

四、多个实验结果的英文表述 ……………………………………… 181

五、"Results"写作中的一些常见错误 ………………………… 186

六、练习 …………………………………………………………… 187

第七章 医学论文英文摘要"Conclusion"写作 ………………………… 190

一、"Conclusion"写作内容 ……………………………………… 191

二、"Conclusion"句与语篇连接 ………………………………… 200

三、功能篇："可能性"表示法 …………………………………… 207

四、"Conclusion"句中几个常用动词特殊用法及其结构 ……… 209

五、其他常用表达法 ………………………………………………… 213

六、"Conclusion"句中动词形式的确定和语态 ……………… 216

七、练习 …………………………………………………………… 220

第八章 医学论文英文摘要写作中的数值表达 ……………………… 223

一、整合数量的表达 ………………………………………………… 223

二、平均数的表达 …………………………………………………… 224

三、百分数、比例及率的表达 ……………………………………228

四、数量增减的表达 ………………………………………………238

五、极限数的表达 …………………………………………………240

六、倍数的表达 ……………………………………………………242

七、其他数值表达 …………………………………………………244

八、练习 ……………………………………………………………256

第九章　医学论文英文摘要语法修辞 …………………………………259

一、主谓一致 ………………………………………………………259

二、非谓语动词 ……………………………………………………270

三、平行结构 ………………………………………………………282

四、复合句 …………………………………………………………285

五、省略与替代 ……………………………………………………289

六、简明与冗余 ……………………………………………………294

七、离散与集合 ……………………………………………………301

八、摘要写作常用比较结构 ………………………………………303

九、写作基本句型及其扩展 ………………………………………311

十、倒装结构及其应用 ……………………………………………314

十一、语态与人称 …………………………………………………316

十二、中英文标点符号 ……………………………………………321

十三、量、单位与符号 ……………………………………………324

十四、练习 …………………………………………………………327

第十章　英文摘要汉译英的原则与方法 ………………………………331

一、医学论文英文摘要的文体特征 ………………………………331

二、翻译的实质 ……………………………………………………331

三、英文摘要翻译标准 ……………………………………………331

四、英文摘要翻译方法 ……………………………………………332

五、练习 ……………………………………………………………353

第十一章　英文摘要写作中常见错误分析 ……………………………355

一、词法、词义类错误 ……………………………………………355

二、句法、语篇、逻辑类错误 ……………………………………371

三、关键词列举不当 ···································· 382

四、练习 ··· 384

附录 1 致谢（Acknowledgement） ············· 389

附录 2 投稿信（Cover letter） ················· 391

附录 3 研究论文文后参考文献书写 ············· 395

附录 4 典型摘要例证 25 篇 ···················· 398

练习参考答案 ································· 415

主要参考文献 ································· 416

第一章 概　　论

一、医学论文英文摘要的撰写意义

21 世纪是生命科学和信息科学的世纪，医学科学迅猛发展，新的医学知识快速积累，新理论、新技术不断涌现，几乎每天都有大量论著问世。同时，医学期刊的数量也在不断上升。以国内文献数据库为例，万方医学网与中国知网（CNKI）分别独家收录了医药卫生类出版物各 1200 余种（不考虑交叉收录比例）。中文生物医学期刊文献数据库（CMCC）收录的数量为 1400 余种，中国生物医学文献数据库收录了 2900 余种，约占科技期刊总量的 1/4。中华医学会主办的医学期刊已达 144 种。从国际范围看，PubMed 为公认的全球最大、最权威的生物医学数据库，收录了近万种生物医学期刊（据粗略统计，收录中国出版的期刊 100 余种），而 SpringerLink 则更为庞大。这些数字足以表明当今医学科学的发展。

为扩大科技信息交流范围，促进国际间科技合作，联合国教科文组织规定，全世界公开发表的科技论文，不论其文种，都必须附有短小精悍的英文摘要。我国国家标准局于 1982 年发布了《科技学术期刊编排规则》（GB 3179—82），1986 年又发布了《文摘编写规则》（GB 6447—86），提出生物医学论著须附有英文摘要。此后，国内大多数公开发行的医学刊物都附有论文的英文摘要。随着全球学术交流不断加强，为繁荣医学教育，提高医疗水平，传播医学知识，推动医学科学进步，撰写高质量的医学论文英文摘要显得尤为重要。

摘要（Abstract）是以提供文献内容梗概为目的，用客观、精练、简明的文字，将该文献重要内容呈现在正文之前，因此，摘要具有独立性（independent）与自含性（self-contained）的特点。其作用有三点：第一，为读者快速获取所需信息提供方便；第二，为文献编辑、杂志索引和情报检索提供直接的信息，尤其是目前国际上主要检索机构的数据库对英文摘要的依赖性日益增强；第三，为文献数据库的建立提供方便。读者无论是计算机检索还是翻阅期刊，通过摘要即可了解全文的主要内容，省时省力，事半功倍。不仅如此，结构完整、语言精练的英文摘要对于增加期刊和论文被检索和引用的机会、吸引读者、扩大学术影响起着不可估量的作用。

二、英文摘要分类

　　科技文摘的出现可追溯至 19 世纪 30 年代，当时科学技术的快速发展使得自然科学领域内学科越分越细，越分越多，科技期刊也日益增多。为促进科技信息交流，让读者及时掌握更多的科研信息，1830 年，在德国创刊了世界上第一部专业文摘杂志——《医学总览》，它就是著名文摘刊物《化学总览》的前身，*Canadian Medical Association Journal*（*CMAJ*，《加拿大医学会杂志》）亦率先在期刊上刊登摘要，随后 *The Journal of the American Medical Association*（*JAMA*，《美国医学会杂志》），*The Lancet*（*Lancet North Am Ed*，《柳叶刀》），*Annals of Internal Medicine*（*Ann Intern Med*，《内科学纪事》），*The New England Journal of Medicine*（*N Engl J Med*，《新英格兰医学杂志》）等多家杂志相继使用摘要。20 世纪 60 年代初，文摘开始出现在生物医学期刊上。20 世纪 70 年代，国外大部分生物医学期刊要求论文附有摘要项。

　　在我国，最早出现的科技文摘是 1934 年中国化学学会编印的《化学》杂志，其中辟有"中国化学摘要专栏"。早在 1973 年《中华医学杂志》率先在中国医学期刊中刊登论著类文章的英文摘要，随后，由中华医学会主办的中华系列医学杂志亦纷纷刊附论文的文摘项。1986 年，国家标准局颁布的《文摘编写规则》（GB 6447—86），对文摘（摘要）的编写提出了明确的规范，即规范了文摘的形式、文摘的详简度（文摘字数的限制）及文摘的要素（结构式摘要的四要素）等。

　　医学研究的内容与方法上的差异通常决定着摘要的结构，按格式分类，摘要可分为非结构式摘要（non-structured abstracts）和结构式摘要（structured abstracts）。若按文摘性质分类，生物医学摘要文体大致可分为报道性摘要、指示性摘要、报道-指示性摘要、结构式摘要四种。步入 21 世纪，随着学术期刊数量的急剧增加及互联网广泛应用于文献联机检索，前三种摘要均显示出一定的局限性，结构式摘要因此脱颖而出。结构式摘要由加拿大 McMaster 大学临床流行病学和生物统计学教授 R. Brian Haynes 博士及 *Annals of Internal Medicine* 杂志 Huth 主编于 1985 年共同倡导和提议。1987 年 4 月，*Annals of Internal Medicine* 杂志率先刊出结构式摘要的使用建议，并于同期开始使用。迄今，结构式摘要已被国际生物医学期刊普遍采用，我国也不例外。现将报道性摘要、指示性摘要、报道-指示性摘要和结构式摘要依次做一简要介绍，以便读者对四种摘要的优缺点有所了解。

（一）报道性摘要

　　报道性摘要（informative abstract），亦称资料性摘要，这类摘要通常是一篇完整的短文，属于传统性摘要（traditional abstract），其层次与正文内容一致，层层展开。内容包括研究目的及范围，使用的材料和方法，研究的结果、结论及对未来的展望。写作格式上不分段、节，字数一般不超过 250 个实词。特点：较完整地浓缩和概括论文的主要内容，尽可能多地提供定量和定性信息。因此，这类摘要语言精练、简明、准确，是一篇正文的微型化。涉及内容丰富，信息量大，参考价值高，使读者不阅读全文也能掌握其实质内容。

例一： **Abstract** Lichen planus (LP) of the lips is a rare condition that is generally associated with other parts of the oral mucosa. Lip localization has an increased risk, since external trauma, smoking and ultraviolet light trigger malignant transformation. Only a few cases of isolated LP of the lips have been reported up to now, but results of larger series on oral LP suggest that it might be underestimated. Treatment of oral LP is usually difficult and lesions are generally resistant or recur, so that novel therapy alternatives are necessary. Here we report four cases of isolated LP of the lip successfully treated with imiquimod 5% cream. It was applied twice daily, 5 days a week, for 2 weeks. Two weeks after therapy, complete clinical and histopathological resolution was observed. No recurrence was observed during the 5, 10 and 18 months' follow-up period in cases 4, 3 and 1, respectively. Clinical and histopathological cure was also observed in case 2, but the patient showed clinical activation after 6 months. We suggest that imiquimod 5% cream is a safe and effective therapeutic treatment for oral LP.

唇扁平苔藓（LP）是罕见病，常累及口腔其他部位黏膜。本病局限于唇部，发病风险会因外伤、吸烟、紫外线辐射诱发恶变后而增加。单发性唇扁平苔藓病例报道较为少见，但较大规模系列口腔扁平苔藓病例研究结果提示，人们低估了单发性唇扁平苔藓。口腔扁平苔藓治疗难，病损常顽固或复发，因此需要找到新的治疗方案。本文报道了应用 5%咪喹莫特软膏成功治疗 4 例单发性唇扁平苔藓。每天用药 2 次，每周 5 天，疗程 2 周。治疗 2 周后，临床病理显示完全治愈。病例 4、病例 3、病例 1 在 5、10、18 个月的随访期内未见复发。病例 2 亦达到临床病理治愈，但 6 个月后出现临床复发。研究结果显示，5%咪喹莫特软膏治疗口腔扁平苔藓安全有效。

【析】该摘要首先简要地介绍了相关研究背景，紧接着交代了研究方法和研究发现（结果），最后给出研究结论。整个摘要层次分明，即使不读全文，读者亦可了解整个研究脉络：研究背景→研究方法（药物临床疗效观察）→研究结果→结论。

引自：*J Dermatolog Treat*, 2011, 22(1): 55

例二： Tobacco smoking is the leading preventable cause of death worldwide. Both donor and recipient smoking have been shown to increase graft loss and mortality in solid organ transplant recipients in many studies. Only in lung transplants is smoking a universal contraindication to transplantation. Transplant centers implement different policies regarding smoking recipients and allografts from smoking donors. Due to scarcity of available allografts, the risks of smoking have to be weighed against the risks of a longer transplant waitlist period. Although transplant centers implement different strategies to encourage smoking cessation pre- and post-transplant, not many studies have been published that validate the efficacy of smoking cessation interventions in this vulnerable population. This article summarizes the results of studies investigating prevalence, impact on outcomes, and cessation interventions for smoking in the transplant population. We report herein a review of the elevated risks of infection, malignancy, graft loss, cardiovascular events, and mortality in solid organ transplant populations.

吸烟虽为全球主要致死原因，但可预防。许多研究表明，供体和受体双方有吸烟史都会增加实体器官移植受者的移植物失效和死亡率，只有在肺移植中，吸烟被普遍视为禁忌。移植中心对吸烟者和来自吸烟捐赠者的同种异体移植实施不同的策略。由于大量缺乏可用同种异体移植物，必须权衡吸烟的风险和更多需要接受移植者长期等待供体的风险。尽管移植中心在移植前和移植后实施了不同的策略来鼓励戒烟，但并没有多少研究来验证戒烟干预在这一易感人群中的有效性。本文综述了前期对吸烟人群的研究结果，包括吸烟流行率，吸烟对移植结果的影响，以及戒烟干预效果，同时报道了实体器官移植人群中感染的高风险因素、发生恶性肿瘤情况、移植物失效概率、心血管疾病发病情况和死亡率。

【析】该摘要分为两个层次。第一层介绍研究背景，即吸烟对移植的影响，以及目前存在的主要问题；第二层介绍了研究性质及研究主题，读者通过阅读摘要，可轻松知晓这是一篇综述类文献及其研究内容。

引自：*Am J Med*, 2019, 132(4): 413

（二）指示性摘要

指示性摘要（indicative abstract），也称为说明性摘要、描述性摘要（descriptive abstract）或论点摘要（topic abstract）。许多专业杂志在其目录页的标题下都有一个指示性摘要，特别是编者认为较重要的一些文章标题后。指示性摘要一般不涉及实质性材料，只做概括性介绍。它的内容和结构比较简单，一般只是说明论文的主题范围，不具体介绍研究方法和结果（An indicative abstract usually tells readers what information the paper contains, outline the purpose, methods, scope of the paper, and introduces the subject），通常只用两三个句子表达，多用于综述、会议报告等；其特点：指示文献的主题及取得成果的性质和水平，以使读者对该研究内容有大概的了解。其作用是给读者一个指示性的概括了解，以帮助读者决定是否需要进一步查阅原文。

例一： This review discusses current and future pharmacological approaches to the treatment of obesity, with a focus on the biological control of energy balance.

本综述讨论了目前和未来治疗肥胖的药理学方法，重点是能量平衡的生物控制。

【析】本摘要仅用一个句子概述了全文研究的主题是什么，简单明了。

引自：*Sci Transl Med*, 2016, 8(323): 323rv2

例二：Atherosclerosis is an inflammatory disease. Platelets can "inflame" the vascular wall by various mechanisms and thereby initiate and support the development of atherosclerosis. Platelet interaction with leukocytes, endothelial cells, and circulating progenitor cells triggers autocrine and paracrine activation processes, leading to inflammatory and atherogenic cascades at the vascular wall. This review highlights the molecular key components and pathways used by platelets to trigger and accelerate inflammation at the vascular wall and, thereby, atherosclerosis.

动脉粥样硬化是炎性疾病。血小板通过不同机制使血管壁"发炎"，由此诱发并促成动脉粥样硬化。血小板与粒细胞、内皮细胞和循环的前体细胞相互作用，触发自分泌和旁分泌过程，导致血管炎症和致动脉粥样硬化的级联反应。本文对血小板在血管触发和促进炎症进而形成动脉粥样硬化的分子结构的关键部分和途径进行重点综述。

【析】该摘要共用了 4 个句子。第 1 句介绍了研究主题，即动脉粥样硬化，第 2、3 句介绍了该病的病理生理机制，第 4 句重点提示该主题所涉及的范围。

引自：*Arterioscler Thromb Vasc Biol*, 2008, 3: 56

例三：Endothelial and smooth muscle cells interact with each other to form new blood vessels. In this review, the cellular and molecular mechanisms underlying the formation of endothelium-lined channels (angiogenesis) and their maturation via recruitment of smooth muscle cells (arteriogenesis) during physiological and pathological conditions are summarized, alongside with possible therapeutic applications.

内皮细胞和平滑肌细胞相互作用形成新的血管。本文主要综述了细胞和分子的潜在机制，即在生理或病理状态下，内皮通道的形成（血管生成）和因平滑肌细胞募集促其成熟过程（动脉生成），以及潜在的医疗价值。

【析】这是一篇文献综述摘要。第 1 句介绍相关背景（文献主题），第 2 句概括了综述的内容（主题范围），并同时指出该研究主题的应用价值。

引自：*Nat Med*, 2000, 6(4): 389

（三）报道-指示性摘要

报道-指示性摘要（informative-indicative abstract）是一种综合性摘要。虽然内容结构分为两个层面，但仍属于非结构式。其特点是对文献中信息价值较高的、重要的部分以报道性形式表达，而对其余的次要部分仅以指示性形式概括。报道-指示性摘要适用于在论文摘要类型和长度受到限制时对论文的重要部分做资料性介绍，而对次要部分仅做概括性介绍。

例一：A 60-year-old black man with poorly differentiated lymphocytic lymphoma presented with generalized lymphadenopathy and marked eosinophilia. Extensive evaluation of the eosinophils revealed them to be normal morphologically and functionally. The patient responded to corticosteroid therapy with resolution of the lymphadenopathy and reversion of the peripheral blood counts to normal limits. Recurrence of the original clinical picture within months prompted institution of systemic chemotherapy. Response was transient, and the patient expired after an unremitting downhill course. Recent advances in our knowledge of mechanisms of eosinophilia and eosinophil function are reviewed. The relationship of lymphoma to eosinophilia is discussed.

患者，黑色人种，60 岁，诊断为低分化淋巴细胞型淋巴瘤，伴全身性淋巴结肿大，嗜酸性粒细胞明显增多。对嗜酸性粒细胞进行全面检查研究发现，其形态与功能均属正常。经皮质素治疗后，患者淋巴结肿消退，周围血细胞计数恢复至正常范围。病情稳定数月后再次复发，随即施予全身化疗，但疗效维持短暂。患者病情再次恶化并最终死亡。本文综述了嗜酸性粒细胞增多症的发病机制和嗜酸性粒细胞功能研究的最新进展，并探讨了淋巴瘤与嗜酸性粒细胞增多症的关系。

【析】这篇摘要原文共 7 个句子。第 1、2 句介绍了患者的病名、主要症状及检查结果；第 3～5 句概括了治疗过程和效果；第 6 句是患者的结局；第 7 句是论文探讨的主要内容。

引自：*Cancer Res*, 2000, 14: 237

例二：Gastroenteropancreatic neuroendocrine tumors (GEP-NETs) are usually sporadic, however, familial (inherited) syndromes, such as the multiple endocrine neoplasia 1 (MEN-1) syndrome, von Hippel-Lindau (VHL) syndrome, neurofibromatosis (NF-1), as well as tuberous sclerosis, may be associated with proximal intestinal and pancreatic NETs. For example, 25% of gastrinoma patients have MEN-1 syndrome. Over the last two decades, the genetic basis of tumorigenesis for these familial syndromes has been clearly identified, providing clinicians with useful screening tools for affected families. Also, over the last few years, advanced molecular genetic techniques, such as comparative genomic hybridization (CGH) and loss of heterozygosity (LOH) analyses, have detected some differences in genomic aberrations among various types of NETs. Whether these chromosomic alterations have implications in the treatment of patients and the outcome of the disease is still unclear.

胃肠道胰腺神经内分泌肿瘤（GEP-NETs）通常表现为非广泛扩散，然而，如多发性内分泌肿瘤综合征 1 型（MEN-1）、von Hippel-Lindau 综合征（VHL）、神经纤维瘤（NF-1）和结节性硬化症等家族性遗传综合征和近端肠道，以及胰腺的神经内分泌肿瘤存在相关性。例如，25%的胃泌素瘤患者并发 MEN-1 综合征。过去 20 年中，这些家族性综合征肿瘤形成的遗传机制得到阐明，并且为医师提供了对这些家庭进行有效筛查的工具。此外，近年来，如比较基因杂交（CGH）和杂合性丢失（LOH）分析等先进分子遗传学技术可以检测到不同类型神经内分泌肿瘤中存在的基因改变。这些染色体改变对于疾病治疗和预后是否有意义目前仍不清楚。

【析】该摘要一共用了五个句子，前四句以报道性摘要的形式提示了文献中具有较高价值的信息，第五句则以指示性摘要的形式表述了这一研究的现状。

引自：*Am J Gastroenterol*, 2008, 103(3): 729

（四）结构式摘要

传统的摘要多为一段式，在内容上大致包括引言（Introduction）、材料与方法（Materials and Methods）、结果（Results）和讨论（Discussion）等主要方面，即 IMRAD（Introduction，Methods，Results and Discussion）结构的写作模式。

结构式摘要（structured abstract）实质上是报道性摘要的结构化表达，这一摘要写作形式出现于 20 世纪 80 年代中期。结构式摘要与传统摘要的差别在于，前者便于读者了解论文的内容，印刷版面中通常用醒目的字体（黑体、全部大写或斜体等）直接标示出"目的、方法、结果和结论"等标题。写作时，此类摘要按顺序列出项目的内容，一般包括目的、设计、地点、对象、处理方法、测试项目、结果、结论等，但可根据需要有所增减。较统一的项目包括"目的、方法、结果及结论"。其优点是内容简洁、完整、信息量大；观点明确，便于阅读；符合计算机数据库的存储和使用要求。本书主要介绍结构式英文摘要的写法及注意事项。

三、结构式英文摘要写作内容及格式

结构式英文摘要应写得简明扼要，清楚具体，表达确切，引人入胜。力求做到短、精、完整。短，是要求语言精练，一般为 150～400 个英文单词（不同期刊对摘要的字数有不同限制要求，如 *JAMA* 要求不超过 350 词；《中华医学杂志》规定中文摘要为 250 字左右，英语摘要 400 个实词左右）。精，是指摘要应集中原文的精华和要点，要选择论文中新颖、具有特色的内容进行缩写；完整，是指要全面反映原文内容，包括研究目的、范围、方法、结果、数据、主要发现和结论。目前，一般期刊的英文摘要，包括我国的绝大多数学术期刊均根据国际《向生物医学期刊投稿的统一要求》（*Uniform Requirements for Manuscripts Submitted to Biomedical Journals*）的规定（注：2014 年更新为 *Recommendations for the Conduct, Reporting, Editing and Publication of Scholarly Work in Medical Journals*《学术研究实施与报告和医学期刊编辑与发表的推荐规范》，简称 ICMJE 推荐规范），采用 OMRAC 或 AMRAC 格式，即主要包括目的（Objective/Purpose/Aim）、方法（Methods）、结果（Results）及结论（Conclusion）四部分内容。例如：

Abstract: Objective To investigate the long-term outcomes of off-pump coronary artery bypass grafting (OPCAB) in patients aged over 75 years and analyze the risk factors affecting the outcomes of the procedure. **Methods** Clinical data were reviewed for 97 consecutive patients aged 75 years or above receiving OPCAB at our center between November, 2000 and November, 2013. The perioperative data including length of ICU stay, duration of mechanical ventilation, incidence of postoperative complications and mortality rate of the patients were analyzed. The follow-up data of the patients were also analyzed including all-cause mortality rate and major adverse cardiac and cerebral events (MACCE, including myocardial infarction, cerebrovascular event, and repeated revascularization). **Results** The perioperative mortality rate was 3.09% (3/97) in these patients. Of the 97 patients analyzed, 91(93%) were available for follow-up for 29-192 months (with a median of 95.61±34.07 months). The10-year survival rate of the patients was 62% with a 10-year MACCE-free survival rate of 47.4%. During the follow-up,6 (6.8%) patients underwent repeated revascularization procedures,12(12.37%) had cerebrovascular accidents and 5 (5.15%) had myocardial infarction. Logistic regression analysis showed that hypertension (OR=1.388, P=0.043) and diabetes (OR=1.692, P=0.017) were independent predictors of MACCE, and incomplete revascularization did not increase the risk of postoperative MACCE. **Conclusion** OPCAB is safe and effective in elderly patients with good long-term outcomes. Hypertension and diabetes are independent risk factors of MACCE, and adequate control of blood pressure and blood glucose can reduce the incidence of postoperative MACCE. Incomplete revascularization is not detrimental to the long-term outcomes of OPCAB in elderly patients.

摘要：目的 分析 75 岁以上高龄患者在非体外循环下行冠状动脉旁路移植术（OPCAB）的远期疗效及其危险因素。**方法** 2000 年 11 月至 2013 年 11 月，97 例 75 岁以上高龄患者由同一术者完成 OPCAB。统计留重症监护病房时间、机械通气时间、术后并发症发生率及死亡率等围术期结果。出院后随访包括全因死亡及主要心脑血管不良（MACCE）事件（心肌梗死、脑血管事件、重复再血管化）。**结果** 围术期死亡 3 例，在院死亡率 3.09%，随访成功率 93%，随访时间为 29～192 个月 [（95.61±34.07）个月]。10 年生存率为 62%，10 年 MACCE 事件免除率为 47.4%。随访期间 6 例（6.8%）患者进行了重复再血管化，12 例（12.37%）患者出现脑血管事件，5 例（5.15%）出现心肌梗死。Logistic 回归分析显示术前合并高血压（OR=1.388，P=0.043）、糖尿病（OR=1.692，P=0.017）是高龄患者 OPCAB 术后远期 MACCE 事件的独立风险预测因素，而不完全再血管化并不会增加术后主要 MACCE 事件发生率。**结论** 高龄冠心病患者行

OPCAB 是一种安全有效的手术方法，远期效果满意。高血压、糖尿病是高龄患者 OPCAB 术后发生 MACCE 事件的危险因素，但术后良好地控制血压及血糖可以有效降低 MACCE 事件的发生率，而不完全再血管化并不会对远期疗效产生不良影响。

引自：南方医科大学学报, 2017, 37(1): 75-78

这是一篇由 4 个层次构成的结构式摘要。由于不同杂志对结构式摘要的写作有其项目上的差异，因此，这类摘要也称为半结构式（semi-structured）摘要。采用何种摘要形式要根据各杂志的具体要求而定。例如：《新英格兰医学杂志》（*The New England Journal of Medicine*）自 1990 年开始即采用这类摘要。

另一种格式是全结构式（full-structured）摘要。1974 年 4 月，加拿大 McMaster 大学医学中心的 R. Brian Haynes 博士首先提出建立临床研究论文的结构式摘要。在 Edward J Huth 博士倡导下，美国《内科学纪事》（*Annuals of Internal Medicine*）在国际上率先采用了全结构式摘要。当今较具影响力的一些学术刊物，如《英国医学杂志》（*British Medical Journal*，*BMJ*）、《美国医学协会杂志》（*The Journal of the American Medical Association*，*JAMA*）等均采用这类摘要。Haynes 所提出的全结构式摘要主要包含以下 8 个要素。

（1）目的（aim/objective/purpose）：说明论文要解决的问题，其中包括研究设想、目的、提出问题的缘由、研究的范围及重要性。

（2）设计（design）：说明研究课题的基本设计，包括所使用的材料与方法（materials and methods），如何分组、对照、数据获得的途径、样本的选择及研究性质。

（3）环境（setting）：说明进行研究的地点和研究机构的等级。

（4）对象（patients/participants/subjects）：说明参加并完成研究的患者或受试者的性质、数量及挑选方法。

（5）处置方法（interventions）：说明确切的治疗或处理方法，如方法的选择、持续时间、借鉴还是自创等。

（6）主要测定项目（main outcome measures）：说明为评定研究结果而进行的主要测定项目，如主要结果是如何测定的，与预期结果的误差等。

（7）结果（results）：说明主要客观结果，包括研究的主要发现，确切的置信度和统计学显著性检验值等。

（8）结论（conclusion）：说明主要结论，包括直接临床应用意义，其理论价值或尚待解决的问题等。

尽管如此，某些期刊在其投稿要求中同时也指出作者可根据需要将相关项目合并。这一灵活处置原则，实质上是符合作者的写作习惯及语篇逻辑关联要求的。

例一：

Early revascularization and long-term survival in cardiogenic shock complicating acute myocardial infarction

Context: Cardiogenic shock remains the major cause of death for patients hospitalized with acute myocardial infarction (MI). Although survival in patients with cardiogenic shock complicating acute MI has been shown to be significantly higher at 1 year in those receiving early revascularization *vs.* initial medical stabilization, data demonstrating long-term survival are lacking.

Objective: To determine if early revascularization affects long-term survival of patients with cardiogenic shock complicating acute MI.

Design, Setting, and Patients: The Should We emergently Revascularize Occluded Coronaries for Cardiogenic Shock (SHOCK) trial, an international randomized clinical trial enrolling 302 patients from April 1993 through November 1998 with acute myocardial infarction complicated by cardiogenic shock (mean [SD] age at randomization, 66[±11] years); long-term follow-up of vital status, conducted annually until 2005, ranged from 1 to 11 years (median for survivors, 6 years).

Main Outcome Measures: All-cause mortality during long-term follow-up.

Results: The group difference in survival of 13 absolute percentage points at 1 year favoring those assigned to early revascularization remained stable at 3 and 6 years (13.1% and 13.2%, respectively; hazard ratio [HR], 0.74; 95% confidence interval [CI], 0.57-0.97; log-rank P=0.03). At 6 years, overall survival rates were 32.8% and 19.6% in the early revascularization and initial medical stabilization groups, respectively. Among the 143 hospital survivors, a group difference in survival also was observed (HR, 0.59; 95% CI, 0.36-0.95; P=0.03). The 6-year survival rates for the hospital survivors were 62.4% *vs.* 44.4% for the early revascularization and initial medical stabilization groups, respectively, with annualized death rates of 8.3% *vs.* 14.3% and, for the 1-year survivors, 8.0% *vs.* 10.7%. There was no significant interaction between any subgroup and treatment effect.

Conclusions: In this randomized trial, almost two thirds of hospital survivors with cardiogenic shock who were treated with early revascularization were alive 6 years later. A strategy of early revascularization resulted in a 13.2% absolute and a 67% relative improvement in 6-year survival compared with initial medical stabilization. Early revascularization should be used for patients with acute MI complicated by cardiogenic shock due to left ventricular failure.

早期血运重建与急性心肌梗死并发心源性休克患者远期生存率的关系

背景： 心源性休克仍然是因急性心肌梗死（MI）住院患者的主要死亡原因。尽管在急性 MI 并发心源性休克患者中接受早期血运重建者比早期保守治疗者的 1 年生存率显著提高，但仍缺乏长期生存率的相关数据。

目的： 确定早期血运重建对急性 MI 并发心源性休克患者长期生存率影响。

设计、地点和参与者： 闭塞冠状动脉急诊血运重建治疗心源性休克（SHOCK）试验是针对 1993 年 4 月至 1998 年 11 月间 302 例急性 MI 并发心源性休克患者[随机化时的平均年龄为（66±11）岁]的一项国际性随机临床试验，对生存状况进行每年 1 次的长期随访，直至 2005 年，随访时间持续 1～11年（生存者的中位随访期为 6 年）。

主要观察指标：长期随访期间的全因死亡。

结果：与接受早期药物保守治疗的患者相比，接受早期血运重建并在术后 3 年和 6 年保持稳定的患者生存率绝对增高约 13%（分别为 13.1% 和 13.2%；HR 0.74，95% CI，0.57～0.97，对数秩检验，P=0.03）。6 年时，接受早期血运重建与早期保守治疗的急性 MI 患者的总生存率分别为 32.8% 和 19.6%。在 143 例院内生存患者中，生存率仍存在组间差异（HR 0.59，95% CI，0.36～0.95，P = 0.03）。早期血运重建组与早期药物保守治疗组之间院内生存者的 6 年生存率分别为 62.4% 和 44.4%，年死亡率分别为 8.3% 和 14.3%；两组的 1 年存活者年死亡率分别为 8.0% 和 10.7%。任何亚组与治疗效果并无显著的交互作用。

结论：本随机化试验中，约有 2/3 接受早期血运重建的心源性休克院内生存患者 6 年后仍存活。与早期药物保守治疗相比，早期血运重建使 6 年生存率绝对增高 13.2%，相对增高 67%。由左心室衰竭致心源性休克的急性 MI 患者应接受早期血运重建治疗。

引自：*JAMA*, 2006, 295: 2511-2515

注：该刊现行结构式摘要标题词变更为 "Importance；Objective；Design，Setting，and Participants；Interventions；Main Outcomes and Measures；Results；Conclusions and Relevance"。

例二：

Therapeutic Angiogenesis Using Tissue Engineered Human Smooth Muscle Cell Sheets

OBJECTIVE: Peripheral arterial disease (PAD) can have severe consequences on patient mortality and morbidity. In contrast to approaches using growth factor administration or isolated cell transplantation, we attempted to develop an alternative method for ischemic therapy using the transplantation of tissue engineered cell sheets with angiogenic potential. **METHODS AND RESULTS:** Human smooth muscle cell (SMC) and fibroblast cell (FbC) sheets were harvested from temperature-responsive culture dishes and transplanted into ischemic hind limbs of athymic rats. ELISA showed significantly increased *in vitro* secretion of angiogenic factors by SMCs in comparison to FbCs. Twenty-one days after transplantation, laser doppler analysis demonstrated significantly increased blood perfusion in the SMC group. Perfusion with Indian ink and immunohistochemistry also revealed significantly greater numbers of functional capillaries in the SMC group. Finally, cell tracing experiments revealed that some SMCs from the transplanted cell sheets migrated into the ischemic tissues, contributing to newly formed vessels. **CONCLUSIONS:** SMC sheet transplantation allows for controlled and localized delivery of cells that possess angiogenic potential directly to ischemic tissues. Through the secretion of angiogenic factors, as well as cell migration and integration with newly formed vessels, SMC sheet transplantation provides an effective method for the revascularization of ischemic tissues.

应用组织工程人类平滑肌细胞片进行新生血管治疗

目的: 外周血管疾病（PAD）可以增加患者的死亡率。与使用生长因子或分离细胞移植不同，我们尝试应用移植具有新生血管潜能的组织工程人类平滑肌细胞片移植进行局部缺血治疗。**方法和结果:** 人类平滑肌细胞（SMC）和成纤维细胞（FbC）从温度敏感培养皿中获得移植到无胸腺鼠的缺血下肢。与 FbCs 相比较，ELISA 法检测到体外 SMC 导致血管生成因子分泌显著增加。移植后 21 天，多普勒分析显示在 SMC 组血液灌注显著增加。墨汁染色和免疫组化也显示有功能的毛细血管在 SMC 组显著增加。最后，细胞示踪试验显示一些移植的 SMC 迁徙至缺血组织，这有助于新生血管的形成。**结论:** SMC 片移植可以控制并移植具有新生血管潜能的细胞到局部缺血组织，通过血管生成因子的分泌、细胞迁徙和形成新生血管，SMC 片移植为缺血组织的血管再生提供了一个有效的方法。

引自: *Arterioscler Thromb Vasc Biol*, 2008, 28(4):637-643

第一例为全结构式摘要，而第二例则为简化式摘要。与非结构式摘要相比，全结构式摘要观点更明确，信息量更大，差错更少，同时也更符合计算机数据库的建立和使用要求。但其缺点也是显而易见的，即烦琐、重复、篇幅过长，而且不是所有研究都能按以上 8 个要素分类的。于是更多的杂志扬长避短，采用半结构式（semi-structured）摘要。无论撰写的摘要是何种格式，但有一点要特别注意，就是英文摘要的完整性。在我国，大多数作者写英文摘要时，都是把论文前面的中文摘要（一般都写得很简单）翻译成英文。这种做法忽略了这样一个事实：由于论文是用中文写作的，中文读者在看了中文摘要后，不详之处还可以从论文全文中获得全面、详细的信息，但由于英文读者一般看不懂中文，英文摘要成了他唯一的信息源。因此，这里要特别提出并强调英文摘要的完整性，即英文摘要所提供的信息必须是完整的。这样，即使读者看不懂中文，通过英文摘要也能对论文的主要目的，解决问题的主要方法、过程，以及主要结果、结论和文章的创新、独到之处，有一个较为完整的了解。注重定量分析是科学研究的重要特征之一，这一点也应该体现在英文摘要的写作中。因此，在写英文摘要时，要避免过于笼统的、空洞无物的一般论述和结论。要尽量利用文章中的最具体的语言来阐述你的方法、过程、结果和结论，这样既可以给以非汉语为母语的读者一个清晰的思路，又可以使你的论述言之有物、有根有据，使读者对你的研究工作有一个清晰而全面的认识。当然，这并不意味着中文摘要就不必强调完整性。事实上，在将中文摘要单独上网发布或文章被收入中文文摘期刊时，中文摘要所提供的信息也必须具有完整性。然而，要写好英文摘要，作者可以从英文语篇角度，按下列问题入手。

1）What I want to do?（本文的目的或要解决的问题）

2）How I did it?（解决问题的方法及过程）

3）What results did I get and what conclusions can I draw?（主要结果及结论）

4）What is new and original in this paper?（本文的创新、独到之处）

　　另外，由于东西方文化传统存在很大的差别，我国长期以来的传统教育都有些过分强调知识分子要"谦虚谨慎、戒骄戒躁"，因此我国学者在写论文时，一般不注重（或不敢）突出表现自己所做的贡献。这一点与西方的传统恰恰相反。西方的学者在写论文时总是很明确地突出自己的贡献，突出自己的创新、独到之处。西方的读者在阅读论文时也总是特别关注论文有什么创新、独到之处，否则就认为论文不值得一读。由于中、英文摘要的读者对象不同，鉴于上述两方面的因素，论文中的中、英文摘要不必强求一致。为写出符合要求的英文摘要，现将常用的英文表达分述如下。

（一）目的

　　目的（Objective）：直截了当地说明研究目的或所阐述的问题。若题目已清楚表明，则摘要中可以不重复。亦可以在摘要开始，简要说明提出问题的背景。英文常以动词不定式"To+动词原形"结构。常用英文表达方式："To study…/To obtain…/To investigate…/To explore…/To observe…/To analyze…/To evaluate…/To examine…/To elucidate…/To determine…/To confirm…/To ascertain…/To detect…/To describe…/To report…/To compare…/To judge…/To establish…/To understand…/To provide…/To clarify…/To know…"等。此部分内容的具体写法及注意点详见本书的有关章节。

（二）方法

　　方法（Methods）：对研究的基本设计予以描述，包括分组情况、诊断标准及随访时间；研究对象的数量及特征，在研究中因副作用或其他原因而撤销的研究对象数目；观察的主要变量及主要的研究方法；治疗手段，包括使用方法及作用时间等。若为临床研究，需说明是前瞻性随机对照研究还是回顾性分析。方法学研究要说明新的或改进的方法、设备、材料，以及被研究的对象（动物或人）。英文常需要用完整的被动或主动结构句子，动词用过去时态。常用英文表达方式："…technique was used to detect…；…were selected as experiment groups…；…were in the control groups…；…methods was used to detect…；…were determined by PCR in…；A randomized, double blind, placebo controlled trial was performed…；A case control study…；A prospective clinical study…；We retrospectively analyzed…；We studied…"等。此部分内容的具体写法及注意事项详见本书的有关章节。

（三）结果

　　结果（Results）：为摘要的重点部分。提供研究所得出的主要结果，列出重要数据，指出新方法与经典方法比较而表现出的优缺点，并说明其可信度及准确性的统计学数据处理结果。英文需采用完整句子，谓语动词用过去时态，研究所得数据如百分数、血压等数据采用临床病历书写形式，不必用书面英文表达。常用英文表达方式："…was (were)…; We found…; There was…; …was significantly different among…; …the result did not show any…; …showed significant difference…"等。此部分内容的具体写法及注意事项详见本书的有关章节。

（四）结论

结论[Conclusion(s)]：是把研究的主要结论性观点，用一两句话简明表达，不必另分段落或设小标题。结论应该有直接依据，避免推测和过于笼统。英文采用完整句子表达，动词时态用一般现在时或现在完成时。建议直接写结论，也可用某些常用句型引出结论。常用英文表达方式："…probably…; Our conclusion is that…; This study shows that…; This study suggests that…; This study confirms that…; These observations support…"等。此部分内容的具体写法及注意事项详见本书的有关章节。

（五）关键词或主题词

紧随摘要之后，必须附有关键词（Key Words）或主题词（Subject Heading）。关键词，顾名思义就是关键性的词语。从语言学上来讲，关键词就是能描述文章本质的词语，而信息检索领域将关键词理解为能表示文献实质意义的那些名词或词组，常出现在文献篇名或文献正文中。它是编辑进行各种索引编写时的选择。关键词不仅可以区别于其他文档，还能方便读者使用各种检索工具查找感兴趣的文献。尤其是互联网上，读者在适当的搜索引擎中输入适当的关键词，可以快速找到自己需要的文献。因此，关键词的选择得当与否，与作者的文献被引频次直接相关。主题词为一组术语或词组，用以表达文献主题概念，又称叙词（descriptors）或受控词（controlled vocabulary）。众所周知，概念是由语词表达的，但是概念和语词之间并不是一一对应的，为保证语词和概念的一一对应，就必须对主题词的词义进行控制。因此，无论是选择关键词还是主题词，均应注意下述三点：①所选择的主题词应能够满足标引文献和检索文献的要求；②所选择的主题词应能够准确地表达概念的含义；③应选择通用的为人们普遍接受的词语作为主题词。

综上所述，关键词是表达论文内容特征的关键性单词或词组，是论文中最能反映中心内容的名词或词组，是最能说明全文含义的词。遴选关键词时，首先以文题为基础，参考摘要和前言，提炼出若干个最能代表论文主要内容的、有实质意义的词，再逐一推敲、斟酌，筛选出其中的若干个词（一般3～8个词，但不同期刊有不同要求，作者投稿前应注意相关信息）。关键词可以是单词，也可以是短语，必须注意的是，这些词或短语必须是名词形式，动词、形容词、副词等不可作为关键词使用。

目前，国内外医学期刊大多要求用美国国立医学图书馆所规定的医学主题词（Medical Subject Headings, MeSH）作为关键词来引用。但 MeSH 中出现的词汇有时滞后于最新研究中的词汇，所以作者有可能会选择一些 MeSH 尚未收录的新的专业术语作为关键词（自由词）。此外，选择关键词时，应尽量选择具体的词汇。例如，有关粉螨的一篇论著，关键词就应该是"acaroid mites"或"粉螨"，而不是笼统的词"mites"或"螨"。国内的期刊除了参照 MeSH 外，还可参照《汉语主题词表》、《医学主题词注释字顺表》和《中医药主题词表》。

有关关键词列举的几点提示：

（1）美国国立医学图书馆 Index Medicus 的主题词表免费查询网址是 https://www.nlm.nih.gov/mesh/meshhome.html。

（2）关键词匹配问题：关键词是专业术语，若该主题词表中尚无相应的匹配词可选用直接相关的几个主题词组配，即借助副主题词（Subheadings/Qualifiers）与主题词进行组配，如运动疗法（exercise therapy）、超声诊断（ultrasonic diagnosis）。若无法组配则可选用最直接的上位主题词（概念上外延更广的主题词），如五硫化物（MeSH 中无），可以用硫化物类（sulfides）。必要时可用适当的习用自由词（自然语言中的词或词组），如肝癌，可以用"liver cancer/carcinoma/neoplasm/tumor/hepatic cancer/carcinoma/neoplasm/tumor"。

（3）关键词词性：一般为名词或名词性词组。

（4）关键词大小写问题：英文关键词首字母大小写，应遵从期刊版式要求，包括关键词与关键词之间的分割符号，如使用"，"还是"；"或其他分割形式。即使某些期刊规定关键词首字母采用小写形式，但以下几种情况首字母必须大写。

1）人名或含有人名的词组，如 Alzheimer's dementia（阿尔茨海默病）；Alstrom-Hallgren syndrome（阿尔斯特伦-海尔格伦综合征）。但以人名为词根构成的名词，首字母一般不用大写，如 roentgen ray（X 线）。

2）种属名称：微生物、植物（草药）等拉丁学名。

3）化学元素符号等。

（5）单复数问题：英文名词除必须用复数者外，一般用单数。

（6）正斜体问题：正常情况下用正体，用斜体的大致有以下两种情况：

1）生物学中属以下（含属）的拉丁学名，如 *Atractylodis macrocephalae Koide*（白术）；*Schistosoma*（裂体吸虫属，血吸虫属）；*Candida albicans*（白念珠菌）；*Enterococcus faecalis*（粪肠球菌）。

2）包含变量的词变量用斜体，如 *P*-value（*P* 值）。

（7）英语单词拼写问题：同一词汇可有英、美两种不同的拼写形式：如贫血[anaemia（英）；anemia（美）]；雌激素[oestrogen（英）；estrogen（美）]。除向英国期刊投稿外，建议首选美式英语拼写。

（8）版式：一般常见版式如下所述。

1）单词间以黑方块或实心圆点相隔，如 *Circulation* 所用的形式为"cardiac arrest ▪ myocardial infarction"；*J Exp Med* 所用形式为"stroke ● heart failure"。

2）用破折号相隔，如"*J Stroke Cerebrovasc Dis*"所用形式为"Dysphagia—Stroke—Diet。

3）用逗号或分号相隔，如 *Annals of Otology，Rhinology and Laryngology* 和 *Cancer*

所用形式为："cell culture，interstitial collagenase"；而 *Brain* 和 *British Journal of Cancer* 等则采用如下形式，如 "transplantation；spinal cord；injury"。

　　国内外期刊均有不同的要求，无论采用何种版式，作者必须认真阅读拟投稿期刊的"稿约"，标出符合该刊风格特色的关键词，这不仅体现出作者对该刊的尊重，也是作者严谨科学态度的一种反映。

　　（9）关键词位置：关键词一般置于文章摘要之后，但也有期刊置于摘要之前，如 *Throax*、*The Oncologist*。为了使作者更好地熟悉和了解关键词的取舍，特选取国内一些主流医学期刊摘要和关键词范例，以供参考。

　　例一:【摘要】目的 观察乐果染毒对大鼠大脑纹状体和血清中多巴胺-β-羟化酶（dopamine-β-hydroxylase，DβH）活性变化的影响，对乐果中毒机制作进一步的探讨。**方法** 56 只雄性 SD 大鼠随机分为对照组（生理盐水，$n=8$）和乐果染毒低（38.9 mg/kg，$n=8$）、中（83.7 mg/kg，$n=8$）和高（180 mg/kg，$n=32$）3 个剂量组，腹腔一次注射染毒。高剂量组大鼠分别在给药后 0.5、2、8、24 h 断头处死取血制备血清待测，并分离脑组织纹状体，生理盐水匀浆待测。其他组动物在给药后 2 h 断头处死，同样方式取样供分析。利用 DβH 将酪胺代谢为真蛸胺原理检测 DβH 活性。另取正常大鼠血清和纹状体匀浆，体外乐果染毒，观察其对 DβH 抑制状况。**结果** 给予不同剂量乐果对大鼠纹状体和血清 DβH 活性均有抑制作用，并随剂量增加而加深，存在剂量-效应关系（$r=-0.996\,7$，$P<0.05$）。乐果高剂量（180 mg/kg）染毒后大鼠大脑纹状体和血清中 DβH 活性与对照组相比，在不同时程观察点差异均有统计学意义（$P<0.05$），随时程增加抑制也加深，24 h 内时程效应关系（$P<0.05$）明确。体外乐果对纹状体和血清 DβH 活性均有抑制作用，并随剂量增加而加深，有剂量-效应关系（$r=-0.891$，$P<0.05$），但存在高浓度有饱和现象。**结论** 大鼠大脑纹状体和血清中 DβH 水平有随染毒剂量和时程的增加而抑制加深的趋势，存在剂量效应和时程效应关系。

　　【关键词】乐果；大脑纹状体；血清；多巴胺-β-羟化酶；大鼠

　　【Abstract】Objective To observe the effect of dimethoate (DM) on dopamine-β-hydroxylase (DβH) activity in rat serum and striatum, and to further discuss the mechanism of dimethoate-induced poisoning. **Methods** Fifty-six male SD rats were randomized into control group (saline, $n=8$)and DM-treated groups with 3 dosages of low(38.9 mg/kg, $n=8$), medium(83.7 mg/kg, $n=8$) and high (180 mg/kg, $n=32$)level, respectively. A poisonous injection was given into celiac. The rats in group of high-level DM treated were decollated respectively at 0.5, 2, 8, and 24 hours after administrating DM to collect blood and brain striatum samples. The rats in the other groups were decollated at 2 hours. Serum and saline homogenate of striatum were prepared for measurement of DβH activity. Moreover, the inhibitive effect of DM on serum and striatum DβH activity *in vitro* were also observed. **Results** The levels of DβH activity in rat serum and striaturn were decreased by administrating dimethoate in dose-dependent manners ($r = -0.996\ 7$, $P<0.05$). Compared with controlled group, DβH activities in serum and striatum of 180 mg/kg dimethoate rats differed at different time points and showed a significant decrease over time ($P<0.05$). The time-effect relationships were definited in 24 h ($P<0.05$). The inhibition effect also existed *in vitro* with a dose-response relationship ($r=-0.891$, $P<0.05$), however, there was saturation effect at high dose. **Conclusions** These findings indicate that DM-induced toxic effects can alter DβH activity in rat serum and striatum, suggesting that some non-cholinergic mechanisms are involved in DM intoxication.

【Key words】dimethoate；striaturn; serum; dopamine-β-hydroxylase；rat

引自：《复旦学报（医学版）》, 2011, 38(3): 194

例二：【摘要】目的：应用 Meta 分析评价内置法与外置法商环包皮环切术的临床疗效与安全性。方法：检索国内外有关比较商环内置法与外置法包皮环切术的随机对照试验，由 2 名评论者分别按 Cochrane 系统评价方法对纳入文献进行质量评价和提取资料数据后，采用 RevMan 5.1.0 统计软件进行 Meta 分析。结果：共纳入 7 篇文献，1200 例患者 Meta 分析结果显示，与外置式相比，商环内置术式具有总并发症率低（RR=0.40, 95% CI: 0.18, 0.87, $P=0.02$），术后伤口水肿率低（RR=0.28, 95% CI: 0.09, 0.81, $P=0.02$），同时可以减轻患者术后 24 h 疼痛（MD=−0.35, 95% CI：−0.55, −0.14, $P<0.001$）的优点。结论：商环内置式包皮环切术相比外置式，具有减少术后总并发症率和术后伤口水肿率、降低术后 24 h 疼痛度等优点。由于纳入文献较少，需要更多大样本量的随机对照试验进一步证实我们的结论。

【关键词】商环；内置法；外置法；包皮环切术；Meta 分析

【Abstract】 **Objective:** To compare the effect and safety of the no-flip method *versus* the external method in ShangRing circumcision. **Methods:** We searched relevant randomized controlled trials published in China and abroad comparing the no-flip method and external method of ShangRing circumcision. Based on the Cochrane Handbook for systematic review of interventions, two reviewers independently evaluated the quality of the included studies and abstracted relevant data, followed by a meta-analysis using the statistical software Review Manager 5.1.0. **Results:** Totally 7 studies with 1 200 cases were included. Compared with the external method, the no-flip method was associated with a lower total rate of complications (RR=0.40, 95% CI: 0.18, 0.87, $P=0.02$), a lower incidence of postoperative edema (RR=0.28, 95% CI: 0.09, 0.81, $P=0.02$),and a lower 24 h postoperative pain score (MD=−0.35, 95%

CI:−0.55, −0.14, *P*<0.001). **Conclusion:** The no-flip method of ShangRing circumcision was superior to the external method for its advantages of fewer complications, lower incidence of postoperative edema, and mild postoperative pain. However, our findings need further support by more high-quality randomized controlled trials.

【**Key words**】ShangRing; no-flip method; external method; circumcision; meta-analysis

引自:《中华男科学杂志》, 2014, 20(12): 1113

例三:【摘要】**目的** 通过报告 6 例血管壁淀粉样蛋白沉积型淀粉样变性肾病（VADAN）的临床和病理特性,以提高对 VADAN 的诊治水平。**方法** 收集 6 例 VADAN 患者行免疫病理、光镜及电镜检查,并进行淀粉样蛋白的分型。**结果** 6 例患者均为中老年（52～73 岁）患者,男女各 3 例。其中 2 例为多发性骨髓瘤。多数病例仅呈轻度的蛋白尿和血尿。1 例因合并微小病变型肾病,呈现肾病综合征表现;1 例因合并 IgA 肾病,呈现蛋白尿和血尿;1 例因骨髓瘤管型肾病,呈现急性肾衰竭。经肾活检证实,淀粉样蛋白仅沉积于小叶间动脉。6 例患者均为原发性系统性淀粉样变性肾病,2 例多发性骨髓瘤继发者,为 κ 型,其余为 λ 型。**结论** VADAN 属于少见的淀粉样变性肾病类型,临床表现不同于常见的淀粉样变性肾病,肾活检有助于其鉴别诊断。

【关键词】淀粉样变性;肾疾病;病理学;临床;淀粉样蛋白

【**Abstract**】**Objective** To analyze clinical and pathologic features of a rare vascular amyloid deposits of amyloid nephropathy（VADAN）in 6 patients, so as to improve its diagnosis and treatment. **Methods** All patients receiving immunopathology, microscopy and electron microscopy examination, and amyloid types were analyzed. **Results** There were 3 males and 3 females with ages ranging from 52 to 73 years. Two patients suffered from multiple myeloma. Majority patients had slight albuminuria and hematuria. One patient combined with minimal change glomerular disease presented nephrotic syndrome. One patient combined with IgA nephropathy had albuminuria and hematuria. And one patient had myeloma cast nephropathy with acute renal failure. Kidney biopsy proved amyloid deposits along interlobular'arterial wall only in all 6 patients.Two cases secondary from multiple myeloma were κ amyloid，and the rests were λ amyloid. **Conclusions** VADAN is a rare type of amyloid nephropathy. Its clinical manifestation is different from common amyloid nephropathy. Kidney biopsy will benefit its differential diagnosis.

【**Key words**】amyloidosis; kidney diseases; pathology; clinical; amyloid

引自:《中华内科杂志》, 2011, 50(7): 576

附：文献分类及二次发表

根据文献的性质、内容及出现的频率，文献通常分为以下三种类型。

一次性文献：是指医学论著，亦即人们习惯上所称的原著或论著。它是创造性的学术成果，主要包括临床论著、医案医话、专利说明书、会议资料及公报等。

二次性文献：是将多种同性质的期刊和图书中那些散在的大量一次性文献资料，按设计要求加工整理，精练简化而成的有科有目、便于查阅、负载储存信息的检索工具书，如中文科技资料目录、国外医学目录索引等。

三次性文献：是以二次性文献提供的信息为线索，有目地地收集一次性文献，在全面广泛的阅读基础上，进行消化吸收、综合分析、归纳对比，将其重要内容重新组织，加工撰写而成的医学论文，即综述类文章。

二次发表（secondary publication）不同于重复发表（duplication submission）。按国际惯例，二次发表是指同一论文用另一种语言再次发表，其宗旨是让更多的读者受益。二次发表的前提是需要取得首次发表论文的期刊和准备二次发表的期刊的认可与授权同意书，首次发表的期刊向二次发表期刊提供论文首次发表的版本。此外，二次发表的论文应在文题页脚注中对发表信息予以声明，其目的是让读者、同行和文献检索机构知道该论文已全文或部分发表过。脚注中的声明标注格式，如："本文首次发表在《皖南医学院学报》，2019, 39(2): 103-106"，英文为 "This article is based on a study first reported in the *Journal of Wannan Medical College*, 2019, 39(2): 103-106. Article in Chinese"

四、练 习

1-1 阅读下列英文摘要，尝试写出关键词

Nitric oxide homeostasis as a target for drug additives to cardioplegia

Abstract The vascular endothelium of the coronary arteries has been identified as the important organ that locally regulates coronary perfusion and cardiac function by paracrine secretion of nitric oxide (NO) and vasoactive peptides. NO is constitutively produced in endothelial cells by endothelial nitric oxide synthase (eNOS). NO derived from this enzyme exerts important biological functions including vasodilatation, scavenging of superoxide and inhibition of platelet aggregation. Routine cardiac surgery or cardiologic interventions lead to a serious temporary or persistent disturbance in NO homeostasis. The clinical consequences are "endothelial dysfunction", leading to "myocardial dysfunction": no- or low-reflow phenomenon and temporary reduction of myocardial pump function. Uncoupling of eNOS (one electron transfer to molecular oxygen, the second substrate of eNOS) during ischemia-reperfusion due to diminished availability of L-arginine and/or tetrahydrobiopterin is even discussed as one major source of superoxide formation. Therefore maintenance of normal NO homeostasis seems to be an important factor protecting from ischemia/reperfusion (I/R) injury. Both clinical situations of cardioplegic arrest as well as hypothermic cardioplegic storage are followed by reperfusion. However, the presently used cardioplegic solutions to arrest and/or store the heart, thereby reducing myocardial oxygen consumption and metabolism, are designed to preserve myocytes mainly and not endothelial cells. This review will focus on possible drug additives to cardioplegia, which may help to maintain normal NO homeostasis after I/R.

1-2　尝试将以下中文摘要翻译成英文

【摘要】男性包皮环切能降低男性阴茎-阴道性交获得性 HIV 感染风险大约 60%，被 WHO 和联合国艾滋病规划署（UNAIDS）推荐作为 HIV 预防策略中的一个重要干预措施。寻求一种更加安全、有效和可接受的男性包皮环切器械和手术方法，以便能够满足加快执行扩大包皮环切预防 HIV 感染项目的需求，已经成为相关国际组织，特别是非洲国家政府公共卫生事业的当务之急。2008 年中国商环（ShangRing）包皮环切标准化手术方案建立，应用这个标准化手术方案和手术培训在中国及 2009 年和 2010 年在肯尼亚实施中国商环成人包皮环切手术获得有用的和有意义的临床数据，证明了中国商环包皮环切术的诸多优势。手术培训手册和教学视频的多次修订为培训医护人员提供了更加准确的教学指南。经过多家相关国际机构专家的考察和评估，中国商环包皮环切技术已经成为支持在非洲 HIV 高发地区扩大包皮环切服务预防 HIV 感染项目最具潜力的候选包皮环切工具之一。可以预计，中国商环包皮环切技术的成功应用将会在改变数百万非洲人的生活方式的同时，也为中国男科学与泌尿外科学医生在包皮环切与 HIV 预防和生殖健康相关的临床研究领域提供了丰富的机会。本文报告了 2008 年 2 月至 2010 年底期间中国商环包皮环切技术临床应用的国际和国内研究进展。

第二章　医学论文英文标题写作

　　标题也称题目、题名、篇名、文题等，是以最恰当、最简明的词语反映论文中最重要的、最具特定内容的文字逻辑组合，是对论文主要内容与中心思想的高度语言概括，也是论文主题和中心思想最精粹的浓缩。突出研究结果的论著标题应能明确表达自变量、因变量、实验对象、变化特点及特定方法等；突出研究方法的论著标题能清楚表达方法的名称、适用范围和主要特点等。读者在阅读摘要之前通常先浏览标题，因此标题应语言精练、表达清楚、引人注目。

　　一篇论文的标题是给读者的第一印象，对论文应能起到画龙点睛的提示、评价、吸引和检索的作用，因此，标题在论文写作中具有举足轻重的地位。一个好的医学论文标题应该具有以下特征。①醒目：虽然论文题目居于首先映入读者眼帘的醒目位置，但仍然存在题目是否醒目的问题。题目所用字句及其所呈现的内容是否醒目，其产生的效果是相距甚远的。所谓醒目，即首先要确定文题的中心词，中心词是标题的基础和骨架，其他词围绕着它做进一步阐明，以丰富中心词内涵，使标题独具特色。如"Thresholds for normal blood pressure and serum cholesterol"（正常血压和血清胆固醇的临界值）和"Hysterectomy for benign conditions"（良性妇科疾病的子宫切除术）中的 thresholds 和 hysterectomy，分别突出了文题的中心；②简明：医学论文写作（medical manuscripts）注重对事实的描述，因此，医学论文英文的标题因其科学性而无须使用诗一样的语言。过于烦琐会使读者却步。尽可能删繁就简，用最少的文字或词汇提供最多的信息。例如，肝移植治疗急性肝衰竭的英文表达"Treatment of acute hepatic failure by liver transplantation"，表面看似乎比较得体，但若将其英文改为"Liver transplantation for acute hepatic failure"就要简明多了。又如，"重症多形红斑和中毒性表皮坏死松解症 35 例临床分析"的英文表达"Clinical analysis of Stevens-Johnson syndrome and toxic epidermal necrolysis in 35 cases"可以简化为"Stevens-Johnson syndrome and toxic epidermal necrolysis：Clinical analysis in 35 cases"；③准确：论文题目要确切而有特异性，即突出论文中特别有独创性、有特色的内容。文题应准确地表达论文的特定内容，实事求是地反映研究的范围和深度，防止小题大做，名不符实。除此之外，标题写作还应符合目录编制、文献标引和检索的要求；标题中的数字应用阿拉伯数字，尽量避免使用作者个人独创的、非公知公认的缩略语，化学分子式、结构式及化学方程式。

　　因此，但凡有经验的论文写作者对标题都是字斟句酌，常在写初稿时就先拟出若干个题目，在论文修改过程中，随着认识的深化再做最后的修改、选定。也有作者把位于文章之首的题目放在全文最后来完成，写好正文后写摘要，再结合摘要和文章内容提炼出与文章所述相匹配的文题。

一、英文标题组成

医学论文英文标题通常由三部分组成：正标题、副标题及分标题，医学论文标题究竟使用何种格式主要由论文内容和杂志要求而定。

正标题最常见，是标题的主体部分，原则上须简短明了，但究竟多少个字为宜，大多数医学期刊都要求简短，却没有严格的限制。我国国家标准局颁布的《科学技术报告、学位论文和学术论文的编写格式》（GB 7713—87）则规定题名一般不宜超过 20 字，外文题名一般不宜超过 10 个实词。另有些杂志对标题的长短、行数甚至惯用字都有一些具体的规定，如美国的 *Journal of National Cancer Institute*（*J Natl Cancer Inst*，《美国国立癌症研究所杂志》）规定标题不得超过 14 个英文单词，*Archives of Internal Medicine*（*Arch Intern Med*，《内科学文献》）规定标题字数不得超过 42 个印刷符，长短不得超过 2 行，其中包括副标题、空白间隔和标点符号。尽管如此，现代医学研究与传统研究相比，仍有着本质上的差异，即使是针对单病种研究，也常涉及多学科、多方法联合交叉。于是，某些文题可能比常规要求略长，使用的字数稍多。例如："Culprit-only or multivessel revascularization in patients with acute coronary syndromes: an American College of Cardiology National Cardiovascular Database Registry report" 急性冠脉综合征患者单支或多支血管病变血管形成术：美国心脏病学会心血管数据库注册研究［引自：*Am Heart J*, 2008, 155(1) :140］；"Randomised controlled trial to compare surgical stabilization of the lumbar spine with an intensive rehabilitation programme for patients with chronic low back pain: the MRC spine stabilization trial" 比较腰椎稳定手术与强化康复训练治疗慢性下腰痛患者：多中心随机对照脊柱稳定实验（引自：*N Engl J Med*, 2005, 352:238）。总而言之，无论标题长短与否，标题内容应包含研究命题、研究结果或研究方法。英文文题格式规范必须满足如下要求。

数字：*Scientific Style and Format*（《科学文体与格式》）一书明确规定，不能用阿拉伯数字作为一个完整句子的开头。文题若以数字开始，则不应选用阿拉伯数字，而要用英文拼写的数词。如："89 female patients with…"，正确的写法："Eighty-nine female patients with…"。

标点符号：如果需要用引号，要用单引号。

药名：应使用药品的通用名，不用商品名或异名，如 aspirin（阿司匹林），esomeprazole（埃索美拉唑）。

种属名称：微生物、植物（草药）等学名用斜体字，如 *Streptococcus pneumoniae*。

缩略语：尽可能少用或不用。尤其不要用那些非公知公认的或有一型多解的缩略语，如 MAC，其对应的词义可能有 mac conkey（agar），麦康基（氏）（琼脂）；machupo virus，马秋波病毒；macrophage surface antigen，巨噬细胞表面抗原。

副标题是对正标题实质内容的必要补充和说明，与正标题是正与副、主与从的关系。国内论文标题一般不主张使用副标题，有时作者为了使标题涵盖更多的内容，或反复斟酌标题，却难以概括文章的中心内容时，也可加设副标题，但一般须用不同的字号或字体以示与正标题的区别，也可用破折号、圆括号或冒号导出副题名。相对于国内期刊，国外期刊使用副标题的现象要普遍得多，如著名学术期刊 *Science*，*The Lancet* 和 *Nature*。医学论文中使用副标题的作用主要有下述几种。

（一）突出病例数

无论是在中文还是英文检索条件下，病例数均不作为文题检索条件，为突出文章主题，提高文献检索率，通常不将病例数列入正标题中，而是置于副标题。

例一： Suppression of Ventricular Tachycardia With Dronedarone: A Case Report
决奈达隆抑制室性心动过速：1 例病例报告
引自：*J Cardiovasc Electrophysiol*, 2011, 22(2): 201

例二： Nosocomial Infection: A Transverse Section Survey on 1483 Inpatients
1483 例住院患者医院感染横断面调查及分析
引自：《中华医院感染学杂志》, 2010, 20(17): 2566

例三： Cryptogenic organizing pneumonia: Serial high-resolution CT findings in 22 patients
22 例患者连续高分辨率 CT 结果
引自：*AJR Am J Roentgenol*, 2010, 195 (4): 916

（二）突出研究方法

医学研究中，介绍一种新的研究方法，或改进已有研究方法，或对定量数据分析方法进行研究、评估或讨论，这类文章都属于方法学论文。研究方法或数据分析方法是这类文章的重点，因此，为方便读者检索，研究方法可置入副标题。

例一： Telemonitoring and self-management in the control of hypertension (TASMINH2): A randomised controlled trial
高血压控制中的远程监控和自我管理（TASMINH2）：随机对照实验
引自：*Lancet*, 2010, 376(9736): 163

例二： Daily left prefrontal transcranial magnetic stimulation therapy for major depressive disorder: A sham-controlled randomized trial
每日经左前额叶磁力刺激治疗严重抑郁：一项假对照随机临床试验研究
引自：*Arch Gen Psychiatry*, 2010, 67(5): 507

例三： Effect of calcium supplements on risk of myocardial infarction and cardiovascular events: Meta-analysis
补钙对心肌梗死和心血管疾病发生风险的影响：荟萃分析
引自：*BMJ*, 2010, 341: c3691

例四： Real-Life Benefits of Statins for Cardiovascular Prevention in Elderly Subjects: A Population-Based Cohort Study

他汀类药物对老年受试者心血管预防的实际益处：一项基于人群的队列研究

引自： *Am J Med,* 2019, 132(6): 740

（三）突出重点内容

此类副标题与上述两种副标题有着本质上的差异。突出病例数是为了强调研究样本，以增强对某种特定疾病研究的说服力，或者是为了强调某种疾病的罕见性；突出研究方法，一是为了评估某种方法的优劣，二是强调某种方法在特定研究中的重要性。而突出重点内容，顾名思义，则是强调同类事物中的重要的、核心部分。

例一： Functional gastrointestinal disorders：History, pathophysiology and clinical features

功能性胃肠疾病：病史、病理生理学及临床特征

引自： *Gastroenterology*, 2016, 150(6): 1262

例二： Feasibility of FDG imaging of the coronary arteries: Comparison between acute coronary syndrome and stable angina

冠状动脉氟脱氧葡萄糖（FDG）成像的可行性：急性冠状动脉综合征和稳定型心绞痛比较

引自： *JACC Cardiovasc Imaging*, 2010, 3(4): 388

例三： Mode of death in patients with heart failure and a preserved ejection fraction: Results from the Irbesartan in heart failure with preserved ejection fraction study (I-Preserve) trial

射血分数正常的心力衰竭患者的死亡归因：厄贝沙坦对射血分数正常的心力衰竭患者的作用的试验（I-Preserve）结果

引自： *Circulation*, 2010, 121(12): 1393

（四）表示同位关系

所谓同位关系是指由两个或两个以上同一层次的语言单位组成的结构，其中前项与后项所指相同，句法功能也相同；后项即是前项的同位语（完整结构）或同位关系语（简略结构）。例如："Evaluation of nutritional indices: Prognostic indicators in the cancer patient"（营养指数——癌症的预后指标）可以表示为"Evaluation of nutritional indices may serve as prognostic indicators in the cancer patient." 或 "Prognostic indicators in the cancer patient are related to evaluation of nutritional indices."。

例： Platelets: Inflammatory Firebugs of Vascular Walls

血小板：血管炎症反应的"煽动者"。

引自： *Arterioscler Thromb Vasc Biol*, 2008, 28(3): 403

（五）提出疑问

鉴于医学研究总是在提出问题，解决问题，争论与质疑，共同探讨，从而推动医学研究向前发展。因此，对于值得商榷的问题，通常采用副标题来表达。

例一： Determinants of coronary calcium conversion among patients with a normal coronary calcium scan: What is the 'warranty period' for remaining normal?
冠状动脉钙化扫描检查结果正常的患者发生冠状动脉钙化的决定因素：其冠状动脉保持正常的'保险期'有多长？

引自：*J Am Coll Cardiol*, 2010, 55(11)：1110

例二： Immunosuppression in Autoimmune Hepatitis: Is There an End Game?
自身免疫性肝炎的免疫抑制：研究何时方休？

引自：*Am J Gastroenterol*, 2020, 115(4): 498

例三： Coronary heart disease in postmenopausal recipients of estrogen plus progestin therapy: Does the increased risk ever disappear?
绝经后患者接受雌激素和孕激素治疗：增加的冠心病风险是否消失？

引自：*Ann Intern Med,* 2010, 152(4)：211

（六）提示研究时间跨度

医学研究与流行病学有着密不可分的联系。医学研究中，人们通常借助疾病的"三间分布"（地区、时间、人群）来探讨某一疾病的分布规律。疾病的时间分布是其中的一个重要因素，它反映出某一特定疾病是短期波动、呈季节性变化、周期性还是长期趋势。因此，这类研究与时间跨度密切相关。例如：

例一： Epidemiological characteristics of measles in Guangxi, 2005-2009
广西壮族自治区 2005～2009 年麻疹流行病学特征

引自：《中国预防医学杂志》, 2010, 11(10): 1012

例二： Monitoring Analysis and Controlling Countermeasures of Nosocomial Infection in ICU: 2008-2009
2008～2009 年 ICU 医院感染监测分析与控制对策

引自：《中华医院感染学杂志》, 2010, 20(14): 2030

例三： Typhoid fever in the United States, 1999-2006
1999～2006 年美国伤寒流行

引自：*JAMA*, 2009, 302 (8): 859

例四： Increasing incidence of zygomycosis (mucormycosis), France, 1997-2006
法国 1997～2006 年间接合菌病（毛霉菌病）发生率上升

引自：*Emerg Infect Dis*, 2009, 15 (9): 1395

（七）表示长篇连载论文各分篇的主题

报告、论文分册出版，或是一系列工作分几篇报道，或是分阶段的研究结果，一般分篇的内容以副标题表示，在副标题前可加上罗马数字Ⅰ、Ⅱ、Ⅲ、Ⅳ、Ⅴ等，以示连续性。

例一： Clinician's guide to the updated ABCs of cardiovascular disease prevention: A review Part 1

Clinician's guide to the updated ABCs of cardiovascular disease prevention: A review Part 2

最新 ABCs 心血管疾病预防临床医生指南：综述第 1 部分

最新 ABCs 心血管疾病预防临床医生指南：综述第 2 部分

引自：*Am J Med*, 2019, 1329(6): 569

例二： Medical treatment of early breast cancer. Ⅰ: Adjuvant treatment

Medical treatment of early breast cancer. Ⅱ: Endocrine therapy

Medical treatment of early breast cancer. Ⅲ: Chemotherapy

Medical treatment of early breast cancer. Ⅳ: Neoadjuvant treatment

早期乳腺癌的内科治疗（Ⅰ）：辅助治疗

早期乳腺癌的内科治疗（Ⅱ）：内分泌治疗

早期乳腺癌的内科治疗（Ⅲ）：化疗

早期乳腺癌的内科治疗（Ⅳ）：新辅助治疗

引自：*BMJ*, 2006, 5: 135

二、英文标题句式

众所周知，句子（sentence）是相对完整而独立的语言单位，在一定的语境中，句子能够表达完整的思想，起到交流的作用，而且可以独立运用，因此，从英语语法分析的角度来看，句子是最高一层的语言单位。一个语言片段可以分解为若干层的语言单位，最高一层的语言单位是句子，次一层是词组/短语（phrase）。句子不是词的序列，而是词组的序列。从词组的构成分析，可以分为名词词组/短语（noun phrase），动词词组/短语（verb phrase）等。由于医学论文英文标题必须达到简明扼要、突出重点、引人注目、便于编写索引等要求，根据对国内外医学学术刊物的检索分析结果，医学论文英文标题表达主要有三种句式结构，即词组/短语型、陈述句型和疑问句型。国外期刊文题使用完整句较为多见，国内期刊则以短语型为主，而词组/短语型则以名词短语为主。

（一）词组/短语型标题

构成名词词组的中心词可以是单字名词（single-word noun），如 cord blood（脐带血）；也可以是复合名词（compound noun），如 screw-driver teeth（旋凿状齿）。英文标题句式多为词组/短语型，即主要由一个名词或若干并列的名词，加上必要的修饰成分构成或由其他词类构成的短语表示，一般没有谓语成分，类似于汉语中的偏正词组或动宾词组，末尾不用句号。其构成及书写方式有以下几种。

1. 常见构成形式

（1）**中心名词+介词短语**：介词短语在标题中可以起到修饰或补充说明作用。例如，可以对标题中的中心词予以原因、目的、方式、手段和工具的阐释等。

例一： Spontaneous Pneumothorax **in** a Young Woman
年轻女性自发性气胸

引自：*Am J Med*, 2019, 132(6): 706

例二： Visual loss **after** silicone oil removal
硅油取出后诱发的视力丧失

引自：*Br J Ophthalmol*, 2005, 89: 5

例三： The impact of anti-HLA antibodies **on** unrelated cord blood transplantations
抗人类白细胞抗原抗体对非血缘脐血移植的影响

引自：*Blood*, 2010, 116(15): 2839

例四： Delirium **after** coronary artery bypass graft surgery and late mortality
冠状动脉旁路移植术后的谵妄和晚期死亡率

引自：*Ann Neurol*, 2010, 67(3): 338

例五： Glucose metabolism **in** nerve terminals
神经末梢的葡萄糖代谢

引自：*Curr Opin Neurobiol*, 2017, 45: 156

（2）**中心名词+分词短语**：分词短语在这一类标题句式中通常采用后位修饰。

例一： Objective cognitive performance **associated** with electroconvulsive therapy for depression: A systematic review and meta-analysis
与抑郁症患者行电休克治疗相关的客观认知能力:系统综述和荟萃分析
【析】名词+-ed 分词短语。

引自：*Biol Psychiatry*, 2010, 68(6): 568

例二： Spherical aberration and contrast sensitivity in eyes **implanted** with aspheric and spherical intraocular lenses: A comparative study
植入非球面和球面晶状体后眼的球面像差和对比敏感度：一项对照研究
【析】名词+-ed 分词短语。

引自：*Am J Ophthalmol*, 2008, 145(5): 827

例三： A Novel Immunoassay **Using** Recombinant Allergens Simplifies Peanut Allergy Diagnosis
应用重组变应原的新型免疫测定法简化花生过敏的诊断

【析】名词+-ing 分词短语。

引自：Int Arch Allergy Immunol, 2010, 154(3): 216

例四：Outpatient pulmonary rehabilitation **following** acute exacerbations of COPD

慢性阻塞性肺疾病急性加重后门诊患者的肺康复

【析】名词短语+-ing 分词短语。

引自：Thorax, 2010, 65 (5)：423

例五：Leukemia-associated minor histocompatibility antigen discovery **using** T-cell clones isolated by *in vitro* stimulation of naive CD8$^+$ T cells

通过刺激体外未致敏 CD8$^+$ T 淋巴细胞产生离体 T 淋巴细胞克隆检测白血病相关次要组织相容性抗原

【析】名词短语+-ing 分词短语。

引自：Blood, 2010, 115(23): 4923

（3）**中心名词+动词不定式**：动词不定式用作后位修饰。

例一：Association of medication attitudes with non-persistence and non-compliance with medication **to prevent fractures**

药物预防骨折与非连续和不顺从的服药态度间的关系

引自：Osteoporos Int, 2010, 21(11): 1899

例二：Helmet continuous positive airway pressure *vs.* oxygen therapy **to improve oxygenation** in community-acquired pneumonia: A randomized, controlled trial

头罩式持续正压气道通气与氧疗对改善社区获得性肺炎患者氧合作用：一项随机对照试验

引自：Chest, 2010, 138 (1)：114

例三：Systematic review: Treatment agreements and urine drug testing **to reduce** opioid misuse in patients with chronic pain

系统性综述：治疗协议和尿液药检可减少慢性疼痛患者阿片类药物的误用

引自：Ann Intern Med, 2010, 152 (11)：712

例四：Aspirin use **to reduce** the risk of sports-related cardiac arrest in high-risk athletes

阿司匹林用于降低高危运动员与运动有关的心搏骤停的风险

引自：Am J Med, 2019, 132(3): e527

（4）**中心名词+同位结构**：由两个或两个以上同一层语言单位组成的结构，其中前项与后项所指相同，句法也相同，这种结构称同位结构（appositive construction）。同位结构的成分称同位成分。由于同位成分的所指相同，句法也相同，即使略去其中某个成分，也不会影响句子结构的完整性。出于标题简洁性的需要，医学论文标题常采用名词（词组）/短语+名词词组/短语这一最为常见结构。

例一：CU-2010：A novel small molecule protease inhibitor with antifibrinolytic and anticoagulant properties

CU-2010：一种具有抗纤溶和抗凝特性的新型小分子蛋白酶抑制剂

引自: *Anesthesiology,* 2009, 110(1): 123

例二：Trimetazidine: a novel protective role via maintenance of Na$^+$, K$^+$-ATPase activity

曲美他嗪：一种新的钠钾 ATP 酶活性保护剂

引自: *Cardiovasc Res,* 2000, 47(4): 637

例三：Splenic Infarction: A Dark Side of the Nephrotic Syndrome

脾梗死：肾病综合征不为人知的一面

引自: *Am J Med,* 2020, 133(3): e106

例四：Cell adhesion molecule 1(CADM1): A novel risk factor for venous thrombosis

细胞黏附分子 1（CADM1）：静脉血栓形成的新危险因素

引自: *Blood,* 2009, 114(14): 3084

例五：Thioguanine nucleotides and thiopurine methyltransferase in immunobullous diseases: Optimal levels as adjunctive tools for azathioprine monitoring

免疫性大疱病的硫鸟嘌呤核苷酸与硫嘌呤甲基转移酶：硫唑嘌呤最佳水平监测的辅助工具

引自: *Arch Dermatol,* 2009, 145(6): 644

（5）**中心名词+从句**：这种标题句式中的从句可以是同位语从句，也可以是形容词从句。采用名词（词组）/短语+名词性限定分句作同位语时，由于这两类结构的引导词相似，注意不要和形容词从句混淆。

例一：What Are the Parameters **That** Should Inform Gestalt as a Clinical Decision Strategy for Pulmonary Embolism?

对于肺栓塞，应该采用哪种参数做临床决策？

【析】名词+形容词从句。

引自: *Am J Med,* 2020, 133(2): e61

例二：Granulocyte colony-stimulating factor (G-CSF) treatment of childhood acute myeloid leukemias **that** overexpress the differentiation-defective G-CSF receptor isoform Ⅳ is associated with a higher incidence of relapse

对分化缺陷的 G-CSF 受体亚型Ⅳ表达水平增高的儿童期急性髓样白血病采用粒细胞集落刺激因子（G-CSF）治疗会使该病复发率升高

【析】名词短语+形容词从句。

引自: *J Clin Oncol,* 2010, 28(15): 2591

例三：Factors **that** predict outcome of abdominal operations in patients with advanced cirrhosis

晚期肝硬化患者腹部手术预后的预测因素

【析】名词+同位结构。

引自: *Clin Gastroenterol Hepatol,* 2010, 8 (5): 451

例四：Medicare's Approach to Paying for Services That Promote Coordinated Care

医疗保险促进协调护理的服务付费方式

【析】名词+同位词从句。

引自：JAMA, 2019, 321(2): 147

（6）**前位修饰语+名词**：英语中能用作前位修饰语的词很多，常见的有形容词、名词或名词词组、分词（-ing、-ed）。无论采用何种前位修饰语，其核心仍然是名词，所以，这类文题表达形式仍属于名词词组（短语）。

> 例一：Fetal Hypertension
> 致死性高血压
> 【析】形容词修饰名词 hypertension。
>
> 引自：Am J Med, 2020, 133(2): e72
>
> 例二：Over-the-counter medicines in Pakistan: Misuse and overuse
> 巴基斯坦的非处方药：滥用和过度使用
> 【析】名词短语 over-the-counter 修饰 medicines。
>
> 引自：Lancet, 2020, 395(10218): 116
>
> 例三：Cytomegalovirus-associated splenic infarction
> 巨细胞病毒导致的脾梗死
> 【析】cytomegalovirus-associated 构成的复合形容词修饰 splenic infarction。
>
> 引自：Am J Med, 2020, 133(3): e104-e105
>
> 例四：Out-of-hospital endotracheal intubation experience and patient outcomes
> （救援者）院外气管插管术经验与患者预后情况
> 【析】形容词短语+名词修饰中心词 experience。
>
> 引自：Ann Emerg Med, 2010, 55(6): 527
>
> 例五：Combined immunodeficiency associated with DOCK8 mutations
> 与 DOCK8 突变相关的联合免疫缺陷
> 【析】形容词修饰名词 immunodeficiency 另加后位修饰。
>
> 引自：N Engl J Med, 2009, 361(21): 2046

（7）**分词短语**：用于标题表达时，常用 V-ing 现在分词。分词与其后的名词或名词短语构成一个动宾短语。这一英文标题表达，句法结构上与汉语文题基本保持一致，均为动宾关系。

> 例一：**Promoting** urinary continence in women after delivery: Randomised controlled trial
> 改善妇女产后尿失禁的随机对照试验
>
> 引自：BMJ, 2002, 324(7348): 1241
>
> 例二：**Turning** placenta into brain: Placental mesenchymal stem cells differentiate into neurons and oligodendrocytes
> 胎盘转变成大脑：胎盘间质干细胞分化成神经元和少突胶质细胞
>
> 引自：Am J Obstet Gynecol, 2010, 202 (3): 294

例三：**Distinguishing** epithelioid blue nevus from blue nevus-like cutaneous melanoma metastasis using fluorescence in situ hybridization

使用荧光原位杂交术鉴别诊断上皮状蓝痣和蓝痣样皮肤黑色素瘤转移瘤

引自：*Am J Surg Pathol*, 2009, 33 (9): 1396

例四：**Predicting** seizure control: Cortical excitability and antiepileptic medication

预测癫痫控制：皮质兴奋性与抗癫痫药物治疗

引自：*Ann Neurol*, 2010, 67 (1): 64

（8）**介词短语**：这类标题表达有别于"名词+介词短语"。介词用法复杂多变，若使用恰当，可删繁就简，明晰主题。尽管英语中有表达各种关系的介词短语，但能用于这一结构句式的主要是介词 on，意义上接近汉语的"探讨、研究"等。

例一：**On** the Pearls and Perils of Sub-Subspecialization

论强调亚专科的利弊

引自：*Am J Med*, 2020, 133(2): 158

例二：**Toward** more accurate measurements of anorectal motor and sensory function in routine clinical practice: Validation of high-resolution anorectal manometry and rapid barostat bag measurements of rectal function

在常规临床实践中更准确地测量肛肠运动和感觉功能：验证高分辨率肛门直肠测压计和快速恒压器测定直肠功能效果

引自： *Neurogastroenterol Motil*, 2014, 26(5): 685-695

例三：**On** the effect of X-ray irradiation on the deformation and fracture behavior of human cortical bone

探讨 X 线照射对人皮质骨变形和破裂的影响

引自：*Bone*, 2010, 46(6): 1475

2. 常见标题书写形式

（1）仅标题第一个词的首字母大写。

例一：Pilot study to estimate the accuracy of mouth self-examination in an at-risk group

初步研究评估高危人群口腔自我检查的准确性

引自：*Head Neck,* 2010, 32 (10): 1393

例二：Effect of splenectomy on mortality and brain water content of rats with brain injury

脾脏切除对颅脑创伤大鼠死亡率及脑含水量的影响

引自：《中华创伤杂志》, 2010, 26(1): 9

例三：Tanslumbar moto-evoked potentials in diagnosis of functional defecation disorder

功能性排便障碍患者经腰刺激运动诱发电位的研究

引自：《第三军医大学学报》, 2013, 35(21): 2292

（2）标题中每个词的首字母都大写，但某些虚词小写，如冠词、3 个字母以内的连词和介词。

例一：Clinical Observation on Tongxinluo Capsule for Treatment of Coronary Heart Disease

通心络胶囊对冠心病治疗效果的临床对照观察

引自：《中西医结合心脑血管病杂志》，2007, 7:575

例二：Dabigatran versus Warfarin in Patients with Atrial Fibrillation

达比加群与华法林治疗心房颤动患者效果的比较

引自：*N Engl J Med*, 2009, 361(12): 1139

例三：Public Awareness and Perceptions of Palliative and Comfort Care

公众对姑息和舒适护理的认识和看法

引自：*Am J Med*, 2019, 132(2): 129

（3）四个字母及以上的虚词多大写，如"with、from、after、before、during、against、between"等。

关于标题中虚词书写格式，不同期刊的处理办法不尽相同，如《美国解剖学杂志》（ *The American Journal of Anatomy* ）就要求标题中的所有介词，不论字母多少，均一律小写。而 I.Griggs 著的 *Guide and Handbook for Writing* 一书中却指出，这类虚词如处于标题中的第一个词时，即使不足 5 个字母，也应大写。

例一：Risk Associated **With** Preoperative Anemia in Cardiac Surgery: A Multicenter Cohort Study

与心脏外科手术前贫血相关的危险因素：多中心队列研究

引自：*Circulation*, 2008, 28(2): 39

例二：Nonlinear Dynamics of Blood Pressure Variability **After** Caffeine Consumption

摄入咖啡因后血压变率非线性动力学研究

引自：*Clin Path*, 2006, 4(2): 79

例三：Advanced Glycosylation End Products Might Promote Atherosclerosis **Through** Inducing the Immune Maturation of Dendritic Cells

深度糖基化最终产物可能通过诱导树突状细胞免疫成熟导致动脉粥样硬化

引自：*Arterioscler Thromb Vasc Biol*, 2005, 25(10): 67

例四：Relation **Between** Red Blood Cell Distribution Width and Cardiovascular Event Rate in People **With** Coronary Disease

冠心病患者红细胞分布宽度和心血管疾病的相关性

引自：*Circulation*, 2008, 28(2): 47

（4）全部大写。标题采用完全大写格式的期刊较少，例如：

例一：P53 AND PCNA EXPRESSION IN THE PREDICTION OF MALIGNANT

POTENTIALS OF PRECANCEROUS CERVICAL LESIONS

P53 和 PCNA 蛋白表达对子宫颈癌前病变恶变潜能预测的意义

引自:《齐鲁医学杂志》, 2005, 20(1): 66

例二: THE EXPRESSION OF hTERT AND PROLIFERATING CELL NUCLEAR ANTIGEN IN HUMAN CERVICAL CANCER

hTERT、PCNA 在人宫颈癌组织中的表达

引自:《中国组织化学与细胞化学杂志》, 2005, (2): 142

例三: EFFICACY OF RECOMBINANT HUMAN FOLLICLE STIMULATING HORMONE AT LOW DOSES IN INDUCING SPERMATOGENESIS AND FERTILITY IN HYPOGONADOTROPIC HYPOGONADISM

低剂量重组人体促卵泡激素（FSH）诱导低促性腺素功能减退症患者精子发生和对生育能力的疗效

引自: *J Endocrinol Invest*, 2010, 33(9): 618

（二）陈述句型标题

医学论文标题一般都是名词性标题。有的医学杂志，如美国的 *Journal of the National Cancer Institute* 及我国编辑出版的 *World Journal of Gastroenterology*，甚至明确规定标题不得写成完整的句子。究其原因，可能是因为人们认为医学科学总是不断创新，不断发展的。陈述句（declarative sentence），即描述某件事实或陈述某人对某一问题的观点看法。尽管如此，有些期刊，如 *The Lancet* 等英国、美国医学杂志中常可见由完整句子构成的标题句式。这类标题句式分为两类：①主-谓-宾/主-谓型陈述句，句末不用句号；②疑问句句式，句末问号则不可省略。

例一: XIAP expression is post-transcriptionally upregulated in childhood ALL and is associated with glucocorticoid response in T-cell ALL

急性淋巴细胞白血病患儿 X 连锁凋亡抑制蛋白转录后上调与急性 T 淋巴细胞白血病糖皮质激素耐药相关

引自: *Pediatr Blood Cancer*, 2010, 55 (2) : 260

例二: Poststroke Constipation Is Associated With Impaired Rectal Sensation

卒中后便秘与直肠感觉受损有关

引自: *Am J Gastroenterol*, 2020, 115(1): 105

例三: Tribbles pseudokinase 3 inhibits the adipogenic differentiation of human adipose-derived mesenchymals

Tribbles 同源蛋白 3 抑制人脂肪间充质干细胞成脂分化

引自:《北京大学学报（医学版）》, 2020, 52(1): 1

例四: In situ vaccination with a TLR9 agonist induces systemic lymphoma regression: a phase Ⅰ/Ⅱ study

用 Toll 样受体 9 激动剂原位疫苗诱导系统性淋巴瘤消退：Ⅰ/Ⅱ期临床研究

引自：*J Clin Oncol,* 2010, 28(28): 4324

例五： Gamma-secretase activating protein is a therapeutic target for Alzheimer's disease

γ 分泌酶激活蛋白是阿尔茨海默病的治疗靶点

引自：*Nature,* 2010, 467 (7311): 95

（三）疑问句型标题

疑问句，就其句法结构和交际功能来说，分为一般疑问句（general questions）、特殊疑问句（special questions）、选择疑问句（alternative questions）和附加疑问句（tag questions）。一般疑问句通常用来询问一件事情或一个情况是否属实，其答案通常是 yes 或 no。而特殊疑问句则就某一特殊部分提出疑问，其答案通常是开放性的。事实上，任何一个具有严谨态度的科学工作者对于其研究领域总会有这样或那样的困惑。鉴于此，科研论文中并不乏以疑问句式作标题的研究论文。根据句法语义功能，用来作标题的疑问句有一般疑问句和特殊疑问句，其目的都是为了提出研究者的疑问或商榷。但也有另一种情况，即作者出于谨慎角度考虑，即使对某一研究结论能做出定性，也会使用疑问式标题。由于标题应简洁，重点突出等特性的要求，采用疑问句作标题时也可省略作用词。例如："(Is) Aggressive treatment of low grade prostate cancer unnecessary?"低度恶性前列腺癌不需要积极治疗？；"Why (do) some people go blind from glaucoma?"为什么有些人因青光眼而失明？。因此，做标题的疑问句可以是完整结构，也可以是省略结构。无论是哪种结构，切记句末一般用问号。然而，在英语中，有一类结构值得注意，即疑问代词或疑问副词加动词不定式结构。这类结构通常在复合句中起名词性短语作用，如用此类结构作标题时，可不用问号。例如："What to look for in rib fractures and how"肋骨骨折时应检查什么及如何检查。

1. 省略作用词式标题

例一： A Genetic Origin? Purpura Fulminans

遗传起源？普普拉·富民族

引自：*Am J Med,* 2019, 132(3): 327

例二： Pelvic packing or angiography: Competitive or complementary?

骨盆填塞或造影：相互竞争还是相辅相成？

引自：*Injury,* 2009, 40 (4): 343

例三： The metabolic syndrome: useful concept or clinical tool? Report of a WHO Expert Consultation

代谢综合征：有用的概念还是临床工具？WHO 专家的磋商报告

引自：*Diabetologia,* 2010, 53 (4): 600

2. 完整结构式标题

例一： Does *Helicobacter pylori* eradication therapy for peptic ulcer prevent gastric cancer?

幽门螺杆菌根除疗法治疗消化性溃疡是否能预防胃癌？

引自：*World J Gastroenterol*, 2009, 15 (34): 4290

例二： Why is laparoscopic surgery underutilised?

为何腹腔镜手术没有得到充分利用？

引自：*Lancet*, 2020, 395(10217): 3

例三： Is sclerotherapy better than intralesional excision for treating aneurysmal bone cysts?

硬化疗法治疗动脉瘤样骨囊肿优于病灶内切除吗？

引自：*Clin Orthop Relat Res*, 2010, 468 (6)：1649

例四： Are red blood cell transfusions associated with nosocomial infections in pediatric intensive care units?

红细胞输注与儿科重症监护病房医院感染相关吗？

引自：*Pediatr Crit Care Med*, 2010, 11 (4): 464

三、英、汉标题比较

文章标题具备信息功能（提供文章的主要内容）、祈使功能（吸引读者阅读和购买）、美感功能（简单明了、新颖、醒目）和检索功能（方便读者和科技工作者检索、查阅及引用）。医学论文的标题还有其自身的特点，即有较多的专业术语和较长的字数。由于绝大多数作者的研究论文是用汉语写作的，写英文标题时常受汉语表达的影响，基本上按完全对等的方式来写出英文标题。这样的英文标题是难以满足上述要求的。更为重要的是，英文标题和摘要，其根本目的是对外交流，因此，英文表达必须能传旨达意。尽管英、汉语言表达方式存在着很大差异，但在医学论文标题用词方面，英语和汉语也有许多相同之处，对于它们的翻译，既要照顾中英文题名的一致性，又要保持其英文题名与中文题名内容上一致。然而，中英文题名的一致性并不等于词语要一一对应。例如：

例一： Study of transcranial moto-evoked potentials in the patients with functional constipation

功能性便秘患者经颅磁刺激运动诱发电位的研究

引自：《南京医科大学学报（自然科学版）》, 2011, 31(11): 1674

例二： Genetic Diagnosis of RHD and RhCE Bloodgrouping

RHD 和 RhCE 血型基因诊断

引自：《中国实验诊断学》, 2010, 14(8): 1242

例三： Study on insulin resistance, glycolipid metabolism, and sex hormones in patients with polycystic ovary syndrome

多囊卵巢综合征患者胰岛素抵抗与糖脂代谢及性激素的研究

引自:《中华内分泌代谢杂志》, 2020, 36(3): 213

例四: Modified method of human islet isolation and purification for clinical transplantation

成人胰岛细胞的分离纯化与应用

引自:《中国现代医学杂志》, 2010, 20(17): 2626

对于一种语言里面的每一个字词,我们不一定在其他语言里找到精确对应的词。也就是说,由一种语言的字词所描述的总体概念并非与另一种语言的字词所表达的总体概念一模一样,即使有些概念也确实能对应。从上述例句可知,如果标题采用单纯性名词短语结构表达,即单一型概念标题,其词序和汉语基本对应。然而,多概念组成的标题,由于英汉两种语言在某些限定修饰语词序位置上的差异,英、汉标题在词序和语序上差异十分明显(如上述例四)。除上述差异之外,还有一种因素会导致英、汉题名不对应现象,即内容与形式。唯物辩证法认为,任何事物都具有内容和形式两个方面。在二者的辩证关系中,内容决定形式,形式必须适合于、服从于内容,有什么样的内容,就要求有什么样的形式。医学论文题名既要简洁明了,同时还应兼顾忠实原则,能直接反映论文内容及意义。如上述例四,中文标题中并未出现"改良方法",而英文标题中却增加了"modified method of..."。众所周知,胰岛细胞产量和纯度与所采用的不同分离纯化方法密切相关,该文主要探讨了这一方法的改良结果,因此,英文标题在概念表达上就与中文标题产生了不一致现象。又如:中文标题"天然虾青素缓解体力疲劳作用的实验研究"与英文标题"Alleviative effect of natural astaxanthin on physical fatigue"[引自:《中国现代医学杂志》, 2010; 20(17): 2567]也同理。

然而,用英文表达文题时要尽可能做到删繁就简,避免出现冗词,即剩余信息(redundancy)。通常情况下,为了使交际渠道通畅,保证理解,人们在交际过程中总是给予超过实际需要量的信息,这是因为学习者在英语习得过程中未能真正驾驭其所学习的语言,从而导致其使用英语时套用母语的模式,甚至滥用所学语言的模式。现就英、汉两种语言表达方式的差异从语用学和句法结构方面做简要分析对比。

(一)"Study of..." "Report of..."等冗词的省略

汉语和英语是两种截然不同的语言,有着迥异的语法、词汇、曲折变化。语言表达方式差异不仅存在于世界各国和不同民族之间,即使是同一个民族,同一种语言,在不同时代也会存在不同的表达风格。现代英语演变的最大特点之一是简洁性,如医学论文英文标题在18世纪时常用"Some thoughts on..." "A few observations on..."的格式,当今却较少见。而现代医学论文英文标题为适应网络的需要,越来越趋向于简短、扼要,甚至连以"Study of..." "Investigation of..." "A report of..."开始的句式也逐渐减少。这是因为上述这些句式中的"Study of..." "Investigation of..." "A report of..."等并无实质性内容，在用论文标题制作检索文件时，它们在某种意义上已成为垃圾信息，所以作者或编者常将这类冗词略去。例如：

例一： Clinical and ECG features of arrhythmogenic right ventricular cardiomyopathy: A retrospective analysis of 31 cases

31例致心律失常性右心室心肌病的临床研究

引自：《中华心血管病杂志》，2007, 35(1): 25

例二： The Relation between Vascular Remodeling in Patients with Essential Hypertension and Syndrome Identified by Traditional Chinese Medicine

原发性高血压病人血管重构与中医证型相关关系的研究

引自：《中西医结合心脑血管病杂志》，2007, 5(1): 11

例三： Study of local anesthetic effect and safety of lidocain using in common bronchoscopy

利多卡因局部麻醉用于清醒支气管镜检查的效果和安全性研究

【析】本标题中的 study of 完全可以略去，而不会影响到标题信息传递。

引自：《国际呼吸杂志》，2014, 34(18): 1390-1392

例四： Pneumoconiosis among underground bituminous coal miners in the United States: Is silicosis becoming more frequent?

美国地下烟煤矿工中发生尘肺病的研究：硅肺的发生是否日益增多？

引自：*Occup Environ Med,* 2010, 67(10): 652

例五： Application value of different lymph node staging system in predicting prognosis of patients with intrahepatic cholangiocarcinoma

不同淋巴结分期指标评估肝内胆管癌患者预后的价值探讨

【析】标题中略去了"探讨"一词。

引自：《中华外科杂志》，2020, 58(4): 295

在上述标题中，基本将冗词省去了。因为，从语用学角度，这些概念和意义本身在标题和论文中已有体现，除掉上述冗词也不会引起读者误解，因此遇到汉语题目带有上述字样时均可省略不译。例如：

例一： The predictive value of TG/HDL-C ratio for coronary heart risk

甘油三酯/高密度脂蛋白胆固醇比值对冠心病的诊断价值的探讨

引自：《中华心血管病杂志》，2000, 28(1): 33

例二： Relevant factors of invasive pituitary adenomas

侵袭性垂体瘤的相关因素分析

引自：《中华外科杂志》，2001, 39(6): 455

例三： Perioperative complications in children with pulmonary hypertension undergoing general anesthesia with ketamine

关于肺动脉高压症患儿围手术期并发症的发生与氯胺酮全麻的相关性研究

引自：*Paediatr Anaesth,* 2010, 20(1): 28

　　国外刊物中也有英文标题上带有 study 等字样的，如"Studies of the lymphatic pathway of bone and bone marrow"（译：骨及骨髓淋巴回路的研究；引自 *J Bone Joint Surg*，1960，42A：716-725），这里 study 如省去不用，丝毫不影响整个标题的实质性内容。但 study 等词之前若有限定性成分，起解释说明作用时，study、analysis、report 等就有了具体的内容，则不可省略，如 "Genetic epidemiological study on non-insulin dependent diabetes mellitus" 非胰岛素依赖型糖尿病的遗传流行病学研究，〔引自：《中华预防医学杂志》，2000，（02）：18〕。即使这样，在英文中，这种带定语的 study 通常也只是被置于副标题中，而较少用于正标题。产生这种现象的原因是标题不仅应简单明了，而且应便于编写索引。正、副标题一分开，编写或查阅索引，只要看正标题，就一目了然。但国内医学期刊和国外医学期刊在这一形式的题名表达上有较大差异。例如：

例一：Comparative Study of the Incidence in Collagen-Induced Arthritis Rats of Different Gender and Species
　　　不同品系、不同性别对大鼠 CIA 发病情况的比较研究
　　　　　　　　　　　　引自：《中国中医基础医学杂志》，2010，16(9): 761

例二：The Experimental Study of IL-8 in Rattus norvegicus AFE pathogenesis
　　　IL-8 在大鼠羊水栓塞发病机制中的实验研究
　　　　　　　　　　　　引自：《中国实验诊断学》2010, 14(9): 1370

例三：Pathogenesis and Imaging Study of Pulmonary Tuberculosis Cavity
　　　现代肺结核空洞性病变的发病及影像学研究
　　　　　　　　　　　　引自：《临床放射学杂志》，2010, 29(5): 603

例四：A randomized, double blind, and parallel controlled multicenter clinical trial of reboxetine in treatment of depression
　　　瑞波西汀治疗抑郁症的随机、双盲、平行对照、多中心临床试验
　　　　　　　　　　　　引自：《中国新药与临床杂志》，2010, 29(7): 490

例五：Simvastatin and disease stabilization in normal tension glaucoma: A cohort study
　　　辛伐他汀与正常眼压性青光眼稳定作用的队列研究
　　　　　　　　　　　　引自：*Ophthalmology,* 2010, 117 (3)：471

例六：A population-based questionnaire survey on the prevalence of peanut, tree nut, and shellfish allergy in 2 Asian populations
　　　两个亚洲人群的花生、坚果及贝类过敏发生率：一项基于人群的问卷调查
　　　　　　　　　　　　引自：*J Allergy Clin Immuno*, 2010, 126 (2): 324

例七：Analysis of the relationship between the number of lymph nodes examined and prognosis for curatively resected gallbladder carcinoma: a multi-institutional study
　　　胆囊癌根治术中淋巴结清扫数目与预后关系的多中心临床研究
　　　　　　　　　　　　引自：《中华外科杂志》，2020, 58(4): 303

（二）as 在标题中的应用

关于英文科技论文标题中是否可以用完整句这一问题，众说纷纭，莫衷一是。不过，据有关对国际著名三大期刊 *Science*、*The Lancet* 和 *Nature* 的统计分析表明，用完整句子作标题的情况十分常见，句式一般为主-谓-宾结构，且多采用陈述句形式。然而，为了标题的简洁，如果标题中心结构蕴含着汉语的主谓关系，即相当于英语的表语结构（含有表示状态的系动词 be）时，通常可以用介词 as 来替代 be，从而将陈述句句式简化为短语式。介词 as 意为"in the function of"或"the same as"，即"以……功能的；如同"。例如：

例一： Homocysteine **as** a Predictive Factor for Hip Fracture in Elderly Women with Parkinson's Disease (=Homocysteine serves as a Predictive Factor for Hip Fracture in Elderly Women with Parkinson's Disease)
同型半胱氨酸作为帕金森病老龄女性患者髋部骨折的预测因子

引自：*Am J Med*, 2018, 131(3): e109

例二： Identification of oxidative stress and Toll-like receptor 4 signaling **as** a key pathway of acute lung injury (=Identification of oxidative stress and Toll-like receptor 4 signaling serve as a key pathway of acute lung injury)
氧化应激和 Toll 样受体 4 信号是急性肺损伤的关键通路

引自：*Cell*, 2008, 133(2): 235-249

例三： Combination antibiotics **as** a treatment for chronic Chlamydia-induced reactive arthritis (=Combination antibiotics serves as a treatment for chronic Chlamydia-induced reactive arthritis)
联合应用抗生素治疗慢性衣原体诱导的反应性关节炎

引自：*Arthritis Rheum,* 2010, 62(5): 1298

例四： The complex nature of serum C3 and C4 **as** biomarkers of lupus renal flare (=The complex nature of serum C3 and C4 serves as biomarker of lupus renal flare)
血清 C3 和 C4 作为狼疮性肾炎发作标志物的复杂特性

引自：*Lupus*, 2010, 19(11): 1272

例五： Ustekinumab **as** Induction and Maintenance Therapy for Crohn's Disease (=Ustekinumab serves as Induction and Maintenance Therapy for Crohn's Disease)
Ustekinumab 作为克罗恩病的诱导和维持治疗

引自：*N Engl J Med*, 2016, 375(20): 1946

例六： Complement regulator factor H **as** a serum biomarker of multiple sclerosis disease state (= Complement regulator factor H serves **as** a serum biomarker of multiple sclerosis disease state)

补体调节因子 H 可以作为多发硬化疾病的血清生物标志物

引自: *Brain*, 2010, 133(6): 1602

（三）and 在标题中的应用

论文标题中有时会出现多概念并列情况，即由两个或两个以上具有独立完整概念的词组并列组成。由于词或词组之间没有说明或被说明、修饰或被修饰的关系，而是无主次的并列关系，因此，标题的英文结构可按各个概念的词或词组的先后顺序借助英语的并列连词 and 来表达。and 在英文标题中的语义关系为 "together with or along with; in addition to; as well as"，即 "和、与、及、同、又、也、加上"。

例一：Diagnosis **and** Management of Obstructive Sleep Apnea: A Review
　　　阻塞性睡眠呼吸暂停的诊断与治疗：综述

引自: *JAMA*, 2020, 323(14): 1389

例二：Clinical characteristics **and** analysis of prognostic factors of 222 patients diagnosed with Hodgkin's lymphoma
　　　222 例霍奇金淋巴瘤患者临床特征及预后分析

引自:《中华医学杂志》, 2019, 99(48): 3792

例三：Genetic Diagnosis **and** Testing in Clinical Practice
　　　基因诊断与临床校验

引自: *Clin Path*, 2006, 4(2): 123

医学论文汉语标题中常出现 "关系" 一词，词组 "关系" 在语义层面表示 "事物之间相互作用、相互影响的状态；两个或更多的事物之间逻辑或自然的联系（a logical or natural association between two or more things; relevance of one to another）"。用语言的理性意义来衡量，and 本身在语篇平面上就提示了事物之间的关联性，因此，也可采用这一句式，从而省略冗词以简化文题。以下列中文期刊标题为例，可以进行相应简化：

例一：Relationship between the CT features of colorectal cancer metastases calcification and tumor response to chemotherapy
　　　化疗后结直肠癌转移瘤钙化 CT 影像学表现与化疗反应之间的关系
　　　【析】本标题可略去 Relationship between，将文题简化为 "CT features of colorectal cancer metastases calcification and tumor response to chemotherapy"。

引自:《北京大学学报（医学版）》, 2019, 51(6): 1078

例二：A study for the relationship between serum calcitionin gene-related peptide and coronary arteriopathy
　　　降钙素基因相关肽与冠状动脉病变关系的探讨
　　　【析】本标题可简化为 "Serum calcitionin gene-related peptide and coronary

arteriopathy"。

引自:《中华内科杂志》, 2001, 40(11): 750

例三: The relationship between smoking and bone mineral density in 386 healthy adult men

386 例健康男性骨密度与吸烟的关系

【析】此标题较为简洁的说法为 "Smoking and bone mineral density in 386 healthy adult men"。

引自:《中华预防医学杂志》, 2001, 35(3): 149

例四: Dose-response relationship between respirable dust and pneumoconiosis in geological exploration industry

地质勘探作业呼吸性粉尘与尘肺病的剂量-反应关系

【析】该文题可简化为 "Dose-response between respirable dust and pneumoconiosis in geological exploration industry"。

引自:《中华预防医学杂志》, 2001, 35(4): 258

例五: Study of relationship between large artery distensibility and left ventricular hypertrophy in patients with essential hypertension

高血压大动脉扩张与左心室肥厚关系的探讨

【析】原标题中 study 和 relationship 都可视为冗词,可以略去。简化后的标题为 "Large artery distensibility and left ventricular hypertrophy in patients with essential hypertension",虽然简化了,但未影响信息传递。

引自:《中华心血管杂志》, 2000, 28(3): 177

例六: Relationship between leptin and liver fibrosis in patients with nonalcoholic fatty liver disease

非酒精性脂肪性肝病患者瘦素与肝纤维化的关系

【析】题名可简化为 "Leptin and liver fibrosis in patients with nonalcoholic fatty liver disease"。

引自:《世界华人消化杂志》, 2010, 18(19): 2055

试比较国外期刊:

例一: Fatty acid oxidation and malonyl-CoA decarboxylase in the vascular remodeling of pulmonary hypertension

肺动脉高压的血管重塑中脂肪酸氧化和丙二酰-CoA 脱羧酶的关系

引自: *Sci Transl Med*, 2010, 2(44): 44ra58

例二: Glucose Metabolism and Coronary Heart Disease in Patients with Normal Glucose Tolerance

糖耐量正常患者葡萄糖代谢与冠心病的关系

引自: *JAMA*, 2004, 291(15): 1857

例三: Family poverty over the early life course and recurrent adolescent and young adult anxiety and depression: A longitudinal study

早年家庭贫困和青少年反复焦虑抑郁之间关系的纵向研究

引自：Am J Public Health, 2010, 100 (9) : 1719

例四： Maintenance of sinus rhythm and survival in patients with heart failure and atrial fibrillation

心力衰竭伴心房颤动患者窦性心律的维持与患者生存率的关系

引自：J Am Coll Cardiol, 2010, 55(17): 1796

例五： Vasomotor symptoms, estradiol levels and cardiovascular risk profile in women

女性血管收缩症、雌二醇水平与心血管风险之间的关系

引自：Maturitas, 2010, 66 (3): 285-90

但同时也要注意：①汉语中的"关系"并非与英语中的词完全对应，因此，英译标题时要具体问题具体对待，如下例六；②若"关系"前有说明性词语时，英译标题时，则 relationship 不宜省略，如下例七。

例六： The **interaction** between perinatal factors and childhood abuse in the risk of developing anorexia nervosa

神经性厌食症的发展危险中围产期因素与儿童期虐待之间的关系

【析】本文题提示的是因果关系，interaction 意为"the act or process of interacting"。

引自：Psychol Med, 2010, 40(4): 657

例七： **Epidemiologic relationships** between A1C and all-cause mortality during a median 3.4-year follow-up of glycemic treatment in the ACCORD trial

ACCORD 试验（降糖治疗的随访时间中位数为 3.4 年）中糖化血红蛋白（A1C）和全因死亡率之间流行病学关系的研究

【析】relationships 之前有 epidemiologic 限定特定"关系"。

引自：Diabetes Care, 2010, 33(5): 983

（四）病例数的处理

国内外医学期刊对于标题中病例数的处理有较大差异。

1. 国内医学期刊由于受母语因素的干扰和汉语表达习惯的影响，病例数通常置于正标题，而较少置于副标题中。例如：

例一： The clinical characteristics and airway inflammatory phenotypes in 35 patients with severe asthma

35 例重症支气管哮喘患者临床特征和气道炎症表型

引自：《中华内科杂志》, 2019, 58(9): 680

例二：Clinical characteristics of Kaposiform lymphangiomatosis: A report of 8 cases

　　　　卡波西样淋巴管瘤病八例临床分析

引自:《中华外科杂志》, 2019, 57(12)：921

例三：Factors influencing prognosis of 90 polymyositis and dermatomyositis patients

　　　　90 例多发性肌炎和皮肌炎预后影响因素随访研究

引自:《第三军医大学学报》, 2010, 32(8): 842-845

例四：Nosocomial Infection: A Transverse Section Survey on 1483 Inpatients

　　　　1483 例住院患者医院感染横断面调查及分析

引自:《中华医院感染学杂志》, 2010, 20(17): 2566

例五：Analysis of 668 Import Infected Malarias in Shanghai

　　　　上海市 668 例输入性疟疾病例流行病学分析

引自:《热带医学杂志》, 2010, 10(8): 988-990

2. 国外期刊中，为了突出论文中心，常将病例数置于副标题中，作为对主标题的补充。国内期刊也有类似处理方法。例如：

例一：Spitz nevus: A clinicopathological study of 349 cases

　　　　349 例斯皮茨痣临床病理研究

引自: *Am J Dermatopathol,* 2009, 31 (2)：107

例二：Circumcision with the Chinese ShangRing in Children: Outcomes of 824 cases

　　　　应用中国商环行儿童包皮环切 824 例疗效分析

引自:《中华男科学杂志》, 2010, 16(3): 35

例三：Laparoscopic pancreaticoduodenectomy: A report of 233 cases by a single team

　　　　腹腔镜胰十二指肠切除术单中心 233 例临床经验总结

引自:《中华外科杂志》, 2017, 55(5): 354

在国内出版的中文医学期刊中，95%左右的期刊都要求附英文标题和摘要，其目的是为了让不懂汉语的同行了解我们的研究现状以提高论文的浏览率和摘引率。论文标题是提供给读者的第一信息源，因此，英文标题表达应突出研究的主题和研究的目的。如果在英译标题时采用完全对等的翻译方式，标题中会充满不必要的次要信息，这就破坏了英文的简洁性。英汉表达过程中的"对等（equivalence）"和"不对等（non-equivalence）"是相对而非绝对。医学论文英文标题表达可以从**概念意义**（即主题意义，它是语言信息的核心和主体，包括词、词组、句子及语段等四个层次的语义内容。概念意义的对等就是双语的语义对等）、**语境意义**〔即从上下文（context）中获得的特殊意义，它是由语言的交际目的、交际对象、交际场合所决定的〕、**形式意义**（即语言以形式作为外部表现方式，使语言符号所承载的内容成为被感知的实体。在双语表达中，以源语为依托，将源语的全部意义忠实地表达到目的语之中）等三个方面来斟酌，从而保持与英语的表达习惯和特征上的一致。据此，标题"提升自我效能感对老年脑卒中患者吞咽功能康复护理的临床应用"，可英译为"Outcomes of rehabilitation nursing based on improving self-efficacy in elderly stroke patients with dysphagia"。

（五）中文标题中一些高频词的英文表达

汉、英两种语言既存在对等又有不对等现象。本节就语言的概念意义、语境意义和形式意义三方面来比较中文标题中一些高频词在英文表达中的异同。

1. "探讨"的意义表示

词组"探讨"的中心在于"探"，意即试图发现（隐藏的事物或情况）或穷本之源。汉语中与之意义接近的词组有"探索、探究、探明"等。英语中可用于表达"探讨"意义的名词有"exploration, study, discussion, approach, investigation, evaluation, detection, survey"等，但措辞时要注意英语对应词词义的内涵和外延，如 exploration 意为"the act of making a careful examination for diagnostic purpose"（为诊断目的而做的调查或检查）；discussion 表示"consideration of a subject; exposition"（讨论；阐述）。"探讨"一词在标题中也可省略翻译。

例一：Exploration of the mechanism of skin expansion
　　　皮肤扩张术机理探讨
　　　　　　　　　　　　　　　　引自：《中华整形外科杂志》，2000, 16(2): 84

例二：Discussion on pT3 staging in TNM staging of AJCC 8th edition gallbladder
　　　carcinoma
　　　关于 AJCC 第八版胆囊癌 TNM 分期中 pT3 期分期的探讨
　　　　　　　　　　　　　　　　引自：《中华外科杂志》，2019, 57(11): 834

例三：A pilot study in treatment of systemic lupus erythematosus by autologous
　　　bone marrow transplant
　　　自身骨髓移植治疗系统性红斑狼疮初探
　　　　　　　　　　　　　　　　引自：《中华内科杂志》，2001, 40(4): 229

例四：Preliminary Study of Enhancement Pattern Changes in the Assessment of
　　　Nonsurgical Treatment in Bronchogenic Carcinoma
　　　强化模式的变化在肺癌非手术治疗疗效评价中作用的初步探讨
　　　　　　　　　　　　　　　　引自：《临床放射学杂志》，2010, 29(10): 1336

例五：Clinical study on endovascular treatment for symptomatic atherosclerotic
　　　stenosis of basilar artery
　　　经皮血管内治疗症状性基底动脉粥样硬化性狭窄的探讨
　　　　　　　　　　　　　　　　引自：《中华外科杂志》，2010, 48(19): 1466

"探讨"这一概念也可用介词 on 来表达。可是，在多数情况下，"探讨"一词可略去不译。例如：

例一： High vaginal uterosacral ligament suspension for treatment of uterine prolapse

经阴道子宫骶骨韧带高位悬吊术治疗子宫脱垂的临床探讨

引自:《中华妇产科杂志》, 2007, 42(12): 797

例二： Surgical treatment of colorectal liver metastases

结直肠癌肝转移外科若干热点问题探讨

引自:《中华外科杂志》, 2017, 55(7): 491

例三： Measurement and significance of the pulmonary capillary wedge pressure in children with nephrotic syndrome

肾病综合征肺毛细血管楔压测定及其临床意义初探

引自:《中华儿科杂志》, 2001, 39(12): 726

例四： Associations between breast milk viral load, mastitis, exclusive breast-feeding, and postnatal transmission of HIV

探讨母乳病毒载量、乳腺炎、纯母乳喂养及产后艾滋病病毒传播间的关系

引自: *Clin Infect Dis*, 2010, 50 (5) : 762

例五： Arteriosclerosis Obliterans of the Lower Extremities: Indications and Strategies of Surgical Therapy

下肢动脉硬化性闭塞症的规范化治疗探讨

引自:《中国医学科学院学报》, 2007, 29(1): 12

例六： "Liver and pancreas oriented" strategies for minimally invasive surgery of biliary malignant tumors

胆道恶性肿瘤"上肝下胰"的微创手术策略探讨

引自:《中华外科杂志》, 2019, 57(1): 16

2. "体会、经验、总结"的译法

"体会"的中心在于亲身经验、体察（personally do or experience sth.；experience and observe），即通过躬亲践行体察认识某种特定事物的性质、特征；"经验"意为从多次实践中得到的知识或技能；"总结"是指把一定阶段内的有关情况分析研究，做出有指导性的结论。对应的英语表达均用 experience，有时在标题中也可省略不译（注意观察对比以下例句）。另有一点需要注意的是，题名中的"总结"非 summary（summary 意为 "presenting the substance in a condensed form; concise" 概括；扼要地叙述）。例如："2009 年精神分裂症 PORT 心理药理学治疗推荐以及概要陈述[The 2009 schizophrenia PORT psychopharmacological treatment recommendations and summary statements；引自:*Schizophr Bull*, 2010, 36 (1) :71]"。此外，应注意 experience 在表达"体会、经验、总结"这一概念时，其为抽象名词。虽然英语中抽象名词可以转换为具体名词，但某些名词转换后，其意义发生较大变化。例如，experiences 表示"经历"；damages 表示"赔偿金"等。

例一： Repeated colonoscopic screening of patients with acromegaly: **15-year experience** identifies those at risk of new colonic neoplasia and allows for effective screening guidelines

结肠镜重复检查肢端肥大症患者：鉴别高危结肠瘤形成和有效检查原则制订的 15 年经验总结

引自：*Eur J Endocrinol*, 2010, 163 (1): 21

例二： **Clinical experience** of placing endocardial temporary pacing wire through the internal jugular vein

经颈内静脉放置心内膜临时起搏导线的临床经验

引自：《复旦学报（医学版）》, 2018, 45(6): 863

例三： Application of fenestration and suction drainage for treatment of large odontogenic mandibular cystic lesions

开窗术后负压引流治疗大型牙源性颌骨囊肿的临床总结

引自：《南方医科大学学报》, 2012, 32(3): 409

例四： The impact of partial biopsy on histopathologic diagnosis of cutaneous melanoma: **Experience** of an Australian tertiary referral service

部分活检对皮肤黑色素瘤组织病理诊断的影响：澳大利亚一家三级转诊中心的经验

引自：*Arch Dermatol*, 2010, 146 (3): 234

例五： **Experience** on increasing the surgical effect of the small primary liver cancer

提高原发性小肝癌手术切除疗效的经验与体会

引自：《中国实用外科杂志》, 2001, 21(8): 485

例六： **Initial experience** with CentriMag extracorporal membrane oxygenation for support of critically ill patients with refractory cardiogenic shock

CentriMag 体外微循环膜氧合器支持难治性心源性休克病危患者的初步研究经验

引自：*J Heart Lung Transplant*, 2010, 29 (1) : 66

3. "问题"的译法

"问题"意指"需要解决的矛盾、疑难或重要之点（crucial point）"，与之对应的英文名词有 problem、aspect、issue，在文题中通常用复数形式。但是，需要注意区分 question（"an expression of inquiry that invites or calls for a reply"，问题征求或要求回答的询问）。对于这三个词的使用应考虑概念和语境。它们的意义分别为 problem（"a question to be considered, solved, or answered"，应该考虑、解决或回答的问题）；aspect（"something can be viewed by the mind"，视点，角度）；issue（"a point or matter of discussion, debate, or dispute or a matter of public concern"，争执的要点，公众关心）。例如：

例一： Prevention and treatment of cerebral ischemia in China: **Problems** and tactics

我国缺血性脑卒中防治研究中存在的问题及对策

引自:《中华医学杂志》, 2000, 80(2): 85

例二： How parents describe the positive **aspects** of parenting their child who has intellectual disabilities: A systematic review and narrative synthesis

父母该如何看待养育智障子女的积极方面：系统回顾和叙述综合

引自: *J Appl Res Intellect Disabil*, 2019, 32(5): 1255

例三： Surgical strategy and relevant **problems** about degenerative spinal deformity

退变性脊柱畸形的手术治疗策略及相关问题

引自:《中华外科杂志》, 2018, 56(9): 653

例四： Stromal vascular progenitors in adult human adipose **tissue**

成人脂肪组织中的间质血管前体问题

引自: *Cytometry*, 2010, 77 (1): 22

例五： Interpersonal **problems** in eating disorders

进食障碍者的人际交往问题

引自: *Int J Eat Disord*, 2009, 43(7): 619

例六： Small intestinal bacterial overgrowth in irritable bowel syndrome: Association with colon motility, bowel symptoms, and psychological distress

肠易激综合征中的小肠细菌过生长：与结肠运动、肠道症状、心理问题相关的研究

【析】在特定语境条件下，"问题"可以略去。

引自: *Neurogastroenterol Motil*, 2008, 20(9): 998

4. "初步"的译法

以"初步"为限定词的医学论文标题，如"初步探讨、初步研究、初步观察、初步小结、初步报告、初步体会"等，国内外期刊中作者用词差异较大。国内作者基本使用Preliminary，而国外作者则使用pilot表达"初步"之意。根据世界权威词典 *Merriam-Webster Collegiate Dictionary* 上的定义，preliminary 的意思是 "coming before and usually forming a necessary prelude to something else, e.g., preliminary studies"；pilot 的意思是 "serving as a tentative model for future experiment or development, e.g., pilot study"。虽然这两个词的汉语定义都是"初步"，但内涵意义还是有区别的，即 preliminary 相当于"入门级"，而 pilot 是为后续希望做的事情提供基础前提。医学科研中初步研究，就是为后续研究提供基础，起到抛砖引玉的作用，所以，使用 pilot 更为合理。

例一： Clinicopathologic criteria for the diagnosis of extranodal anaplastic large-cell lymphoma：A **preliminary** study

淋巴结外间变性大细胞淋巴瘤临床病理诊断要点的初步探讨

引自:《中华肿瘤杂志》, 2000, 22(5): 20

例二： Parotid CT imaging reporting and data system: A **preliminary** study

腮腺 CT 影像报告与数据系统的初步研究

引自:《北京大学学报（医学版）》, 2020, 52(1): 83

例三： **Pilot** study to estimate the accuracy of mouth self-examination in an at-risk group

评估高危人群口腔自我检查的准确性的初步研究

引自: *Head Neck*, 2010, 32 (10): 1393

例四： High-grade soft-tissue sarcomas: Tumor response assessment—**pilot** study to assess the correlation between radiologic and pathologic response by using RECIST and Choi criteria

高级别软组织肉瘤：利用 RECIST 和 Choi 标准进行肿瘤疗效初步判定来评估放射学和病理反应间的相关性

引自: *Radiology*, 2009, 251(2): 447

例五： Effect of sildenafil on digital ulcers in systemic sclerosis: Analysis from a single centre **pilot** study

西地那非对系统性硬化症患者手指溃疡的疗效：单中心初步研究分析

引自: *Ann Rheum Dis,* 2010, 69(8): 1475

5. "分析"及相关概念的译法

所谓"分析"，是指将事物、现象、概念分门别类，离析出本质及其内在联系。对应的英文单词常用 analysis，但根据论文主旨内容，可灵活处理，即选择与语境相吻合的词，如例三。

例一： Clinical **analysis** of laparoscopic anterior resection for 258 cases with rectal cancer

腹腔镜直肠癌前切除术 258 例临床分析

引自:《中华腔镜外科杂志》, 2010, 3(2): 182

例二： **Analysis** of imported falciparum malaria cases in Yangzhou City

扬州市输入性恶性疟疾病例分析

引自:《中国血吸虫病防治杂志》, 2010, 22(2): 196

例三： Dependability **Investigation** of the Risk Factors of Childhood Leukaemia

儿童白血病致病危险因素分析

【析】本例中"分析"使用的是 investigation。

引自:《中国循证医学杂志》, 2010, 10(9): 1037

例四： Epidemiological Characteristics of Human Avian Influenza (H5N1) in China from 2005 to 2009

2005—2009 年中国人禽流感（H5N1）病例流行病学特征分析

【析】"分析"在题名中省略了，但并不影响题名的完整性。

引自:《实用预防医学》, 2010, 17(6): 1070

　　此外，由于研究方法上的差异，医学论文标题中常涉及不同的分析方法。例如：多因素分析（multivariate analysis）；分层分析（stratified analysis）；临床经济/决策分析（clinical economic/decision analysis）；敏感性分析（sensitivity analysis）；生存分析（survival analysis）；荟萃分析（meta-analysis）；回顾性分析（retrospective analysis）；相关性分析（relevant analysis）；临床病理学分析（clinicopathological analysis）；预后分析（prognostic analysis）等。

例一： Early combination antibiotic therapy yields improved survival compared with monotherapy in septic shock: A **propensity-matched analysis**

与单一疗法相比早期联合抗生素治疗可提高脓毒性休克患者生存率：倾向匹配性分析

引自：*Crit Care Med*, 2010, 38 (9)：1773

例二： Doxycycline's effect on ocular angiogenesis: An *in vivo* **analysis**

多西环素对眼球内新生血管生成的影响：一项体内分析研究

引自：*Ophthalmology*, 2010, 117 (9)：1782

例三： Variation in the risk of suicide attempts and completed suicides by antidepressant agent in adults: A **propensity score-adjusted analysis** of 9 years'data

成人服用抗抑郁药物导致自杀倾向和自杀行为的差异因素：一项为期 9 年的倾向评分校正分析

引自：*Arch Gen Psychiatry,* 2010, 67 (5): 497

例四： **International cohort analysis** of the antiviral activities of zidovudine and tenofovir in the presence of the K65R mutation in reverse transcriptase

逆转录酶 K65R 突变时齐多夫定和替诺福韦抗病毒活性：全球队列分析

引自：*Antimicrob Agents Chemother,* 2010, 54 (4)：1520

6. "应用"的译法

　　医学论文题名中的"应用"含"运用、使用、利用"之意，是指把某种东西（通常为技术、方法）用于预期适合的某一目的。常用名词有 application 或动词 apply。在特定语境条件下，application 可以省略，有时也可使用名词或动词 use 表达"应用"这一概念，使用时应注意词性变化，同时注意观察对比我国作者和国外作者在这一概念表达上的差异。

例一： **Application** of three-dimensional reconstruction images of spiral CT in pelvis fractures

螺旋 CT 三维重建技术在骨盆骨折中的应用

引自：《中国组织工程研究与临床康复》, 2010, 14(35): 6529

例二： Preliminary **Application** of a Mosquito Densovirus-Mediated Artificial Intron *in vitro* and *in vivo* of Mosquito

蚊浓核病毒介导的人工内含子在蚊体内外的初步应用

引自：《病毒学报》, 2010, 26(5): 384

例三：Ethosuximide, valproic acid, and lamotrigine in childhood absence epilepsy

乙琥胺、丙戊酸、拉莫三嗪在儿童失神癫痫治疗中的应用

引自：*N Engl J Med*, 2010, 362 (9): 790

例四：Total disc replacement surgery for symptomatic degenerative lumbar disc disease: A systematic review of the literature

人工椎间盘置换术在有症状的退行性腰椎间盘突出症中的应用：文献系统回顾

引自：*Eur Spine J*, 2010, 19 (8): 1262

例五：Amniotic membrane grafting in patients with epidermolysis bullosa with chronic wounds

羊膜移植在大疱性表皮松解症患者慢性创面治疗中的应用

引自：*J Am Acad Dermato*, 2010, 62 (6): 1038

例六：Construction of a recombinant lentiviral vector of p38 MAPK and establishment of a human prostatic carcinoma cell line stably expressing p38 MAPK

p38 丝裂原激活蛋白激酶基因重组慢病毒载体的构建及其在建立人前列腺癌稳定细胞株中的应用

引自：《南方医科大学学报》, 2012, 32(3): 317

例七：Breast Cancer Risk by Breast Density, Menopause, and Postmenopausal Hormone Therapy Use

乳腺密度、绝经及绝经后激素治疗的应用与乳腺癌风险

引自：*J Clin Oncol*, 2010, 28(24): 3830

例八：Allergy or tolerance in children sensitized to peanut: Prevalence and differentiation using component-resolved diagnostics

花生敏感儿童的过敏或耐受性：使用成分分辨诊断的患病率和差异性

引自：*J Allergy Clin Immunol*, 2010, 125(1): 191-7e1-13

上述例三至例八均省略了 application，但完整的语境仍然可以提示文题中所蕴含的"应用"之意，同时也使得文题更为简洁。

四、英文标题中冠词省略及常见名词与介词搭配

（一）冠词的省略

冠词（articles），属于虚词，是最主要、最典型的限定词，放在名词之前，用来说明名词所指的人或事物。由于汉语中没有冠词，所以，对于冠词的用法就显得特别难以把握。英语中冠词有两个形式：不定冠词 a/an 和定冠词 the。不定冠词与数词 one 同源，相当于汉语中的"一"，但与数目概念关联不大，通常用来表示泛指关系；定冠词与 this、that 同源，用来表示特定的对象或事物。医学论文英文标题表达应以简洁为本，据相关

统计研究分析表明，国内医学期刊的论文题名常以冠词开头，而国外医学期刊则很少使用冠词开头，如 *The Lancet*，*Journal of the American Medical Association* 等。题名（包括副标题）中名词前的冠词在下列情况下常可以省略。

1. 标题题首一般不用冠词

例一： Optimal timing of endovascular treatment for uncomplicated Stanford type B aortic dissection

非复杂性 Stanford B 型主动脉夹层腔内修复术的时机选择

> 引自：《中华外科杂志》, 2018, 56(10)：741

例二： Pesticides and Human Reproduction

农药和人类生殖

> 引自：*JAMA Intern Med*, 2018, 178(1)：26

例三： The drug resistance of pathogenic bacteria of nosocomial infections in surgical intensive care unit

普通外科重症加强治疗病房获得性感染的耐药性监测

> 引自：《中华外科杂志》, 2006, 44(17)：1189

例四： The Diagnosis of CT, MRI, MRV and DSA in Cerebral Venous Sinus Thrombosis during Pregnancy and Puerperium

孕产妇颅内静脉窦血栓形成的 CT、MRI、MRV、DSA 诊断

> 引自：《中华医学影像学杂志》, 2009, 17(2)：142

例五： A prospective multicenter study of adrenal function in critically ill children

对重症患儿的肾上腺功能进行的前瞻性多中心研究

> 引自：*Am J Respir Crit Care Med,* 2010, 182 (2)：246

至于英文标题题首是否使用冠词，同一期刊所刊载的论文标题也存在一定差异，有省略的，也有带定冠词或不定冠词的情况（如例三、例四、例五），但绝大多数标题基本上是省略冠词的。事实上，题首冠词完全可以省略，而不影响题名所反映的主旨内容。

2. 标题中的疾病名称前一般不用冠词

例一： Relationship between ER α gene polymorphisms and endometriosis

雌激素受体 ER α 基因多态性与子宫内膜异位症的相关性研究

【析】endometriosis 前省略了冠词。

> 引自：《中国病理生理杂志》, 2010, 26(9)：1828

例二： Advances in counselling and surveillance of patients at risk for pancreatic cancer

对胰腺癌高危患者咨询和监测方面的进展

【析】pancreatic cancer 前省略了冠词。

> 引自：*Gut*, 2007, 56(10)：1460

例三： Vasovagal syncope in the older patient

老年患者的血管迷走性晕厥

【析】Vasovagal syncope 前省略了冠词。

引自：*JACC*, 2008, 51(6): 599

例四： Minimal residual disease-directed therapy for childhood acute myeloid leukaemia: Results of the AML02 multicentre trial

儿童急性髓性白血病以最小残留病变为目标的治疗：AML02 多中心试验结果

【析】myeloid leukaemia 即使与形容词连用，同样省略了冠词。

引自：*Lancet Oncol*, 2010, 11 (6): 543

例五： A new rating instrument to assess festination and freezing gait in Parkinsonian patients

一种新的评价帕金森病慌张步态和冻结步态的分级方法

【析】虽然 Parkinsonian 为形容词，修饰 patients，但其义仍然表示疾病，故省略冠词。

引自：*Mov Disord*, 2010, 25 (8): 1012

例六： Gluten-sensitive enteropathy (celiac disease): Controversies in diagnosis and classification

关于谷蛋白敏感性肠病（乳糜泻）的诊断与分类争议

【析】gluten-sensitive enteropathy 前冠词省略。

引自：*Arch Pathol Lab Med*, 2010, 134(6): 826

3. 标题中的手术名称前一般不用冠词

例一： Hysterectomy for benign conditions

良性妇科疾病的子宫切除术

【析】hysterectomy 表示手术名称。

引自：*BMJ*, 2005, 330(7506): 1457

例二： Perioperative nursing of 86 patients undergoing tricuspid valve replacement

86 例三尖瓣置换术的围手术期护理

【析】tricuspid valve replacement 表示手术名称。

引自：《中华护理杂志》, 2013, 48(4): 297

例三： Radiofrequency ablation of atrial fibrillation: Is the persistence of all intraprocedural targets necessary for long-term maintenance of sinus rhythm?

心房颤动的射频消融：是维持持久性窦性心律所需的术中靶点？

【析】Radiofrequency ablation 表示手术名称。

引自：*Circulation*, 2008, 117(2): 136

例四： Short-term outcomes of lung transplant recipients using organs from brain death donors

脑死亡供者肺移植近期预后分析

【析】lung transplant 代表手术名称。

引自:《中华外科杂志》, 2016, 54(12): 894

例五: Risk Assessment in Cholelithiasis: Is Cholecystectomy Always to be Preferred?

行胆囊切除术前必须对胆石症进行风险评估吗?

【析】cholelithiasis 代表手术名称。

引自: J Gastrointest Surg, 2010, 14 (8) : 1271

例六: Influence of corneal collagen crosslinking with riboflavin and ultraviolet-A irradiation on excimer laser surgery

角膜胶原交联核黄素/紫外线 a 辐射对准分子激光手术的影响

【析】excimer laser surgery 代表手术名称。

引自: Invest Ophthalmol Vis Sci, 2010, 51(8): 3929

4. 标题中专有名词之前一般不使用冠词

英语中专有名词是表示人、地方、事物等特有的名词。专有名词的第一个字母要大写。医学领域中有大量的专有名词,这些专有名词一般都与人名有关,或与微生物种群有关,如 Seldinger technique(Seldinger 技术)、Doppler effect (多普勒效应)、Apgar score (阿普加评分)、*Dermatophagoides farina*(粉尘螨)等。例如:

例一: Psychosocial impact of implantable cardioverter defibrillators(ICD)in young adults with Tetralogy of Fallot

植入式心脏复律除颤器(ICD)对青壮年法洛四联症患者的心理社会影响

引自: Clin Res Cardiol, 2012, 101(7): 509

例二: Small-bowel imaging in Crohn's disease: A prospective, blinded, 4-way comparison trial

克罗恩病小肠成像检查:前瞻、盲法、四种检查途径对照实验

引自: Gastrointest Endosc, 2008, 68(2) : 255

例三: Radical Surgery for Budd-Chiari Syndrome through Exposure of the Whole Hepatic Segment of Inferior Vena Cava

肝段下腔静脉全程显露的布-加综合征根治术

引自:《中国医学科学院学报》, 2007, 29(1): 47

例四: A phase Ⅰ trial of deep brain stimulation of memory circuits in Alzheimer's disease

深部刺激阿尔茨海默病患者大脑记忆环路的Ⅰ期临床试验

引自: Ann Neurol, 2010, 68(4): 521

例五: Prevalence of Growth Hormone Deficiency in Hashimoto's Thyroiditis

生长激素缺乏症在桥本甲状腺炎中的发病率

引自: J Clin Endocrinol Metab, 2010, 95(5): 2266

5. 标题中复数名词前一般不用冠词

无论处于题首还是在题名中间其他位置，标题中复数名词前一般不用冠词，因为复数名词具有类属性质或泛指功能。例如：

例一： **Changes** of coagulation-related parameters in normal pregnant women
妊娠期血凝指标的变化
引自:《上海交通大学学报（医学版）》, 2008, 28(5): 561

例二： Evaluation on quality of life instrument for **patients** with diabetes mellitus
糖尿病患者生命质量量表研制及评价
引自:《中国公共卫生》, 2012, 28(5): 588

例三： **Effects** of angiotensin-converting enzyme inhibition in low-risk patients early after coronary artery bypass surgery
低危患者行冠状动脉旁路移植手术后早期应用 ACEI 的作用
引自: *Circulation*, 2008, 117(1): 24

例四： Perioperative **complications** in children with pulmonary hypertension undergoing general anesthesia with ketamine
肺动脉高压症患儿围手术期并发症的发生率与氯胺酮全麻相关性研究
引自: *Paediatr Anaesth,* 2010, 20(1) : 28

（注：上述标题实例中复数名词前均省略了冠词。）

6. 标题中普通名词前若带有修饰词通常省略冠词

例一： Effects of nerve growth factor on expression of **apoptosis-related genes** in experimental retinal detachment
实验性视网膜脱离时神经生长因子对凋亡相关蛋白表达的影响
引自:《上海交通大学学报（医学版）》, 2008, 28 (6): 630

例二： Acute hepatitis B after the implementation of universal vaccination in Italy: Results from **22 years** of surveillance
意大利实行乙型肝炎疫苗普遍接种后 22 年的监测结果分析
引自: *Clin Infect Dis*, 2016, 62 (11): 1412

例三： Hepatitis C eradication with **direct-acting anti-virals** reduces the risk of variceal bleeding
用直接作用的抗病毒药物根除丙型肝炎可降低静脉曲张出血的风险
引自: *Aliment Pharmacol Ther*, 2020, 51(3): 364

7. 标题中药物名称前通常使用零冠词

例一： Anesthetic Efficacy of Articaine Versus Lidocaine for Irreversible Pulpitis: A Meta-analysis

阿替卡因与利多卡因对不可逆转性牙髓炎麻醉效果比较：Meta 分析

　　　　　　　　　　引自：《中国循证医学杂志》, 2010, 10(9): 1058

例二： Linezolid in the treatment of multidrug-resistant tuberculosis

利奈唑胺治疗多药耐药性结核病

　　　　　　　　　　引自：*Clin Infect Dis*, 2010, 50 (1): 49

例三： Comparison of two doses of imatinib for the treatment of unresectable or metastatic gastrointestinal stromal tumors: A meta-analysis of 1,640 patients

两种不同剂量伊马替尼治疗不能切除或转移性胃肠间质瘤比较——对 1640 例患者的荟萃分析

　　　　　　　　　　引自：*J Clin Oncol*, 2010, 28 (7) : 1247

8. 物质名词在题名中表示一般概念时通常不加定冠词（包括基因、蛋白、抗体、抗原等）

例一： Hypertonic saline improves the LCI in paediatric patients with CF with normal lung function

高张生理盐水可以改善肺功能正常的囊性纤维化患儿的肺清除指数（LCI）

　　　　　　　　　　引自：*Thorax*, 2010, 65(5): 379

例二： Toll-like receptor 2 signaling in CD4$^+$ T lymphocytes promotes T helper 17 responses and regulates the pathogenesis of autoimmune disease

CD4$^+$T 淋巴细胞 Toll 样受体 2 信号促进辅助性 T17 应答并调控自身免疫性疾病的发病

　　　　　　　　　　引自：*Immunity*, 2010, 32(5): 692

例三： Chlorhexidine-Alcohol versus Povidone-Iodine for Surgical-Site Antisepsis

氯己定酒精与聚维酮碘用于手术部位消毒的比较

　　　　　　　　　　引自：*N Engl J Med*, 2010, 362 (1) : 18

例四： Preparation of antibody against human S100A7

抗人 S100A7 抗体的制备

　　　　　　　　　　引自：《中国实验诊断学》, 2010, 14(8): 1330

例五： Antigenic modulation limits the efficacy of anti-CD20 antibodies: Implications for antibody selection

抗原调整限制抗 CD20 抗体的效果——抗体选择的重要性

　　　　　　　　　　引自：*Blood*, 2010, 115(25): 5191

例六： Genomic and genic deletions of the FOX gene cluster on 16q24.1 and inactivating mutations of FOXF1 cause alveolar capillary dysplasia and other malformations

FOX 基因簇在 16q24.1 的基因缺失和 *FOX* 基因的失活突变导致肺泡毛细血管发育异常及其他畸形

　　　　　　　　　　引自：*Am J Hum Genet*, 2009, 84 (6): 780

例七： C3d immunohistochemistry on formalin-fixed tissue is a valuable tool in the diagnosis of bullous pemphigoid of the skin

福尔马林液固定组织行C3d免疫组织化学染色有助于皮肤大疱性类天疱疮的诊断

引自：*J Cutan Pathol*, 2010, 37(6): 654

9. 标题中由两个名词构成的并列对称结构中，名词之前均省略冠词

例一： Circulating osteogenic cells: Characterization and relationship to rates of bone loss in postmenopausal women

外周血成骨细胞特性及其与绝经后妇女骨丢失的关系

引自：*Bone*, 2010, 47(1): 83

例二： Bisphosphonates and Fractures of the Subtrochanteric or Diaphyseal Femur

双膦酸盐与股骨粗隆及股骨干骨折的关系

引自：*N Engl J Med*, 2010, 362(19): 1761

例三： Hearts and minds: Coordination of neurocognitive and cardiovascular regulation in children and adolescents

心与脑——儿童和青少年的神经认知和心血管调节间的联系

引自：*Biol Psychol*, 2010, 84(2): 296

例四： Bioinformatics analysis of ulcerative colitis and its malignant complications and screening of potential therapeutic drugs

溃疡性结肠炎及其恶性并发症的生物信息学分析和潜在治疗药物筛选

引自：《上海交通大学学报(医学版)》, 2020, 40 (3): 317

（二）医学论文英文标题中常见名词语义特点及其介词搭配

介词（或称前置词）属于虚词，在句子结构中表示词与词或有关句子成分之间的关系，它虽然不能独立作为句子的成分出现，但前置词和前置词构成的短语，在句子中起着非常重要的作用。它的数量虽不甚多，但在英语中属于最活跃的词类，用法也相当复杂。在医学论文英文标题的写作中，特别要注意一些常见名词和介词在使用中的相互搭配问题。

1. 医学论文英文标题中一些高频名词和介词搭配

（1）study：医学论文英文标题中常用study这一词，其后可搭配介词of、on或in，意义相同。studies与study在意义上没有什么区别，但studies表示"研究"的范围要广些。例如：

例一： EBV positive mucocutaneous ulcer—a **study of** 26 cases associated with various sources of immunosuppression

皮肤黏膜溃疡EB病毒阳性——26例不同因素所致免疫抑制患者研究

引自：*Am J Surg Pathol*, 2010, 34 (3)：405

例二： **Study on** expression of mineralocorticoid receptor in human atria during atrial fibrillation

心房颤动患者心房肌盐皮质激素受体表达研究

引自：《中华心血管病杂志》,2007, 35(2): 114

例三： Prospective **study on** occupational stress and risk of stroke

关于职业应激与卒中危险性的前瞻性研究

引自：*Arch Intern Med*, 2009, 169(1): 56

例四： New-onset heart failure due to heart muscle disease in childhood: A prospective **study in** the United kingdom and Ireland

儿童心肌病引起的新发心力衰竭：一项在英国和爱尔兰进行的前瞻性研究

引自：*Circulation*, 2008, 117(1): 79

在英译标题时，中文文题中研究（study）属于冗词，从语境角度看，论文本身就是研究性质的，一般可以省略而不会影响意义表达。但当该词前带有表明该项研究的某种特性修饰语时，就不宜省略，如"Comparative study…"（比较研究）；"Retrospective study…"（回顾性研究）；"Prospective study…"（前瞻性研究）；"Randomized study…"（随机性研究）。例如：

例一： Psychological Outcomes of Labiaplasty: **A Prospective Study**

阴唇成形术的心理结果：前瞻性研究

引自：*Plast Reconstr Surg*, 2017, 140(3): 506

例二： **Genome-wide association study** in alopecia areata implicates both innate and adaptive immunity

涉及固有免疫和获得性免疫斑秃的全基因组关联性研究

引自：*Nat Med*, 2010, 466(7302): 113

（2）research：与 research 搭配使用的介词有 on、for、of、into。

例一： Report on initiating clinical **research for** electrical and mechanical synchronism of selective region pacing in the right ventricular

心脏选择性部位起搏的电和机械同步性研究的初步报告

引自：《中华心血管病杂志》, 2007, 35(2): 147

例二： Clinical and Basic **Researches on** HIV/AIDS

艾滋病的临床与基础研究进展

引自：《中国医学科学院学报》, 2006, 28 (5) : 609

例三： Experiment **research of** radioisotope labeling for His-Annexin V and scintigraphy *in vivo*

重组改良型人膜联蛋白的核素标记及体内显像的实验研究

引自：《中国现代医学杂志》, 2010, 20(17): 2579

（3）investigation：其后可接介词 of 或 on。需要注意的是，与介词 of 搭配，仅表示动宾关系；介词 on 强调细节内容。例如：

例一： **Investigation of** Various Fluorescent Protein-DNA Binding Peptides for Effectively Visualizing Large DNA Molecules

不同荧光蛋白-DNA 结合肽用于有效观察 DNA 大分子的研究

引自：*RSC Adv,* 2016, 6:46291

例二： Cross sectional epidemiological **investigation on** the prevalence of gastrointestinal helminths in free range chickens in Narsingdi district, Bangladesh

孟加拉国 Narsingdi 地区散养鸡胃肠道蠕虫流行情况横断面流行病学调查

引自：*J Parasit Dis,* 2016, 40(3): 818

以上三个词均有"研究、探讨、科研"等含义。表示"研究"这一概念时，study 使用最频繁；research 的含义有些抽象，接近常说的"科研"（scientific investigation）；investigation 强调调查研究，详细的查问或系统的检查（A detailed inquiry or systematic examination）。

（4）report：其后可接介词 of 或 on，引出研究的对象，偶尔与 from 连用，后接机构名称。例如：

例一： Late recurrence in pediatric cancer: A **report from** the Childhood Cancer Survivor Study

儿科癌症晚期复发：一项儿童期癌症生存率研究的报告

引自：*J Natl Cancer Inst,* 2009, 101 (24)：1709

例二： Large benign cystic teratoma of mesosigmoid causing intestinal obstruction: **Report of** a case

一例引起肠梗阻的大乙状结肠系膜良性囊肿性畸胎瘤报告

引自：*Surgery Today,* 2002, 32(10): 922

例三： A one-page summary **report of** genome sequencing for the healthy adult

一份关于健康成人基因组测序结果的概要报告

引自：*Public Health Genomics,* 2015, 18(2): 123

（5）survey：强调"综览，从广泛的方面检查或察看（to examine or look at in a comprehensive way）"其后可跟介词 of 或 on，引出研究对象。另外，可与 in 连用，后接地点名词。例如：

例一： Cancer-related pain: A pan-European **survey of** prevalence, treatment, and patient attitudes

癌症相关性痛：患病率、治疗和患者态度的泛欧调查结果

引自：*Ann Oncol,* 2009, 20 (8): 1420

例二： Subjective health status in men and women with congenital adrenal hyperplasia: A population-based **survey in** Norway

患有先天性肾上腺增生男性和女性的主观健康状况：挪威的一份基于人群的调查

引自：Eur J Endocrinol, 2010, 163 (3): 453

例三：Flash **survey on** severe acute respiratory syndrome coronavirus-2 infections in paediatric patients on anticancer treatment

接受抗癌治疗的儿科患者中严重急性呼吸综合征冠状病毒-2感染的快速调查

引自：Eur J Cancer, 2020, 132(7): 11

（6）observation：表示"观察结果"或"观察报告"的含义。其后可搭配介词 of、on 或 in，意义相同。例如：

例一： **Observation of** long-term therapeutic outcome in chronic granulocytic leukemia

慢性粒细胞白血病远期疗效观察

引自：《中华血液学杂志》, 2001, 22(2): 61

例二：Guidelines: The do's, don'ts and don't knows of direct **observation of** clinical skills in medical education

指南："会做、不会做、不知如何做"应用于医学教育中直接观察临床技能

引自：Perspect Med Educ, 2017, 6(5): 286

（7）treatment 与 therapy：两词后接疾病名称时，均可用 for 或 of。偶接介词 with，表示"用……治疗"。therapy 和 treatment 这两个词均有"治疗"之意，但 therapy 有"疗法"的含义，强调治疗的方式方法，包括药物、饮食治疗及以 therapy 为后缀的派生词。如 radium beam therapy（镭射线治疗）、reflex therapy（反射疗法）、replacement therapy（替补疗法）、durg therapy（药物治疗）、diet therapy（食疗）、radiotherapy（放射疗法）、psychotherapy（精神疗法）。treatment 则意为"administration or application of remedies to a patient or for a disease or an injury; medicinal or surgical management"（为患者或为治疗一种疾病或损伤施加或使用药物；药物处理或外科治疗），强调行为、手段。注意通过以下例证仔细体会。例如：

例一：Cognitive behavioral **therapy** for **treatment of** chronic primary insomnia:A randomized controlled trial

认知行为疗法治疗慢性原发性失眠：随机对照实验

引自：JAMA, 2001, 285(14): 1856

例二：Mechanisms, prevention, and **treatment of** atrial fibrillation after cardiac surgery

心脏外科术后心房颤动的机制、预防和治疗

引自：J Am Coll Cardiol, 2008, 51(8): 793

例三： Corticosteroid treatment and intensive insulin **therapy for** septic shock in adults: A randomized controlled trial

　　　成人脓毒性休克患者的皮质类固醇治疗和强化胰岛素治疗的随机对照试验

引自：*JAMA*, 2010, 303 (4): 341

例四： **Treatment with** monoclonal antibodies against *Clostridium difficile* toxins

　　　难辨梭状芽孢杆菌毒素的单克隆抗体治疗

引自：*N Engl J Med*, 2010, 362 (3)：197

　　表示治疗方法和检查方法的名词还可与介词 in 搭配，其意义与后接介词 for 没有区别。例如：

例一： Comprehensive surgical management **in** primary venous reflux disease of lower extremity

　　　下肢原发性静脉反流性疾病的综合性外科治疗

引自：《中华实用外科杂志》, 2001, 21(1): 51

例二： Patterns of diagnosis **for** colorectal cancer: Screening detected versus symptomatic presentation

　　　结直肠癌的诊断模式：筛检诊断或根据症状表现诊断

引自：*Dis Colon Rectum*, 2008, 51(5)：573

例三： Non-surgical septal myocardial reduction by coil embolization **for** hypertrophic obstructive cardiomyopathy: Early and 6 months follow-up

　　　非外科手术线圈栓塞法室间隔心肌消融治疗肥厚梗阻型心肌病：早期和 6 个月随访研究

引自：*Eur Heart J*, 2008, 29(3): 296

2. 医学论文英文标题中常见介词的搭配用法

　　医学论文英文标题中，一些常见的用于表示"范围、用途、原因、先后"等介词，在使用中有一些相对比较固定的搭配模式，如 in、due to、after、following 等。

　　（1）in 的搭配及使用范围较广。常见搭配模式有 in 后接生物名词、动源性名词、各种疾病名称等。例如：

例一： Colonic adaption **in** short bowel syndrome

　　　短肠综合征时结肠的代偿研究

引自：《中华外科杂志》, 2001, 39(4): 313

例二： The feasibility of wireless capsule endoscopy **in** detecting small intestinal pathology in children under the age of 8 years: A multicentre European study

　　　无线胶囊内镜在检查 8 岁以下的儿童小肠病理学方面的可行性：欧洲多中心研究

引自：*Gut*, 2009, 58 (11)：1467

例三：Contribution of the local and referred pain from active myofascial trigger points **in** fibromyalgia syndrome

活动肌筋膜触发点局部痛和牵涉痛在纤维肌痛综合征中的作用

引自：*Pain*, 2009, 47(1-3): 233

例四：Ferric carboxymaltose **in** patients with heart failure and iron deficiency

应用静脉补铁药物纠正心力衰竭合并贫血患者的缺铁状态

引自：*N Engl J Med*, 2009, 361(25): 2436

（2）标题中表示"原因"时，应用 due to，不可用 because of 或 owing to，但可用 caused by 代替。另外，介词 from 也可表示原因。但在汉语中它们有时可以省略不译。例如：

例一：Hereditary angioedema **caused by** missense mutations in the factor XII gene: Clinical features, trigger factors, and therapy

XII因子基因错义突变引起的遗传性血管性水肿：临床特征、诱因及治疗方法

引自：*J Allergy Clin Immunol*, 2009, 124 (1)：129

例二：The projected increase in glaucoma **due to** an ageing population

人口老龄化导致青光眼发病率明显上升

引自：*Ophthal Physiol Opt*, 2003, 23(2): 175

例三：Intellectual outcome **from** preschool traumatic brain injury: A 5-year prospective, longitudinal study

学龄前儿童创伤性脑损伤对智力的影响：为期 5 年的前瞻性、纵向研究

引自：*Pediatrics*, 2009, 124 (6)：e1064

例四：Tolerance rather than immunity protects **from** Helicobacter pylori-induced gastric preneoplasia

个体耐受性而非免疫力可阻止幽门螺杆菌感染诱导的胃癌前病变的发生

引自：*Gastroenterology*, 2011, 140(1): 199

（3）after 和 following 这两个词意义基本相同，但仍然存在一定的差异。after 意为 "behind in place or order" 或 "next to or lower than in order or importance"；following 意为 "coming next in time or order"。在表示"时间或事件"方面可以通用。例如：

例一：Optic disc and visual field changes **after** trabeculectomy

小梁切除术后视盘和视野的变化

引自：*Invest Ophthalmol Vis Sci*, 2009, 50 (10)：4693

例二：Obliterative bronchiolitis **following** lung transplantation: From old to new concepts?

肺移植后闭塞性细支气管炎：从旧观念到新认识的改变？

引自：*Transpl Int*, 2009, 22(8)：771

例三： Predictors and outcomes of a perioperative myocardial infarction **following** elective vascular surgery in patients with documented coronary artery disease: Results of the CARP trial

择期血管外科手术的冠心病患者,围手术期心肌梗死的预测因子与预后：CARP 试验

引自: *Eur Heart J*, 2008, 29(3): 394

例四： Renin-angiotensin blockade is associated with increased mortality **after** vascular surgery

肾素血管紧张素阻断与血管外科手术后死亡率增加有关

引自: *Can J Anaesth*, 2010, 57(8) : 736

五、英文标题概念表达常用句式结构

（一）药物治疗类属概念的表达句式

1. 药物名称+in（或 for）+病名

例一： Osmotic diuretics **in** acute hydrocephalus
渗透性利尿药治疗急性脑水肿

例二： Anisodamine **for** gastrospasm
山莨菪碱治疗胃痉挛

例三： Pirenzepine **in** gastric hyperacidity
哌仑西平治疗胃酸过多

例四： Biofermin **for** flatulent dyspepsia
乳酶生治疗腹胀型消化不良

2. 药物名称+ in the treatment（或 management）+ of+病名

treatment 为通用词，但在英国出版的医学期刊中常用 management。

例一： Gentamycin **in the treatment of** septemia
庆大霉素治疗败血症

例二： Interferon (IFN) **in the management of** melanotic sarcoma
干扰素治疗黑色素肉瘤

例三： Penicillin G **in the treatment of** streptococcus pneumonia
青霉素治疗链球菌型肺炎

例四： Combination of isoniazid and ethambutol **in the management of** pulmonary tuberculosis
异烟肼和乙胺丁醇联合治疗肺结核

3. 药物名称+therapy（或 treatment）+ of +病名

例一：Levamisole **therapy of** system lupus erythematosus
左旋咪唑治疗系统性红斑狼疮

例二：Nitroglycerin **treatment of** acute myocardial infarction
硝酸甘油治疗急性心肌梗死

例三：Berberine **in the treatment of** metabolism-related chronic diseases
小檗碱治疗代谢相关慢性疾病

例四：Coagulation Factor Ⅷ **treatment of** hemophilia A
凝血因子Ⅷ治疗血友病

4. Treatment of+病名+with+药物名称

例一：**Treatment of** glandular phthisis **with** rifampicin
利福平治疗淋巴结核

例二：**Treatment of** polioencephalitis **with** sulfadiazine(SD)
磺胺治疗流行性脑脊髓膜炎

5. Use of+药物名称+in the treatment of+病名

出于简洁为本的英文表达原则，use of 常可以省略，因此，下列例句中若略去 use of 意思也不会改变。

例一：**Use of** chlorpromazine **in the treatment of** expansive delusion
氯丙嗪在治疗扩张性幻想中的应用

例二：**Use of** digoxin **in** the treatment of chronic systolic heart failure
地高辛治疗慢性收缩性心力衰竭

例三：**Use of** carbamazepine **in the treatment of** trifacial neuralgia
卡马西平治疗三叉神经痛

（二）治疗方法类属概念的表达句式

1. 治疗方法+in（或 for）+病名

例一：X-ray **in** gallstone
X 线照射治疗胆结石

例二：Thoracotomy **in** pulmonary metastasis from malignant melanoma
开胸手术治疗恶性黑色素瘤肺转移

例三：Modified maze procedure **for** atrial fibrillation
改良迷宫手术治疗心房颤动

例四：Photodynamic **for** port wine stains using chlorophyl derivative activated by red light

叶绿素光敏剂光动力治疗鲜红斑痣

2. 治疗方法+in the treatment（或 management）+of+病名

management 常见于英国医学期刊。

例一：Combination chemotherapy **in the treatment of** uterine sarcomas

子宫肉瘤的联合化疗

例二：Splenolaparotomy **in the management of** hard-baked spleen

开腹式脾切开术治疗烘硬性脾

例三：Ureteroscope **in the management of** ureteral calculus

经输尿管镜治疗输尿管结石

例四：Clinical application of Amplatzer septal occluder device **in the treatment of** transcatheter closure of secundum atrial septal defect

Amplatzer 房间隔封堵器介入治疗继发孔型房间隔缺损中的临床应用

3. Treatment of+病名+by（或 with）+治疗方法

例一：**Treatment of** nasoseptitis **by** sympathicotherapy

交感神经刺激疗法治疗鼻中隔炎

例二：Operative **treatment of** perforation of duodenal ulcer with highly selective vagotomy **with** hemigastrectomy

十二指肠溃疡穿孔的高选择性迷走神经切断术加半胃切除疗法

例三：**Treatment of** thromboangiitis obliteration **by** negative pressure therapy on limbs

肢体负压法治疗血栓闭塞性脉管炎

例四：**Treatment of** arthrokleisis in knee **with** mobilization

膝关节强直的关节松动疗法

（三）诊断方法类属概念的表达句式

1. 诊断方法+in+病名

例一：Endoscopic retrograde cholangiopancreatograhy **in** acute pancreatitis

内镜逆行胰胆管造影术诊断急性胰腺炎

例二：Ultrosonography **in** amoebic liver abscess

超声诊断阿米巴肝脓肿

例三：Coombs test **in** autoimmune hemolytic anemia

库姆斯试验诊断自身免疫溶血性贫血

2. 诊断方法+in the diagnosis of+病名

例一： Enzyme-linked immunosorbent assay (ELISA) **in the diagnosis of** amebiasis
酶联免疫吸附法诊断阿米巴病

例二： Molecular hybridization **in the diagnosis of** malaria
核酸分子杂交诊断疟疾

例三： Nucleo-scano-thyroidography **in the diagnosis of** Hashimoto's thyroiditis
甲状腺核素显像诊断桥本甲状腺炎

3. Assay（或 detection）of+被检测对象+in+病名

例一： **Assay of** MAO **in** patients with alcoholic cirrhosis of liver
酒精性肝硬化患者单胺氧化酶的检测

例二： **Detection of** immunoglobulin **in** agammaglobulinemia
无丙种球蛋白血症的免疫球蛋白检测

例三： **Assay of** cytochrome b **in** chronic granulomatous disease
慢性肉芽肿患者的细胞色素 b 检测

例四： **Detection of** hepatitis C virus **in** the tissue of hepatocellular carcinoma by multiple detection system
肝细胞肝癌组织中丙肝病毒复合检测系统的检测

4. Diagnosis of+病名+by（或 with）+诊断方法

例一： **Diagnosis of** traumatic disk from semilunar plate **by** arthroscopy
关节镜手术诊断关节盘半月板损伤

例二： **Diagnosis of** pheochromocytoma **with** I-MIBG imaging
嗜铬细胞瘤的 I-MIBG 显像诊断

例三： **Diagnosis of** herpesvirus encephalitis **by** PCR
PCR 诊断疱疹病毒性脑炎

例四： Early **diagnosis of** nasopharyngeal carcinoma **with** recombinant antigens expressed in bacterial
基因工程表达的抗原用于早期诊断鼻咽癌

5. Detection of+病名+by+诊断方法

例一： **Detection of** medulla thyroid carcinoma **by** somatostatin receptor scintigraphy
生长抑素受体显像诊断甲状腺髓样癌

例二： **Detection of** dilate cardiomyopathy **by** radiocardiogram techniques
放射心脏扫描技术诊断扩张型心肌病

例三： **Detection of** diastematomyelia **by** MRI
磁共振显像诊断脊髓纵裂

6. Application of+诊断方法+to the diagnosis of+病名

例一： **Application of** electroencephalogram **to the diagnosis of** meningoblastoma
脑电图在诊断脑膜胚细胞瘤中的应用

例二： Clinical **application of** myocardial perfusion imaging **to the diagnosis of** coronary artery disease
心肌灌注断层显像在诊断冠心病中的临床应用

例三： **Application of** color Doppler echocardiography **to the diagnosis of** ruptured aneurysm of sinus of Valsalva
彩色多普勒超声在诊断主动脉窦瘤破裂中的应用

（四）表示研究结果的标题句式

基本公式是"Effect of X on Y in Z"。Effect 还可用 Involvement、Role 等代替；X 为自变量（处理因素）；Y 为因变量（试验效应）；Z 为试验对象；某些研究，如形态学或某些疾病的观察没有自变量，其公式相应变为"Y in Z"；有时为了突出论著的特点，使之更加醒目，可以将公式稍加变动，将需要突出的要点放在题目开始处。

例一： **Effects of** risedronate **on** bone marrow adipocytes **in** postmenopausal women
利塞膦酸钠对绝经后妇女骨髓脂肪细胞的影响
引自：*Osteoporos Int*, 2011, 22(5): 1547

例二： The **effects of** retinoic acid **on** expression of ASC protein **in** thyroid cancer
维 A 酸对甲状腺癌 ASC 蛋白的影响
引自:《中华内分泌科杂志》, 2012, 6(1): 11

例三： **Effect of** tumor vascular invasion **upon** cardio-pulmonary exercise functions **in** patients with lung cancer
肿瘤侵及血管对肺癌患者心肺功能的影响
引自:《中华医学杂志》, 2010, 90(2): 96

例四： **Effects of** estradiol valerate **on** osteoporosis **in** ovariectomized rats
戊酸雌二醇对去卵巢大鼠骨质疏松的治疗作用
引自:《中华妇产科杂志》, 2001, 36(10): 606

例五： Emotional and behavioral comorbidities and the **impact on** the quality of life **in** epilepsy children
癫痫患儿共患情绪与行为障碍及其对生活质量的影响
引自:《中华儿科杂志》, 2010, 48(5): 346

例六： **Effect of** sildenafil **on** digital ulcers **in** systemic sclerosis: Analysis from a single centre pilot study
西地那非对系统性硬化症患者手指溃疡的疗效：一项单中心初步研究的分析
引自：*Ann Rheum Dis*, 2010, 69 (8) : 1475

例七： **Effect of** acute hypoxia **on** respiratory muscle fatigue **in** healthy humans

急性缺氧对健康人呼吸肌肌肉疲劳的影响

引自: *Respir Res*, 2010, 11(1): 109

六、练 习

2-1 将下列标题改为带有副标题的格式

1) A clinical analysis of 57 cases of abdominal tuberculosis

2) Retrospective study on use of waist circumference to predict insulin resistance

3) Experimental study of laser surgery of the heart

4) Population based nested case-control analysis on risk of myocardial infarction in patients taking cyclo-oxygenase-2 inhibitors or conventional non-steroidal anti-inflammatory drugs

5) Unstable angina and non-ST segment elevation myocardial infarction in acute coronary syndrome

6) Twenty years' experience with hysterectomy for benign conditions

7) Systematic review on value of routine funduscopy in patients with hypertension: systematic review

8) Orphan disease or persistent problem in bronchiectasis in children

9) Evidence-based medicine is a new approach to teaching the practice of medicine

10) Outstanding questions for primary care in estimating cardiovascular risk for primary prevention

2-2 根据逻辑关系，用 and 或 as 改写下列标题

1) Comorbidity and age are predictors of risk for early mortality of male and female colon carcinoma patients

2) p21 (WAF1/Cip1) and p27 (Kip1) are involved in intestinal epithelial cell differentiation

3) High levels of sperm DNA denaturation are the sole semen abnormality in a patient after chemotherapy for testis cancer

4) Prostaglandins serve as mediators of inflammation

5) Influenza pandemics are related to avian flu

6) Occurrence of insomnia is related to the epidemiology and occurrence of insomnia

7) Chronic chlamydia pneumoniae infection is a risk factor for coronary heart disease in the Helsinki Heart Study

8) Red blood cell exchange transfusion serves as an adjunct treatment for severe pediatric falciparum malaria

9) Carbonyl reductase 1 serves as a novel target of (−)-epigallocatechin gallate against hepatocellular carcinoma

10) Basal follicle-stimulating hormone is in relation to peak gonadotropin levels after gonadotropin-releasing hormone infusion shows high diagnostic accuracy in boys with suspicion of hypogonadotropic hypogonadism

2-3 标题改写，删除下列标题中冗余信息而保持原义不变

1) Studies on safety evaluation of cefotetan sodium for injection

2) A clinical investigation of hereditary angioedema with recurrent abdominal pain

3) Discussion on cholesterol precursors and plant sterols in children with food allergy

4) Is folate fortification enough already?

5) A research on standards for statistical models used for public reporting of health outcomes

6) Expression and significance of brain-derived neurotrophic factors and receptors in multiple myeloma

7) The clinical and pathological characteristics and prognosis of pseudomyxoma peritonea

8) A study of antiendothelial cell antibodies in Behcet's disease

9) The relationship between the five β-fibrinogen gene polymorphisms and cerebral infarction

10) Investigate the relation between atrial fibrillation and coronary heart disease in the elderly: An analysis of pathological data of 509 cases

2-4 根据题名所提供的语境，在标题空格处填上适当的词（如名词、代词、介词等）

1) Analysis of peripheral arterial obstructive disease related factors _____diabetic population aged≥50 years

2) Study _____ association of BAFF receptors gene expression and primary biliary cirrhosis

3) _____between LKB1 bene and invasion-related factors of breast cancer cells

4) Secular trends in cardiovascular disease risk factors _____body mass index in US adults

5) Cardiac metabolism _____a target for the treatment of heart failure

6) Age-dependent susceptibility to a viral disease _____decreased natural killer cell numbers and trafficking

7) Hypersensitivity pneumonitis _____molds in a saxophone player

8) Outpatient pulmonary rehabilitation _____acute exacerbations of COPD

9) Impact of obesity on outcomes_____ open surgical and endovascular abdominal aortic aneurysm repair

10) Subfoveal choroidal thickness _____treatment of central serous chorioretinopathy

11) Choice of fluids for resuscitation _____children with severe infection and shock

12) Granulocyte colony-stimulating factor (G-CSF) treatment of childhood acute myeloid leukemias _____overexpress the differentiation-defective G-CSF receptor isoform IV is

associated with a higher incidence of relapse

13) Association between family structure, parental smoking, friends_____ smoke, and smoking behavior in adolescents with asthma

14) The _____of proximal femoral shape and incident radiographic hip OA in elderly women

15) Hereditary angioedema _____missense mutations in the factor XII gene: clinical features, trigger factors, and therapy

2-5 用英语写出下列标题，注意概念及逻辑关系

1）腹腔镜手术改善憩室病术后近期疗效

2）小儿获得性血友病的系统综述

3）改良 SDS 法提取书虱总 RNA 的效果评估

4）江苏丹阳市省级土源性线虫病监测点纵向监测结果

5）边缘系统胶质瘤的临床分型及显微手术治疗

6）紫杉醇脂质体与紫杉醇联合替吉奥一线治疗晚期胃癌的临床疗效观察

7）抗人类白细胞抗原抗体对非血缘脐血移植的影响

8）严重急性呼吸综合征患者冠状病毒总抗体及 N 和 S 蛋白抗体的随访研究

9）大鼠脑缺血再灌注后诱发急性肾损伤模型的建立与评价

10）X 染色体连锁严重联合免疫缺陷的基因治疗效果

11）运动训练强度对肥胖的代谢综合征患者夜间生长激素分泌的影响

12）初始治疗选用联合化疗而非手术的同时患Ⅳ期结直肠癌的患者原发性肿瘤的结局

13）Th17 淋巴细胞对甲型 H1N1 流行性感冒病毒清除作用的探讨

14）幽门螺杆菌根除治疗消化性溃疡是否能预防胃癌？

15）胞嘧啶脱氨酶基因治疗结肠直肠癌

16）吸虫排泄分泌产物成分及其功能的研究进展

17）肠病性肢端皮炎 1 例

18）弥漫大 B 淋巴瘤患者肠道菌群动态分析

19）霍奇金病放射治疗引起的甲状腺癌

20）2005～2014 年厦门市居民白血病死亡特征与趋势分析

第三章　医学论文英文署名与工作单位

一、署　　名

（一）论文署名的意义

每一篇科技论文的标题下应有其作者、整理者和执笔者的署名，这是医学论文中不可或缺的重要组成要素。大体上，作者署名有三个方面的含义：①体现作者的贡献与权利，同时对论文本身的科学性、创造性等负有直接责任；②标明文责人，承担履行相关法律所规定的责任和义务（如著作权人不得损害公共利益）及享受相关法律所赋予的权利，如决定对该作品是否公之于众的权利（发表权），表明作者身份（署名权）等，另外还包括道德责任。③便于编辑联络、读者检索文献或联系沟通。

（二）论文署名的原则条件

论文作者的署名要坚持实事求是的原则。例如，GB 7713—87《科学技术报告、学位论文和学术论文的编写格式》（GB 7713—87）中对学术论文作者资格规范：只限于那些对于选定研究课题和制订研究方案、直接参加全部或主要部分研究工作并做出主要贡献、以及参加撰写论文并能对内容负责的人，按其贡献大小排列名次。国际医学期刊编辑委员会（ICMJE）在《学术研究实施与报告和医学期刊编辑与发表的推荐规范》第 Ⅱ 节 "*Roles and Responsibilities of authors, contributors, reviewers, editors, publishers, and owners*"（作者、贡献者、审稿人、编辑、出版者、期刊所有者的职能和责任）中对于什么样的地位才享受作者资格界定为 "An 'author' is generally considered to be someone who has made substantive intellectual contributions to a published study, and biomedical authorship continues to have important academic, social, and financial implications."。同时详细规定了署名作者应具备的条件：①曾参与论文的构思与设计，或者对资料进行分析与解释；②起草论文或对其中重要理论内容进行修改；③同意定稿论文的发表。对于那些仅参加过局部具体工作，或给予过某些帮助，而又无须列入作者名单的单位或人员，可在文末参考文献前予以致谢。无论是何种标准或规范，其目的都是维护学术尊严和道德规范，杜绝违反学术道德而随意"搭车"署名或"狐假虎威"，假借有影响力的知名人士之名以提高其论文的声誉和影响等欺诈行为，从而保护真实作者的合法权益及其知识产权。对此，国外很多知名学术期刊均要求作者在投稿时填写 Contributions（贡献单），按贡献单所罗列内容项目进行对照如实填写并亲笔签名，如 *Journal of the American Medical Association*，（*JAMA*，《美国医学会杂志》）就"作者的职责、标准和贡献"规定了其具体的衡量标准（详情可参见：其官方网站 http://jama.ama-assn.org/）。除此之外，其他期刊还要求作者声明其所做的研究工作成果是否存在"利益冲突"等。例如，*British Medical Journal*（*BMJ*，《英国医学杂志》），在其刊载的论文正文尾部，参考文献之前所罗列的项目：①关于作者（contributors）：LV，MS，and LL had the idea for the article；LV，MS，AF，and MP performed searches and data collection；LV and LL wrote the article and are guarantors。②资助（funding）：EC 6th Framework IST grant，AMICA，contract number 507048。③利益冲突（competing interests）：None declared。④伦理批准（ethical approval）：Not required.（引自 *BMJ*，2005，331：2635）。

（三）论文署名方式及通信作者

无论是中文还是英文署名，一般均放在标题下方居中的位置。一个以上的作者，中间用逗号"，"分开。个人研究成果署个人的真实姓名；集体研究成果，应按对论文的贡献大小依次署名，或署集体名称，并在文末注明执笔人。但鉴于各类期刊对这类论文署名的要求及作者对其权利主张的要求，集体研究成果论文的署名有一定的差异。另外，国内医学期刊所刊发的论文署名前一般不加学位和职称，但研究生写的论文需要以脚注形式加上指导老师的姓名、职称和职务，以表明该项研究是在具有硕士、博士学位授予权的专家教授指导下完成的。国外期刊的署名，多有在其署名后加学位的现象。

通信作者另起一行，在"通信作者："字样后列出通信作者姓名、邮政编码、单位名称，Email 如有可以列出。通信作者可以在标题下方，也可标注在脚注位置。

例一： 细菌性阴道病诊断试剂盒性能的比较研究

Comparison of the Experimental Diagnostic Reagent Kits for Bacterial Vaginosis

Dong Jing, Li Li, Shi Xia, et al.

引自：《中国计划生育学杂志》，2009, 17(11): 679

例二： 中医综合治疗方案治疗急性缺血性中风阴类证的疗效和安全性评价（英文）

Outcome and safety assessment of an herbal medicine treatment protocol for yin pattern of acute ischemic stroke

Yan HUANG, Jian-we GUO; the Project Group for Demonstration Study of Syndrome Differentiation Protocol and Effect Evaluation of Acute Ischemic Stroke

引自：*Zhong Xi Yi Jie He Xue Bao*, 2010, 8(5): 417

例三： 中国住院冠心病患者糖代谢异常研究——中国心脏调查

中国心脏调查组

Cross-sectional study on the prevalence of abnormal glucose metabolism in patients with coronary artery disease in China—China Heart Survey

China Heart Survey Group, HU Da-yi, PAN Chang-Yu

Corresponding authors: HU Da-yi, Center for Heart, Lung and Blood Vessel, Tongji University, Shanghai 200092

PAN Chang-Yu, Department of Endocrinology, Chinese PLA General Hospital, Beijing 100853

引自:《中华内分泌代谢杂志》, 2006, 22(1): 7

例四： 超声心动图检测右心功能指标对急性肺栓塞不同治疗方法的评价

国家"十五"攻关"肺栓塞规范化诊疗方法的研究"课题组

Evaluation of Right Ventricular Indexes on Echocardiogram in Different Therapy Regimens for Pulmonary Embolism

National Project of the Diagnosis and Treatment Strategies for Pulmonary Thromboembolism (NATSPUTE)

引自:《中国循环杂志》, 2007, 22(1): 41

例五： 商环使得男性包皮环切更加简单快捷

The ShangRing device for simplified adult circumcision

Masson P, Li PS, Barone MA, Goldstein M.

这是一篇刊发在 *Nature* 上的研究论文，在其文末处有如下声明：

Author contributions（做出贡献的作者）

All authors researched data for the article and were involved in discussion of content, as well as writing and reviewing and editing the manuscript before submission.

声明：本文所有作者均参与了该项研究并在本论文投稿之前就其内容进行过集体商讨、审核、修订。

引自: *Nat Rev Urol*, 2010, 7(11): 638

例六： 肥胖症治疗结局分析报告系统：为期 15 年的胆胰分流术治疗效果评估

A 15-Year Evaluation of Biliopancreatic Diversion According to the Bariatric Analysis Reporting Outcome System (BAROS)

Giuseppe M. Marinari, MD; Federica Murelli, MD; Giovanni Camerini, MD; Francesco Papadia, MD; Flavia Carilini, MD; Cesare Stabilini, MD; Gian Franco Adami, MD; Nicola Scopinario, MD

注：该文署名后的 MD 为医学博士

引自: *Obesity Surgery*, 2004, 14: 325

例七： 系统综述：芯针与手术组织活检诊断乳腺疾病效果对比

Systematic Review: Comparative Effectiveness of Core-Needle and Open Surgical Biopsy to Diagnose Breast Lesions

Wendy Bruening, PhD; Joann Fontanarosa, PhD; Kelley Tipton, MPH;

Jonathan R. Treadwell, PhD; Jason Launders, MSc; and Karen Schoelles, MD, SM

Author Contributions: Conception and design: W. Bruening, J.R. Treadwell, K.Schoelles.

Analysis and interpretation of the data: W. Bruening, J. Fontanarosa, J.R. Treadwell, K. Schoelles.

Drafting of the article: W. Bruening, J. Fontanarosa.

Critical revision of the article for important intellectual content: J.R. Treadwell, J. Launders, K. Schoelles.

Final approval of the article: W. Bruening, J. Fontanarosa, J.R. Treadwell, K.Schoelles.

Statistical expertise: W. Bruening, J.R. Treadwell, K.schoelles.

Administrative, technical, or logistic support: W. Bruening.

Collection and assemble of data: J.Fontanarosa, K.Tipton.

【析】本例中，在论文文末处对本文作者所承担的工作（author contributions）做了详细介绍，如 W. Bruening, J. Fontanarosa, J.R. Treadwell, K. Schoelles, 承担数据分析任务；W. Bruening, J. Fontanarosa 承担论文撰稿等。

引自：*Ann Intern Med*, 2010, 152(4)：247

（四）英文摘要中的中文姓名表达

欧美人姓名排列次序与我国不同，且很复杂，不仅牵涉其种族的人文、地理、宗教和习俗，而且涉及族、家等谱系，尤其在复姓人名中常涉及祖、父世系的沿袭关系或部族关系。一般说来，外国人的名称一般先"名"后"姓"，如首次证实微生物存在的荷兰人列文虎克的姓名全称是"Antony van Leeuwenhoek"，Leeuwenhoek 是"姓（surname 或 family name）"，而 Antony 是"名（教名）（Christian name 或 first name）"，van 是"中间名（middle name）或 second name"。又如，美国病理学家立克次的全名是 Howard Talyor Ricketts。

我国是个多民族的国家，有 56 个民族，各民族的姓名由于受其宗教和习俗的影响，排列次序也不尽相同。随着人口的增长，汉语姓名更是种类繁多，从传统上频繁使用的单姓单名、单姓双名、复姓单名，至现在的单姓多名、复姓双名等。采用汉语拼音拼写姓名在一定程度上势必造成混乱。尽管目前国内学术刊物大体上采用中华人民共和国国家标准《汉语拼音正词法基本规则》（GB/T 16159—2012）来处理姓名，但从实际情况看，我国各类医学学术期刊在姓名表达方面差异性较大，如姓名的顺序、字体字形（正斜体、大小写）、拼写规范［缩写、全拼、复名之间的连字符（hyphen）使用与否］通常各随其好。以夏敬医和赵贺为例，中文名形式可能有以下几种：①XIA Jing-yi, ZHAO He, 采用正体印刷，复名之间使用连字符分隔；②*XIA Jing-Yi, ZHAO He*，采用斜体印刷形式，每个音节首字母均大写，复名之间使用连字符分隔；③XIA Jingyi, ZHAO He，复名采用连拼。无论采用何种拼写或印刷形式，但有一点需要作者特别注意，即汉语姓名拼写必须依据现代汉语拼音方案，如"王（Wang）"不能拼写为 Wong，不能将"许（Xu）"拼写为 Hsu；表达形式参照中华人民共和国新闻出版署印发、2006 年 6 月开始实施的《中国学术期刊（光盘版）检索与评价数据规范》*Data Norm for Retrieval and Evaluation of Chinese Academic Journal（CD）*（CAJ-CD B/T 1—2006）。该规范规定中国作者姓名的汉语拼音应采用："姓前名后，中间为空格，姓氏的全部字母均大写，复姓应连写，名字的前字母大写，双名中间加连字符，名字不缩写"。例如，"欧阳连勤"应拼写为 OUYANG Lian-qin，"诸葛鸿"拼写为 ZHUGE Hong。按照现代汉语拼音方案，还有两点需要注意：①在以 a、o、e 开头的音节连接在其他音节后面的时候，如果音节的界限发生混淆，要用隔音符号（'）隔开，避免发生歧义，如"Wang Xi'an（王玺安）"或"Wang Xi-An（王玺安）"，否则就拼成"WangXian（王贤）"了；②在拼音方案 ü 行的韵母，前面没有声母时，写成 yu，或韵母跟声母 j、q、x 连拼的时候，ü 上的两点均省略，如"章语"可拼写为 ZHANG Yu，"张学军"拼写为 ZHANG Xue-jun。但若跟声母 n、l 连拼时，仍然要写成 ü，如"吕德农"应写为 Lü De-nong。

　　除此之外，国外期刊，包括国内出版的英文版杂志，在中文姓名拼写方面一般习惯采用西式表达方式，如张学军可拼写为 Xuejun Zhang 或 Xue-jun Zhang 或名字采用缩写，将其拼成 Zhang XJ。拼写译名时切勿随意乱拼，建议查阅汉语字典，以免译音受乡土音影响而拼出的姓名不规范。

二、工作单位及属地

　　工作单位及属地是指作者所属工作机构及机构所在地，是期刊编辑部或读者与作者之间联系的重要信息源，其位置一般位于论文作者署名的下方，但国内外医学期刊对工作单位的排列次序和排版位置都有一定的格式要求，作者投稿时应就此事先了解具体规范要求。例如，《临床外科杂志》对中英文摘要写作要求中规定："……英文摘要一般与中文摘要内容相对应。英文摘要应包括文题、作者姓名（汉语拼音，其姓的字母均大写）、工作单位、所在省市名、邮政编码及国名。作者应列出前 3 位，3 位以上加 et al；不属同一单位时，只注明第一作者工作单位。"例如，"LIN Xian-ya, WU Jian-ping, QIN Qiong, et al. Department of Pediatrics, First Hospital, Beijing Medical University, Beijing 100034, China"，引自：《临床外科杂志》，2008，16（3）：181。又如，《中华眼耳鼻喉科杂志》[2010，10（3）：99] 在其"读者·作者·编者"中规定"……首先应列出单位名称的全称，如已归属综合大学的单位，应先列出大学名称，之后列出医学院名称或医院名称、科室名称"。由于我国在行政区划上设置和国外有较大差异，因而，机构属地也显得较复杂，特别是基础单位的属地，这给我国作者投稿，尤其向国外期刊投稿时对于工作单位及属地的书写造成了不少的困惑或麻烦。我国早在 1980 年 7 月 1 日就实施了邮政编码区分行政区划，因此，对研究机构所需的过于小的街道名就可以不必列出，只需列出正确的邮政编码即可，对于高等院校、机构应具体到系和教研室。此外，还有以下几点需要注意。

（1）多作者署名，而这些作者又不在同一单位时，应按作者的排列顺序列出他们相应的工作单位。

（2）若作者预计到论文出版时，可能会因工作调动等原因更换到新的工作单位，有必要在脚注中给出新地址（present address）。

（3）如果第一作者不是通信作者，应在该作者名称右上角给出标示符（期刊中多以"*"标示），在脚注中标注通信作者或联系人。

以下为工作单位及属地的英文表示法。

（一）工作单位的排列次序

在英文中，工作单位的排列次序应合乎英文表达规范，习惯上按由小到大的顺序排列，如按组、室、科、院、所、市、省、国的顺序。小的单位单元常涉及如下常用词。

部门、科、处：division　　　　科、系：department

研究所、学院：institute　　　　处、中心：center

部门、处、组：section　　　　实验室：laboratory

部门、处：branch

其中 division、section 和 branch 意义比较接近，均表示分支的含义，因此，基本可以通用。

例一：**Department** of Internal Medicine, **Division** of Endocrinology, Diabetes and Nutrition, University of Maryland School of Medicine, Baltimore

马里兰大学医学院，内分泌、糖尿病和营养学系内科学教研室；巴尔的摩

引自：*Am J Med*, 2019, 132: 408

例二：**Division** of Newborn Medicine, **Department** of Pediatrics, The Mount Sinai School of Medicine, New York, NY, USA

美国蒙坦西奈医学院儿科学系新生儿科

引自：*Am J Med*, 2007, 3: 31

例三：**Division** of Hematology and Internal Medicine

血液学与内科学系

引自：*Blood,* 2010, 116(24): 5126

（二）工作单位的排版位置

1. 国外医学学术期刊

总体上，国外医学期刊中对作者的工作单位处置方式大同小异。大部分采用：①直接置于署名的正下方；②置于脚注位置。置于脚注或其他位置时，单位名称前一般常加用介词 from。对于多位作者，若来自不同机构则采用特殊符号或阿拉伯数字依次标注作者姓名和工作单位，同一单位用相同符号或数字，但标识符号各有不同。例如：

例一：Serum free light chains: Diagnostic and prognostic value in multiple myeloma

血清游离轻链在多发性骨髓瘤中的诊断与预后判断价值

Pavai Sthaneshwar, Veerasekaran Nadarajian, Jayaranee A.S. Maniam, Nani Nordin and Gan Gin Gin

Department of Pathology, University of Malaya, Kuala Lumpur, Malaya

马来西亚大学，病理学系。

【析】本文虽有多位作者，但均来自同一机构，作者单位直接置于署名下方。

引自：*Clin Chem Lab Med*, 2009, 47(9): 1101

例二：Cancer genes and the pathways they control

肿瘤基因及其控制通道

Bert Vogelstein , Kenneth W Kinzler

The authors are at the Howard Hughes Medical Institute and The Sidney Kimmel Comprehensive Cancer Center, The Johns Hopkins University Medical Institutions, Baltimore, Maryland 21231, USA

美国马里兰州，巴尔的摩市，约翰霍普金斯大学医学院，肿瘤综合研究中心

【析】本刊将作者单位地址置于左下脚注处，采用完整结构句式表达。

引自：*Nat Med*, 2004, 10(8): 789

例三：Systematic Review: Gene Expression Profiling Assays in Early-Stage Breast Cancer

早期乳腺癌基因谱表达分析

Luigi Marchionni, MD, PhD; Renee F.Wilson, MSc; Antonio C.Wolff, MD; Spyridon Marinopoulos, MD, MBA; Giovanni Parmigiani, PhD; Eric B. Bass, MD, MPH; and Steven N. Goodman, MD, MHS, PhD

Current Author Addresses: Drs. Marchionni and Wolff: Johns Hopkins University School of Medicine, Oncology Cancer Biology, Baltimore, MD 21287.

Ms. Wilson, Dr. Marinopoulos, and Dr. Bass: Johns Hopkins University, School of Medicine, General Internal Medicine, Baltimore, MD 21287.

Dr. Parmigiani: Johns Hopkins University, School of Medicine Oncology Informatics, Baltimore, MD 21287.

Dr. Goodman: Johns Hopkins University School of Medicine, Oncology Biostatistics, Baltimore, MD 21287.

【析】本文相关作者工作单位全部罗列在论文文末处，并明确使用了 current author addresses（作者现地址），同时在各作者供职机构前加上头衔称呼，如 Drs. Marchionni and Wolff（Drs. 表示这两位作者均为博士），约翰霍普金斯大学医学院分子肿瘤研究所；Ms. Wilson（Wilson 女士），约翰霍普金斯大学医学院大内科系。

引自：*Ann Intern Med*, 2008, 148(5): 358

例四： An ARF-independent c-MYC-activated tumor suppression pathway mediated by ribosomal protein-Mdm2 Interaction

核糖体蛋白 Mdm2 相互作用介导的不依赖于 ARF 的 c-MYC 活化肿瘤抑制通路

Everardo Macias[1,2],Aiwen Jin [1,2],Chad Deisenroth[1,2,4] ,Krishna Bhat[5],Hua Mao[3],Mikael S.Lindstrom[6],and Yanping Zhang[1,2,3*]

[1] Department of Radiation Oncology

[2] Lineberger Comprehensive Cancer Center

[3] Department of Pharmacology

[4] Curriculum in Genetics and Molecular Biology

School of Medicine, the University of North Carolina at Chapel Hill, Chapel Hill, NC 27599, USA

[5] Department of Pathology, The University of Texas, M.D. Anderson Cancer Center, Houston, TX 77030, USA

[6] Department of Oncology-Pathology, Cancer Center Karolinska, CCK 8:05, Karolinska University Hospital in Solna, Stockholm, SE-17176, Sweden

[*] Correspondence: ypzhang@med.unc.edu

【析】这篇论文由多位作者共同完成，采用数字标志分别在署名的右上角标识了作者排序。作者有来自同一机构的，也有来自其他机构。排序 1～4 的作者来自于同一机构，即北卡罗来纳大学教堂山分校医学院（肿瘤放射学系；莱茵博格综合肿瘤中心；药学系；遗传学与分子生物学统一课程教学部）；排序在第 5 位的作者来自于得克萨斯大学，MD 安德森癌症中心病理学系；排位第 6 的作者来自于瑞典卡罗琳斯卡大学。

引自：*Cancer Cell*, 2010, 18(3): 231

例五： Molecular detection and prevalence of porcine caliciviruses in eastern China from 2008 to 2009

2008～2009 年华东地区猪肠道杯状病毒的分子检测及流行情况

Quan Shen • Wen Zhang • Shixing Yang • Yan Chen • Huibo Ning • Tongling Shan • Junfeng Liu • Zhibiao Yang • Li Cui • Jianguo Zhu • Xiuguo Hua

【析】本刊作者与作者之间采用 "•" 分隔，来自同一机构及不同机构的作者及通信地址和电子邮箱放在论文首页脚注分别列出如下：

Q. Shen • W. Zhang • S. Yang • Y. Chen • H. Ning • T. Shan • J. Liu • Z. Yang • L. Cui • J. Zhu • X. Hua(✉)

Shanghai Key Laboratory of Veterinary Biotechnology,

School of Agriculture and Biology, Shanghai JiaoTong

University, 800 Dongchuan Road, Shanghai,

People's Republic of China

e-mail: hxg@sjtu.edu.cn

Q. Shen

e-mail: njnushenquan@yahoo.com.cn

W. Zhang

School of Medical Technology, Jiangsu University,

301 Xuefu Road, 212013 Zhenjiang, Jiangsu,

People's Republic of China

H. Ning

Shanxi Agricultural University, Shanxi, China

引自：*Arch Virol*,2009,154:1625

例六：A Novel Mouse Model of Experimental Asthma

新型大鼠哮喘试验模型的建立

Sampson B. Sarpong [a,b]   Liu-Yi Zhang[b]   Steven R. Kleeberger[b,c]

[a]Department of Pediatrics and Child Health, National Human Genome Center, Howard University, Washington D.C.;

[b]Department of Environmental Health Sciences, Bloomberg School of Public Health, Johns Hopkins University, Blatimore, Md., and [c]Pulmonary Branch, National Institute of Environmental Health Sciences, Research Triangle Park, N.C., USA

【析】作者排序与其对应的机构采用的是字母表示法。

引自: *Int Arch Allergy Immunol*, 2003, 132: 346

例七：Metabolic Syndrome and Ischemic Stroke Risk Northern Manhattan Study

代谢综合征与缺血性卒中发生率——北曼哈顿研究

Bernadette Boden-Albala, MPH, DrPH; Ralph L.Sacco, MD, MS; Hye-Sueng Lee, MS; Cairistine Grahame-Clarke, MRCP, PhD; Tanjia Rundek, MD, PhD: Mitchell V. Elkind, MD, MS: Clinton Wright, MD, MS; Elsa-Grace V. Giardina, MD; Marco R.DiTullio, MD; Shunichi Homma, MD; Myunghee C. Paik, PhD

From the Departments of Neurology (B.B.-A., R.L.S., T.R., M.V.E., C.W.) and Sociomedical Science (B.B.-A), the Sergivsky Center(R.L.S.,M.V.E.), and the Departments of Epidemiology (R.L.S.), Biostatistics (M.C.P.,H.-S.L.), and Medicine, Division of Cardiology (C.G.-C., E.-G.V.G, M.R.D.T., S.H.), Columbia University College of Physicians and Surgeons and the Nailman School of Public Health, New York, NY.

Correspondence to Bernadette Boden-Albala, DrPH, Neurological Institute, 710 W 168 St, New York, NY 10032. E-mail bb87@columbia. Edu

【析】本例与以上其他例证有所不同。首先表达机构名称,采用括号将来自同一机构的作者列举在后，如神经学系（B.B.-A., R.L.S., T.R., M.V.E.,

C.W.）；社会医学系（B.B.-A）等。此外，从机构地址表示可以看出，上述作者均来自同一单位（哥伦比亚大学内科与外科医师学院与 Nailman 公共卫生学院）。作者未做排序，但指定了通信作者（Bernadette Boden-Albala），由此判断，这是一项集体研究，所有作者贡献程度大体相当。

引自：*Stroke*, 2008, 39(1): 30

2. 国内医学学术期刊

1）中文版：作者的工作单位一般被直接置于作者姓名之下，而且不用介词"from"。

2）英文版：一种版式同中文版一致，即直接将作者所属机构地址置于署名下方，另一种参照国外模式，将工作单位置于脚注位置。例如：

例一： 不动杆菌属多重耐药及泛耐药的分子机制研究

Molecular mechanism of multiple-drug and pan-drug resistance among acinetobacter species

WANG Hui[*], SUN Hong-li, NING Yong-zhong, YANG Qi-wen, CHEN Min-jun, ZHU Yuan-jue, XU Ying-chun, XIE Xiu-li. [*]Department of Clinical Laboratory, Peking Union Medical College Hospital, Peking Union Medical College and Chinese Academy of Medical Sciences, Beijing 100730, China

中国医学科学院 中国协和医科大学 北京协和医院检验科

【析】作者单位直接紧跟在署名之后。

引自：《中华医学杂志》, 2006, 86(1): 17

例二： 经内镜逆行胆管造影在肝移植术后胆管并发症中的应用价值

The practical value of endoscopic retrograde cholangiography in biliary complications after liver transplantation

WANG Gen-shu[*], LU Min-qiang, YANG Ying, CAI Chang-jie, ZHENG Feng-ping, WANG Wei-dong, LI Hua, XU Chi, YI Shu-hong, YI Hui-min, CHEN Gui-hua.

[*]Organ Transplantation Institute, Sun Yat-Sen University, Liver Transplantation Center, Affiliated Third Hospital, Sun Yat-Sen University, Guangzhou 510080, China

Corresponding author: CHEN Gui-hua, Email: chgh@gzsums.edu.cn

广州，中山大学附属第三医院肝脏移植中心　中山大学器官移植研究所

【析】作者署名与工作单位随标题后连续排版。

引自：《中华外科杂志》, 2006, 44(21): 1453

例三： 尿激酶型纤溶酶原激活物（u-PA）基因对小鼠实验性肺气肿的影响及其机制

The role of urokinase type plasminogen activator gene in mouse experimental emphysema

Hu Hua, XIAO Yao, TAL Xian-mei, SONG Hou-yan

(Key Laboratory of Molecular Medicine, Ministry of Education-Shanghai Medical College, Fudan University, Shanghai 200032, China)

（复旦大学上海医学院分子医学教育部重点实验室　上海　200032）

引自：《复旦学报（医学版）》，2008, 35(1): 7

例四： 小剂量胺碘酮用于 70 岁以上老年患者冠状动脉搭桥术后预防房颤效果研究

Low-dose amiodarone for the prevention of atrial fibrillation after coronary artery bypass grafting in patients older than 70 years

GU Song, SU Pi-xiong, LIU Yan, YAN Jun, ZHANG Xi-tao and WANG Tian-you

Department of Cardiac Surgery, Beijing Chaoyang Hospital, Capital Medical University, Beijing 100020, China (Gun S, Su PX, Liu Y, Yan J and Zhang XT)

Department of Cardiothoracic Surgery, Beijing Friendship Hospital, Capital Medical University, Beijing 100033, China (Wang TY)

Correspondence to Prof. WANG Tian-you, Department of Cardiothoracic Surgery, Beijing Friendship Hospital, Capital Medical University, Beijing 1000033, China

【析】 这是《中华医学杂志英文版》，作者工作单位置于脚注，首先罗列机构名称，再用括号罗列出来自同一单位的作者名。版式基本与 *Stroke* 相同。

引自：*Chin Med J*, 2009, 122(24): 2928

例五： 中药五倍子对牙釉质深度损伤再矿化影响的体外研究

Effect of Galla chinensis on the *In Vitro* Remineralization of Advanced Enamel Lesions

Lei Cheng, Jacob M. ten Cate

Department of Cariology, Endodontology, Pedodontology, Academic Centre for Dentistry Amsterdam(ACTA), Amsterdam, The Netherlands

荷兰，阿姆斯特丹口腔医学研究中心，龋病、牙髓病及儿童口腔医学系

【析】 这是《国际口腔科学杂志英文版》，作者单位直接置于作者署名下方。

引自：*Int J Oral Sci,* 2010, 2(1): 15

3. 作者单位英译注意的问题

医学论文的写作与发表，其目的是学术交流。这种交流不仅限于国内同行，还包括国际交流。尽管现代通信手段高度发达，但单位名称的英文表达在国际交流中仍然起着至关重要的作用。既然学术成果代表的是一个单位的科研水平，那么，单位名称就是这个机构的"标志物"。我国出版发行的中文医学学术刊物均要求附有英译标题、作者姓名、单位名称及英文摘要，如通过医学检索网站检索"An innovative male circumcision technique in China and HIV prevention"，除了提供英文摘要外，在该标题下方提供了如下信息：【Article in Chinese】；作者署名及作者所属机构地址（Jiangsu Family Planning Research Institute, Nanjing, Jiangsu 210036, China）。提供单位名称及地址，正是为了满足国际交流需要。对于单位名称的表达，目前主要存在两个方面问题：①尽管我们国家对科技论文写作出台了相关标准，如《科学技术报告、学位论文和学术论文的编写格式》（GB 7713—87）；《信息与文献　参考文献著录规则》（GB/T 7714—2015），但对单位机构翻译没有制订相关标准。由于我国单位名称过多且复杂，故无法统一翻译标准，这势必导致英译单位名称五花八门，即使是同一单位名称，在不同的期刊上也存在不一致现象。②单位地址缺乏完整或翻译过于烦琐。因此，书写单位名称时要注意下述几点。

（1）按照作者单位已有的译名。当前，大部分单位为了交流或宣传需要，大体上都有其英译名称，如上海市高血压研究所英译名称为 Shanghai Institute of Hypertension，切勿擅自随意改变固有的英译名称，以免造成不一致现象。

（2）高等学校、医疗单位、研究所等应具体到二级或三机构，如"Department of Preventive Medicine, School of Public Health, Sun Yat-sen University; Department of Radiology, Affiliated Yijishan Hospital, Wannan Medical College; Laboratory of Vascular Biology, Shanghai Institute of Hypertension."

（3）采用汉语拼音拼写名称时，要按《汉语拼音正词法基本规则》（GB/T 16159—2012）规范拼写。

（4）单位所在区域邮政编码需认真核实，防止造成邮件分拣过程出现差错从而导致邮件投递延误。

（5）对于基层医疗机构，虽然有邮政编码可以确认单位所在地，但由于中国的行政区划与国外存在一定的差异，单位名称与地址应尽可能详尽。如要表示某县某乡某卫生所，其表达格式为"＿＿＿Clinic, ＿＿＿County（+邮编），＿＿＿Province, China"。

4. 常见学衔、职称、职务、医疗卫生机构、科研教学单位、医院科室等英语表达方法

（1）学衔

产科硕士	MAO: Master in Obstetrics
产科学士	BAO: Bachelor of Obstetrics
耳科硕士	MChOtol: Magister Chirurgiae Otologicae; Master of Otology
放射学硕士	MRad: Master of Radiology
工业卫生学硕士	MIH: Master of Industrial Health
公共卫生学博士	DrPH: Doctor of Public Health
公共卫生学硕士	MPH: Master of Public Health
骨科硕士	MChOrth: Magister Chirurgiae Orthopaedicae; Master of Orthopaedic Surgery
护理学硕士	MN: Master of Nursing

护理学学士	BN: Bachelor of Nursing
理学博士	DSc/ScD: Doctor of Science
理学硕士	MSc: Master of Science
外科博士	DCh/ChD: Doctor of Chirurgiae; Doctor of Surgery
外科硕士	MCh/ChM: Chirurgiae Magister; Master of Surgery
外科学士	BC/BCh/BChir/BS/ChB: Baccalaureus Chirurgiae; Bachelor of Surgery
卫生学硕士	MHyg: Master of Hygiene
卫生学博士	DHyg: Doctor of Hygiene
卫生学学士	BHyg: Bachelor of Hygiene
牙科博士	DDSc: Doctor of Dental Science
牙科学士	BDSc: Bachelor of Dental Science
牙外科博士	DDS: Doctor of Dental Surgery
药学博士	PharD: Pharmaciae Doctor; Doctor of Pharmacy
药学硕士	PharM: Pharmaciae Magister; Master of Pharmacy
医学博士	DM: Doctor of Medicine
医学学士	BM: Bachelor of Medicine
医学硕士	MB: Bachelor of Medicine
注册护士	RN: Registered Nurse

（2）职称、职务

产科医师	obstetrician
传染病科医师	doctor for infectious disease
儿科医师，儿科专家	pediatrician; pediatrist
耳鼻喉科医师,耳鼻喉科专家	otolaryngologist
放射科医师	radiologist
妇科医师	gynecologist
副教授	associate professor
护师	senior nurse
护士长	head nurse
检验士	laboratory technician
讲师	lecturer
矫形外科医师	orthopedist
教授	professor
精神科医师	psychiatrist
科主任	head/chief of the department
口腔科医师，口腔科专家	stomatologist
理疗科医师	physicotherapist; physicotherapeutist
临床护理专家	clinical specialist

流行病学家	epidemiologist
麻醉医师	anesthetist
门诊部主任	head of the out-patient department
泌尿外科医师, 泌尿外科学家	urological surgeon; urologist
内科医师	internist
内科主任	physician-in-chief
皮肤科医师	dermatologist
全科医生	general practitioner (GP)
神经科医师	neurologist
神经外科医师	neurosurgeon
实习医师	intern
外科医师	surgeon
外科主任	surgeon-in-chief
心脏外科医师	cardiac surgeon
胸科医师	chest physician
胸外科医师	thoracic surgeon; surgeon of thoracic surgery
牙科医师	dentist
眼科医师，眼科学家	eye doctor; oculist; ophthalmologist
药剂师	pharmacist
药剂士	assistant pharmacist
院长	director/president of the hospital
整形外科医师	plastic surgeon
主管护师	supervisor nurse
主任护师	chief superintendent nurse
主治医师	attending doctor/physician
住院医师	resident doctor; house staff/officer
助教	assistant

（3）医疗卫生机构、科研教学单位

艾滋病研究中心	AIDS Research Center
保健站	Health Station
病理解剖学教研室	Department of Pathologic Anatomy; Department of Pathoanatomy
病理生理学教研室	Department of Pathophysiology
病理学教研室	Department of Pathology
不育症研究会	Association fro the Study of Infertility
产妇咨询单位	Maternity Consultant Unit
产院	Maternity Hospital; Prenatal Center; Lying-in Hospital
传染病医院	Infectious Disease Hospital

传染病中心	Communicable Disease Center
催眠疗法诊疗所	Institute fro Research in Hypnosis
地段医院	Local Hospital; Neighbourhood Hospital
地区卫生局	District Health Bureau
地区医院	District Hospital/Regional Hospital
第一人民医院	The First People's Hospital; No.1 People's Hospital
毒理学教研室	Department of Toxicology
儿科医院	Pediatric Hospital
儿童医院	Children's Hospital
法医病理学教研室	Department of Forensic Pathology
防疫站	Anti-Epidemic Station
防治所	Prevention and Treatment Center
放射医学教研室	Department of Radiation Medicine
放射医学研究所	Research Institute of Radiation Medicine
分析化学教研室	Department of Analytical Chemistry
分子生物学实验室	Laboratory of Molecular Biology
分子遗传学实验室	Laboratory of Molecular Genetics
妇产科医院	Obstetrics and Gynecology Hospital; Women's Hospital
妇婴保健院	Maternal and Infant/Child Health Institute
妇幼保健指导站	Consulting Station for Health of Women and Children
妇幼医院	Women and Children's Hospital
附属医院	Affiliated Hospital
工人医院	Workers' Hospital
公共卫生系	Faculty of Public Health
公共卫生学院	School of Public Health
公立医院	Public Hospital
骨科医院	Osteopathic Hospital
护理学院	School of Nursing
核医学实验室	Laboratory of Nuclear Medicine
基础护理学教研室	Department of Basic Nursing
寄生虫学教研室	Department of Parasitology
解剖学教研室	Department of Anatomy
口腔医院	Hospital for Stomatology
科学技术处	Science & Technology Office
矿泉疗养院	Mineral Spring Sanatorium
老年医学协会	Association of Gerontology
老年医院	Hospital for the Aged; Senility Hospital
疗养院	Sanatorium

陆军医院	Army Hospital
麻风病医院	Leprosy Hospital
皮肤病防治研究所	Skin Disease Prevention and Treatment Institute
皮肤性病研究所	Institute of Dermatology and Venereology
区幼保健院	District Maternity and Child Health Hospital
人民卫生出版社	People's Medical Publishing House
人民医院	People's Hospital
生化教研室	Department of Biochemistry
生化试剂实验所	Biochemical Reagent Laboratory
生理学教研室	Department of Physiology
生命科学学院	School of Life Sciences
生物系	Faculty of Biology
生物医学工程研究所	Institute of Biomedical Engineering
生物制品研究所	Institute of Biological Products; Vaccine and Serum Institute
省卫生厅	Provincial Health Bureau; Provincial Bureau of Health
省医院	Provincial Hospital
实验动物中心	Laboratory Animals Centre
食品药品监督管理局	Food and Drug Administration
市卫生局	Municipal Health Bureau; City Health Bureau
市医院	Municipal Hospital; City Hospital
私立医院	Proprietary Hospital
铁路中心医院	Central Railway Hospital
图书情报研究所	Institute of Information and Library
微生物学教研室	Department of Microbiology
卫生部	Ministry of Public Health
卫生防疫站	Anti-Epidemic Station; Hygiene and Anti-Epidemic Centre; Health and Prevention Station
卫生检疫所	Quarantine Service
卫生室	Health Post
卫生所	Health Station
卫生统计学教室	Department of Health Statistics
卫生学教研室	Department of Hygiene
卫生学校	Health School
县医院	County Hospital
献血站	Blood Donor Centre
乡卫生院	Township Clinic
协和医院	Union Medical College Hospital; Union Hospital

协会	Association; Society
心血管病研究所	Institute of Cardiovascular Diseases
心脏病学会	Society of Cardiology
血库	Blood Bank
血吸虫病防治所	Anti-Schistosomiasis Station; Station for Prevention & Treatment of Schistosomiasis
牙病防治所	Dental Disease Prevention and Treatment Clinic
牙科医院	Dental Hospital
药理学教研室	Department of Pharmacology
药品管理处	Drug Enforcement Administration
药品检验所	Institute for Drug Control
药学会	Pharmaceutical Association
药学院	College/School of Pharmacy/ Pharmaceutical Science
医科大学	Medical University
医疗管理处	Medical Service Administration
医学部	Faculty of Medical Sciences
医学考试委员会	Board of Medical Examiners
医学情报研究所	Institute of Medical Science Information
医学院	Medical College
医学专科学校	Medical School
医药工业公司	Pharmaceutical Industrial Company
优生学会	Eugenics Society
针灸推拿诊所	Acupuncture-Massage Clinic
诊所	Clinic
整形外科医院	Hospital for Plastic Surgery
整形医院	Plastic Surgery Hospital
职工医院	Workers' Hospital
职业病研究所	Occupational Medicine Research Institute
制药厂	Pharmaceutical Factory
制药有限公司	Pharmaceutical Co. Ltd.
中国红十字总会	Red Cross Society of China
中国科学院	Chinese Academy of Science
中国人民解放军总医院	Chinese People's Liberation Army General Hospital
中国医疗队	Chinese Medical Team
中国医学科学院	Chinese Academy of Medical Science
中国预防医学科学院	Chinese Academy of Preventive Medicine
中国中医研究院	China Academy of Traditional Chinese Medicine
中华护理学会	Nursing Association of China

中华医学会	Chinese Medical Association
中日友好医院	Sino-Japan Friendship Hospital
中西医结合研究会	Association of Integration of Traditional Chinese and Western Medicine
中心医院	Central Hospital
中医医院	Hospital of Traditional Chinese Medicine
中医诊所	Traditional Chinese Medicine Clinic
肿瘤研究所	Cancer Research Institute
专科医院	Special Hospital
咨询门诊	Consulting Clinic
自治区医院	Autonomous Region Hospital
综合医院	General Hospital
总医院	General Hospital
组织胚胎学教研室	Department of Histology & Embryology

（4）医院科室

CT 室	CT Room
病房	Ward
病理科	Department of Pathology
病理室	Laboratory of Pathology
产房（分娩室）	Delivery Room
产科	Department of Obstetrics
超声波检查室	Sonography Room
超声检查科	Department of Ultrasonography
超声诊断室	Ultrasonic Diagnosis Room
传染（病）科	Department of Infectious Diseases Service
传染病中心	Centre for Infectious Diseases
传染科	Department of Infectious Diseases
创伤外科	Department of Traumatology
磁共振检查中心	MRI Centre
电子显微镜室	Laboratory of Electron Microscopy
儿科	Department of Pediatrics
耳鼻喉科	Department of Otorhinolaryngology; Otolaryngology
放射科	Department of Roentgenology; X-ray Department
放射治疗科	Department of Radiation Therapy; Department of Radiotherapy
肺功能室	Laboratory of Lung Function
妇产科	Department of Obstetrics and Gynecology
妇科	Department of Gynecology

肝病科	Liver Department
肝胆外科	Department of Hepatobiliary Surgery
肛肠外科	Department of Anorectal Surgery
高压氧治疗室	Unit for Hyperbaric Oxygen Therapy
隔离病室	Isolation Ward
供应室	Supply Room
骨科	Department of Orthopaedics
骨髓移植中心	Bone Marrow Transplantation Center
挂号处	Registration Office
核医学科	Department of Nuclear Medicine
颌面外科	Department of Maxillofacial Surgery
候诊室	Reception Room; Waiting Room
呼吸内科	Department of Respiratory Diseases
护理部	Nursing/ Nurses Department
护理系	Faculty of Nursing
护士办公室	Nurses' Office
化疗科	Chemotherapy Department
换药室	Dressing Room
肌电图室	Electromyography Room
急诊室	Emergency Room
检验科	Department of Clinical Laboratories
康复中心	Rehabilitation Centre
口腔科	Department of Stomatology
老年病科	Department of Gerontology
麻醉科	Department of Anesthesiology
门诊部	Out-patient Department
泌尿外科	Department of Urology
免疫学教研室	Department of Immunology
内分泌科	Department of Endocrinology
内镜检查室	Endoscopy Room
内科	Department of Internal Medicine; Department of Medicine
脑电图室	Electroencephalography Room
皮肤科	Department of Dermatology
普通外科	Department of General Surgery
普外科	Department of General Surgery
烧伤科	Department of Burn
神经内科	Department of Neurology

神经外科	Department of Neurosurgery
肾内科	Department of Nephrology
手术室	Operating Room
输血中心	Blood Transfusion Center
碎石中心	Lithotripsy Center
外科	Department of Surgery
显微外科	Department of Microsurgery
消化内科	Department of Gastroenterology; Section of Digestive Diseases
心电图室	Electrocardiography Room
心血管内科	Department of Cardiovascular Diseases
心血管外科	Department of Cardiovascular Surgery
血库	Blood Bank
血液内科	Department of Haematology
血液透析中心	Haemodialysis Center
药房	Department of Pharmacy
医院图书馆	Hospital Library
院内传染科	Division of Hospital Infection
心理健康教育咨询中心	Mental Health Education & Counseling Center
中药房	Department of Chinese Pharmacy
中医科	Faculty of Traditional Chinese Medicine
肿瘤科	Department of Oncology
住院部	In-patient Department

注：除上述参考外，亦可参考《公共服务领域英文译写规范第 7 部分：医疗卫生》（ *Guidelines for the use of English in public service areas-Part7:Health and medicine* ）（ GB/T 30240.7—2017 ）。

三、练　习

3-1　仔细观察并了解下列作者姓名、工作单位及地址表示方法

1) Clinical profile of Saudi children with bronchiectasis

Banjar Hanaa Hasan

Department of Pediatrics, King Faisal Specialist Hospital and Research Centre (KFSH&RC), Riyadh, Saudi Arabia

2) Immunization in urbanized villages of Delhi

Chhabra Pragti, Nair Parvathy, Gupta Anita, Sandhir Meenakshi, Kannan

Department of Community Medicine, University College of Medical Sciences and GTB

Hospital, Delhi, India

  3) Neonatology in developed and developing nations

Garg Pankaj, Bolisetty Srinivas

[1] Department of Pediatrics, Central Hospital, Sector 20A, Faridabad, India

[2] Department of Newborn Care, Royal Hospital for Women, Randwick, NSW 2031, Australia

  4) An Analysis of Why Highly Similar Enzymes Evolve Differently

Fahd K. Majiduddin and Timothy Palzkill

[a] Verna and Marrs McLean Department of Biochemistry and Molecular Biology, Baylor College of Medicine, Houston, Texas 77030

[b] Department of Molecular Virology and Microbiology, Baylor College of Medicine, Houston, Texas 77030

3-2   尝试按下列要求用英语写出你自己的姓名、工作单位和地址

1. 你是独立作者。

2. 你和你的同事是论文合作者，但分别来自两个不同部门/科室。

3. 你的论文合作者分别来自不同单位。

3-3   写出下列工作单位的英文表示

1. 中国医学科学院心血管研究所（阜外医院）心内科

2. 上海交通大学附属第六人民医院内分泌代谢科

3. 上海市糖尿病临床医学中心—上海市糖尿病研究所   上海   200233

4. 第四军医大学生物医学工程系军队卫生装备与计量学教研室，陕西   西安   710033

5. 兰州大学基础医学院病理学教研室

6. 中山大学附属第二医院内分泌科

7. 成都军区总医院核医学科

8. 天津大学材料学院纳米生物技术研究所

9. 中国医科大学附属第一医院艾滋病研究中心

10. 北京市神经外科研究所神经介入科，北京   100050

第四章 医学论文英文摘要"Objective"写作

　　如同中文摘要写作，医学论文英文摘要应紧紧围绕论文的主题，明确研究目的、研究对象、研究所采用的方法、路线、具体的研究结果和结论。因而在"目的"句（Objective or Aim）中应直截了当地提出本研究所要解决的问题，或简要介绍必要的研究背景后阐述整篇论文所要证明的假设或评估、评价的主要问题，有助于使读者一目了然。因此，"目的"句虽然只有短短的一两句话，但作为英文摘要中提纲挈领的部分，其撰写必须具有高度的简明性、完整性、科学性、检索性和准确性。

　　绝大多数结构式英文摘要采用动词不定式短语导入研究目的，偶有个别作者使用完整句子表述研究目的。有关定量研究结果显示，在"目的"项里，完整句子和带 to 的动词不定式短语使用的频率没有显著性差异。尽管如此，从英文摘要的文体风格来看，应尽可能与摘要的类型保持一致。资料性摘要和报道性摘要需要从整个语篇上保持语篇照应，而结构式摘要虽然同样要保持语篇照应，但其中各个项目又自成一体，相对独立。另外，英语语言表达一般强调"经济"原则，即简明性。在结构式摘要中，小标题"目的(Objective、Aim、Purpose)"与"目的"句本身就存在逻辑关联，如 Objective: To evaluate the effect of surgery in cases of rhegmatogenous retinal detachment. 该句的逻辑关系为："(The) objective (is) to evaluate…"。相比而言，前者比后者更为简洁。当然，各类期刊编辑通常有其独特的文体风格，采用短语式还是完整句子表述"目的"，需仔细研究拟投期刊的编辑风格和要求。本章就非动词不定式引导的"目的"句做一简要介绍，在此基础上重点介绍如何撰写借助动词不定式引导的目的句。

一、非动词不定式引导的"Objective"

　　非动词不定式，或者称为完整句。采用该类结构导入研究目的时通常可以借助下列常用词和句型。

（一）purpose

The purpose of the present study is/was to…　　本研究的目的在于……

The purpose of this review is/was to…　　本综述的目的在于……

The purpose of this paper is/was to…	本文的目的在于……
The purpose of this report is/was to…	本文的目的在于……
The purpose of this chapter is/was to…	本章的目的在于……
The purpose of the present work is/was to…	本文的目的在于……
The purpose of this investigation is/was to…	本研究旨在……
The purpose of this study is/was to…	本研究旨在……
The primary purpose is/was to…	本研究的主要目的是……

（二）aim

The aim of this investigation/study/the present study is/was to…	
	本研究旨在……；本文的目的在于……
The aims of this study were to…	本文的目的在于……
Our aim is to…	本文的目的在于……
This study aimed/aims to…	本研究的目的在于……
We aimed to…	本文的目的在于……
This study /research was aimed at…	本研究的目的在于……

（三）object/objective

The objectives of this study were to…	本研究旨在……
The object of this study was to…	本研究旨在……

（四）attempt

The present study is an attempt to…	本研究旨在……
In this study, an attempt was made to…	本研究旨在……；
	在本研究中，我们试图……
Attempts were made to…	我们试图……
In an attempt to…	为了……
In this study, we attempt to…	在本研究中，我们试图……
In a first attempt to…	本文主要的目的旨在……

（五）goal

A major goal is…	本研究的主旨是……

The goal of this study/investigation/research is/was to…　　　本研究的目的在于……

（六）intend/intent

This report/paper is/was intended to…　　　　　　本研究的目的在于……
In brief the article is intended to…　　　　　　本文主要的目的旨在……
In this study we intended to…　　　　　　　本研究中，我们旨在……
It is intended to…　　　　　　　　　　本研究旨在……
The intent of this study is/was…　　　　　　本研究的目的在于……

（七）其他类

The present study was undertaken to…　　　　本研究旨在……
The study here reported was undertaken to…　　　本研究旨在……
The authors undertook a retrospective study to…　　本研究旨在回顾性……
A study was undertaken to…　　　　　　　本研究的目的在于……
A double-blind prospective investigation was undertaken to…

　　　　　　　　　作者做了前瞻性双盲研究，以期……
　　　　　　　　　本前瞻性双盲研究的目的在于……

A retrospective review was undertaken to…

　　　　　　　　　作者进行了回顾性检查，以期……
　　　　　　　　　本回顾性检查的目的在于……

This study/paper was designed/conducted to…　　本研究旨在……

例一： **The purpose of this study was to** characterize early-onset lichenoid GvHD.
本研究的目的在于阐明早发苔藓样移植物抗宿主病的特征。

引自：*J Cutan Pathol*, 2010, 37(5)：549

例二： **The aim of this study was to** develop a clinical rating instrument for short-interval rating of festination and freezing of gait（FOG）.
本研究的目的是为具有复杂分级系统的慌张步态和冻结步态（FOG）制订一个临床分级方法。

引自：*Mov Disord*, 2010, 25(8)：1012

例三： **The goal of this project was to** identify the incidence of and risk factors for the development of behavior change in children after surgery.
本研究的目的确定儿童手术后行为改变的发生率和危险因素。

引自：*Paediatr Anaesth*, 2010, 20(5)：445

例四： **This study was designed to assess** the prevalence of congestion over time and to investigate its impact on outcome in chronic heart failure.

本研究旨在评估一段时间内充血的发生率，并调查其对慢性心力衰竭预后的影响。

引自：Am J Med, 2019, 132(9): e679

例五： **The objective of this study was to** investigate the feasibility of creating tissue engineered heart valves from human mesenchymal stem cells and decellularized porcine heart valve leaflets to obtain viable constructs.

探讨运用组织工程技术以骨髓间充质干细胞和去细胞猪心脏瓣膜支架构建组织工程心脏瓣膜的方法。

引自：《复旦学报(医学版)》, 2007, 34(2): 183

例六： Acute infection increase the risk of arterial cardiovascular events, but effects on venous thromboembolic disease are less well established. **Our aim was to** investigate whether acute infections transiently increase the risk of venous thromboembolism.

急性感染可增加动脉性心血管疾病发病的风险，但其对静脉血栓栓塞性疾病的影响尚不确定。本研究的目的是确定急性感染是否会短暂增加静脉血栓栓塞的风险。

引自：Lancet, 2006, 367(9516): 1075

例七： This review focuses on the potential of nanobiomaterials including biocompatible surface, tissue engineering and regenerative materials, new drug/gene delivery system and bioanalysis system, **with an attempt to** explore their possible applications in clinical practice.

本文主要针对纳米生物医用材料在生物相容性界面、组织再生修复、基因和药物传递及生物诊断上的应用进行评述，并探讨纳米生物医用材料的发展前景。

引自：《中国医学科学院学报》, 2006, 28(4): 472

例八： Peripheral arterial disease (PAD) can have severe consequences on patient mortality and morbidity. In contrast to approaches using growth factor administration or isolated cell transplantation, **we attempted to** develop an alternative method for ischemic therapy using the transplantation of tissue engineered cell sheets with angiogenic potential.

外周血管疾病（PAD）可以增加患者的死亡率。与使用生长因子或分离细胞移植不同，我们尝试应用移植具有血管生成潜能的组织工程人类平滑肌细胞片移植进行局部缺血的治疗。

引自：Arterioscler Thromb Vasc Biol, 2008, 17: 142

例九： **The intent of this study was to** clarify the relationship among metformin exposure, levels of Cbl, Hcy, and MMA, and severity of peripheral neuropathy in diabetic patients.

本研究的目的在于阐明二甲双胍暴露、钴胺素（Cbl）吸收障碍和高同型半胱氨酸（Hcy）及甲基丙二酸（MMA）水平与糖尿病患者周围神经病变的严重性之间的关系。

引自：*Diabetes Care*, 2010, 33(1)：156

二、动词不定式引导的 "Objective"

研究论文的"目的"除了使用完整句表述外，另一种方式是借助动词不定式短语来引导，尤其是在结构式英文摘要的"目的"项中，以这类句式描述"目的"的方式极为常见，且简单明了，其通用格式是"To+verb+所要阐述的内容"。由于不定式引导的"目的"句格式比较固定，所以无需过多叙述。所谓"目的"，指的是"行动和努力最终要达到的地点或境界最终的目的"。一般情况下，结构式摘要中"目的"应直接点题，但是，一些国内外医学杂志，在描述"目的"之前，会加入研究背景描述。如 "Obstructive sleep apnea (OSA) is common and independently associated with atrial fibrillation (AF) in patients with hypertrophic cardiomyopathy (HCM). This study aimed to investigate the relationship between apnea-hypopnea index (AHI), a measure of OSA severity, and prevalence of AF in a large series of patients with HCM." ［阻塞性睡眠呼吸暂停（OSA）是肥厚型心肌病（HCM）患者常见的与心房颤动（AF）独立相关的疾病。本研究通过大样本探讨呼吸暂停低通气指数（AHI，即：OSA 严重度测定）与 HCM 患者房颤发生率之间的关系。*JAHA*，2020，9：e015013］。无论是直接点题还是在背景资料支撑下的点题，研究论文按研究性质及研究背景分类，在语篇、语义关系上，汉、英两种语言既存在一定的对应，又存在非对应现象。此外，严格意义上说，标题词 Objective 应该使用单数形式，但国外部分期刊也有使用 Objectives 的情况（如 *Am J Gastroenterol* 等）。本节就"目的"的英、汉语义对应关系按研究类型加以分类介绍。

（一）研究型

本类型的特点是在中文摘要中常用"研究……的关系、效果、作用、情况、方法、依据、影响、规律或机制"等概念来表达研究论文的属性关系，在英文摘要中通常可用相应的 study、develop、evaluate、obtain、assess、probe、investigate...effect、relationship、method、expression、basis、mechanism 等词与之相对应。例如：

例一： **To study** the different patterns of *Treponema pallidum* distribution in primary and secondary syphilis.

研究梅毒螺旋体在一期及二期梅毒中的不同表现形式。

引自：*Hum Pathol*, 2009, 40(5)：624

例二： **To evaluate** the occurrence of acute renal failure (ARF) and the factors associated with it in cases of neonatal sepsis.

研究急性肾衰竭与新生儿脓毒症的相关因素。

引自：Ind J Pediatr, 2006, 73(6): 499

例三： **To develop** a method for the determination of simvastain in human plasma.

研究健康受试者血浆中辛伐他丁浓度的测定方法。

引自：《中国药科大学学报》, 2001, 32(4): 282

例四： **To obtain** more information **concerning** the thyrotropin receptor (TSHR)gene mutations in the autonomously functioning thyroid adenomas(AFTA).

研究 TSH 受体（TSHR）基因突变在自主性功能性甲状腺瘤（AFTA）发病中的作用。

引自：《中华内分泌代谢杂志》, 2000, 16(3): 153

例五： **To assess** the likelihood ratios of diagnostic strategies for pulmonary embolism and to determine their clinical application according to pretest probability.

评估肺栓塞诊断策略的似然比（likelihood ratios），并通过预测概率（pretest probability）来判定其临床应用价值。

引自：BMJ, 2006, 2: 38

例六： **To probe** the experimental basis for anti-mullerian hormone (AMH) served as a specific tumor label in diagnosis of granulosa cell tumor (GCT) of ovary.

研究抗苗勒管激素在诊断卵巢颗粒细胞瘤中作为特异性肿瘤标志物的实验依据。

引自：《中华妇产科杂志》, 2000, 35(6): 356

例七： **To investigate** the effect and the mechanism of activation of Gs-protein on bilirubin-induced apoptosis of rat cerebellar granule neurons .

研究激活 Gs 蛋白对胆红素诱导的小脑颗粒神经元凋亡的影响及作用机制。

引自：《中华儿科杂志》, 2000, 38: 16

例八： **To assess** angiogenesis and explore the expression and regulation of vascular endothelial growth factor(VEGF), VEGF receptor 1(VEGFR-1), and VEGFR-2, the leading mediators of angiogenesis, in SSc patients and controls.

研究系统性硬化症患者（SSc）和对照者血管生成情况，并探讨血管生成的主要介导物血管内皮生长因子（VEGF）、VEGF 受体 1（VEGFR-1）和 VEGFR-2 的表达和调控。

引自：Arthritis Rheum, 2008, 58(11) : 3550

（二）探讨型

基于研究性质分类特点，医学研究中大量研究属于探讨型研究，这本身体现出了医务工作者和研究人员的严谨科研态度。因此，探讨型"目的"在英文摘要中使用频率颇高。英文中能够表达"探讨"这一语义关系的动词很多，常用的有 investigate、study、 explore、probe into、determine、discuss、evaluate 等词，在某些场合也可以用 analyze、assess、inquire into、measure、review、clarify、ascertain 来表达，关键是要依据概念搭配来选择合适的动词，句法结构多为"动词不定式+宾语+宾语补足语（对宾语进行限定和修饰）"。

例一：**To investigate** the combined association of diet and physical activity with AD risk.

探讨饮食与运动相结合对阿尔茨海默病（AD）患病风险的影响。

引自：*JAMA*,2009, 302(6): 627

例二：**To determine** whether relative abundance of epidermal growth factor receptor (EGFR) mutations in plasma predicts clinical response to epidermal growth factor receptor-tyrosine kinase inhibitors (EGFR-TKI) in patients with advanced lung adenocarcinoma.

探讨晚期肺腺癌患者血浆循环肿瘤 DNA 表皮生长因子受体（EGFR）相对突变丰度与表皮生长因子受体酪氨酸激酶抑制剂（EGFR-TKI）疗效的相关性。

引自：《中华内科学杂志》, 2019, 58(1): 49

例三：**To explore** the influence of anti-tumor necrosis factor (anti-TNF) therapy upon the incidence of cancer in patients with rheumatoid arthritis (RA) and prior malignancy.

探讨抗肿瘤坏死因子（TNF）治疗对之前曾患恶性肿瘤的类风湿关节炎（RA）患者的肿瘤发病率的影响。

引自：*Arthritis Care Res*, 2010, 62(6) : 755

例四：**To study** the therapeutic mechanism of Octreotide in acute necrotizing pancreatitis.

探讨奥曲肽治疗急性坏死性胰腺炎的作用机制。

引自：《中华消化杂志》, 2000, 20(1): 17

例五：**To assess** the clinical significance of radionuclide techniques in differentiating dilated cardiomyopathy (DCM) from ischemic cardiomyopathy (CAD-CM).

探讨核素显像在扩张型心肌病（DCM）和缺血性心肌病（CAD-CM）诊断及鉴别诊断中的作用。

引自：《中华核医学杂志》, 2000, 20(3): 105

例六：**To investigate** the possible role of miR-449a/b in the occurrence of gastric cancer.

探讨 miR-449a/b 在胃癌发生中的可能作用机制。

引自：《南方医科大学学报》, 2020, 40(1): 13

（三）评价型

这类研究目的常用于对某种药物的疗效、某种治疗或实验方法予以评价，以期进一步推广应用。常用的英语表达可用 evaluate、assess、estimate 等动词，其句法结构：动词不定式+被评价对象（如"作用、效果、性能和价值"），与之连用的名词有"the effects of、the value of、the curative effects of"等。

例一： **To evaluate** the safety and efficacy of a novel removable self-expanding metal stent in the management of refractory variceal bleeding.

评估一种新型可移动自膨式金属支架治疗难治性食管静脉曲张出血的安全性和有效性。

引自：*Gastrointest Endosc*, 2010, 71(1)：71

例二： **To assess** the immunization coverage of BCG, DPT, OPV, Measles, MMR and Hepatitis B vaccines in two urbanized villages of East Delhi and study the factors affecting the coverage.

评价德黑兰东部两个城市化村庄 BCG、DPT、OPV、麻疹、MMR 及乙肝疫苗免疫覆盖率和影响覆盖率因素。

引自：*Am J Med*, 2007, 16：21

例三： **To evaluate** the efficacies of lopinavir/ritonavir and arbidol in the treatment of Novel Coronavirus Pneumonia (NCP).

评价洛匹那韦/利托那韦和阿比多尔对治疗新型冠状病毒肺炎的有效性。

（注：新型冠状病毒肺炎英文名称现修订为"COVID-19"）

引自：《中华传染病杂志》, 2020, 38(2)：86

例四： **To estimate** the incidence of nonmelanoma skin cancer (NMSC) in the US population in 2006 and secondarily to indicate trends in numbers of procedures for skin cancer treatment.

评估美国 2006 年非黑色素瘤皮肤癌（NMSC）的发病率，并描述皮肤癌治疗数的趋势。

引自：*Arch Dermatol*, 2010, 146(3)：283

（四）阐明型

在医学论文中，所谓阐明，就是研究者试图把某个问题或事情讲明白，基于其本人的研究发现，对认知模糊的某种机制或某些概念予以澄清或解释说明。表达这类研究论文的"目的"可用 reveal、clarify、elucidate 等。

例一： **To test** the effect of corneal epithelial scrape on myofibroblasts associated with haze and **elucidate** the effect of interleukin-1 and transforming growth factor beta1 on corneal stromal myofibroblasts viability and death *in vitro*.

观察角膜上皮擦伤对肌成纤维细胞及混浊的影响，并且阐明白细胞介素 1 和转化生长因子 β_1 对体内角膜间质成肌纤维细胞活力和死亡的影响。

引自：*Exp Eye Res*, 2009, 89(2)：152

例二： **To clarify** the role of the age-associated dysfunction of…

（为了）阐明与年龄相关的功能紊乱机制……

引自：*Am J Med*, 2007, 74: 25

例三： **To clarify** whether the gas exchange response to prone position is associated with lung recruitability in mechanically ventilated patients with acute respiratory failure.

（为了）明确仰卧位气体交换能力与行机械通气的急性呼吸衰竭患者肺的复张性之间是否存在联系。

引自：*Intensive Care Med*, 2009, 35(6)：1011

例四： **To reveal** the basis of molecular of the phase change of *influenza A (A1N1)* viruses.

阐明甲 1（H1N1）亚型流感病毒相变异的分子生物学基础。

引自：《中华实验和临床病毒学杂志》, 2000, 14(2): 9

例五： **To elucidate** the complexity of common human diseases such as obesity.

为了阐明诸如肥胖等普通人类疾病的发病机制。

引自：*Nature*, 2008, 452(7186)：423

例六： **To further elucidate** the impact of Gynemesh PS polypropylene mesh and MatriStem ECM bioscaffolds on the vaginal smooth muscle in terms of micro-morphology of vaginal smooth muscle.

为了进一步阐明 Gynemesh PS 聚丙烯网片和 MatriStem 细胞基质外生物支架对阴道平滑肌微观形态的影响。

引自：*Am J Obstet Gynecol*, 2019, 221(4):330.e1-330.e9.

（五）比较型

此型常用于对两种或两种以上的药物或实验方法、治疗方法的效果进行对比，以说明各自的优缺点和应用范围。因此，在"目的"句中要说明对比的对象及对比的内容，对比的双方是并列对等的。由于比较的内容在很多情况下可以直接通过语境提示，除了使用 compare 之外，可以用 and 连接两个被比较的对象，也可根据研究性质，使用其他词汇进行表述。需要提醒的是，无论是结构式摘要，还是非结构式摘要，整个语篇都应该具有紧密的逻辑关联。"目的"为了比较什么，"方法"就应该将被比较的对象罗列出来。在这个问题上，我们在审稿过程中经常发现，某些作者对"方法"描述过于笼统，或重要信息丢失，导致"结果"描述给人以极其突兀的感觉。

例一： **To compare** the effect of short-term metformin and fenofibrate treatment, administered alone or in sequence, on glucose and lipid metabolism, cardiovascular risk factors, and monocyte cytokine release in type 2 diabetic patients with mixed dyslipidemia.

比较短期内单独或依次使用二甲双胍和非诺贝特对伴有混合性血脂异常的 2 型糖尿病患者的糖、脂代谢，心血管危险因素，单核细胞释放细胞因子的影响。

引自：Diabetes Care, 2009, 32(8)：1421

例二： **To compare** the clinical efficacy and adverse reaction between Everolimus and Axitinib as the second-line treatment of metastatic renal cell carcinoma （mRCC）.

比较依维莫司与阿昔替尼二线治疗转移性肾细胞癌（mRCC）的临床疗效及不良反应。

引自：《复旦学报(医学版)》, 2020, 47(1)：37-41

例三： **To determine** which protocols work better between cetrorelix and long protocols in older patients in a randomized controlled study.

采用随机对照实验，比较西曲瑞克方案和长方案在老年患者中的治疗效果。

引自：Fertil Steril, 2009, 91(5)：1842

例四： **To study** the effect of supplemental fish oil *vs.* placebo on ventricular tachyarrhythmia or death.

比较研究补充鱼油与安慰剂对室性快速性心律失常发生或死亡的影响。

引自：JAMA 2006, 295：2613

（六）回顾型

医学论文中回顾性研究通常是研究者对其经验进行总结以供他人借鉴。表达此类概念时常用英语动词有 review、summarize、study、investigate 等，但措辞时要注意这几个词在语义上的差异。Review 和 summarize 本身蕴含 "…to consider retrospectively" 之意，因此，使用这两个词中的任何一个来表达此类概念时，无需与 retrospectively 连用，否则就会导致语义重复；而 study 和 investigate 只有其外延意义，因此，在 "目的" 表达中若使用这两个词，应与副词 retrospectively 连用。例如：

例一： **To review** authors institutional experience of congenital cystic lung disease, …

回顾（作者所在医院）治疗先天性囊性肺疾病的临床经验。

引自：Indian J Pediatr, 2007, 74(2)：192

例二： **To review** the current knowledge of persistent visual loss after nonocular surgeries under general anesthesia.

回顾性（分析）当前关于全身麻醉下行非眼科手术后持续性视力丧失的经验。

引自：Am J Ophthalmol, 2008, 145(4)：604

例三： **To retrospectively review** the experience and early clinical results of coronary artery bypass grafting (CABG) for the treatment of coronary artery disease (CAD).

回顾应用冠状动脉旁路移植术治疗冠心病的早期疗效和经验。

【析】本句中副词 retrospectively 与 review 语义重复，retrospectively 应该略去。

引自：《中华心血管病杂志》，2000, 28(1): 36

（七）建立型

建立型用于表达"建立……系统，实验方法，技术"，常用动词为 establish、develop、create、construct 等，常用格式为动词不定式+所建立的系统、实验方法、技术等（如 method，system，technique）。例如：

例一： **To establish** a scoring system predicting the ascites postoperatively by analyzing the variant factors associated with massive ascites after hepatectomy in the patients with hepatocellular carcinoma (HCC).

通过对肝细胞癌患者术后大量腹水形成相关因素的分析，建立一套预测术后大量腹水形成的评分体系。

引自：《中华外科杂志》，2010, 48(20): 1534

例二： **To develop** a genetic test to evaluate the propensity of a chronic ulcer to heal.

创建基因测试方法，以评估慢性溃疡愈合趋势。

引自：*Br J Surg*, 2019, 3(4):549

例三： **To create** a simple, practical, stable, and easy to popularize rCBF quantitative measurement **method.**

建立一种简便、实用、可靠、易于普及的定量测定 rCBF 方法。

引自：《中华核医学杂志》，2000, 20(1): 8

例四： **To establish a noninvasive technique** to determine monocyte trafficking to atherosclerotic lesions in live animals.

建立一种无创技术，观察单核细胞在活体动物动脉粥样硬化病变处的变化情况。

引自：*Circulation*, 2008, 117(3): 388

例五： **To develop** a simple risk stratification score for primary therapy with an implantable cardioverter-defibrillator (ICD).

建立 ICD 一级预防的危险分层系统。

引自：*JACC*, 2008, 51(3): 288

（八）提高型

提高型用于表达"提高……（某种诊疗或检验技术的）水平或是（某种药物的）治疗效果"，常用 increase、improve 等词。例如，在表达提高某种疾病的检出率时，常用"To increase the detection rate of…"。

例一：**To improve** outcomes for patients with high-risk head and neck squamous cell cancer (HNSCC) after surgical resection by testing the feasibility and safety of early postoperative chemotherapy followed by concurrent chemoradiotherapy.

通过评估术后早期化疗和同步放化疗的可行性和安全性，改善高危头颈部鳞状细胞癌（HNSCC）患者手术切除后的预后。

引自：*J Clin Oncol*, 2009, 27(28): 4727

例二：**To increase the detection rate of** primary hepatic carcinoma (PHC) and to diagnose PHC earlier.

探讨提高原发性肝癌（PHC）的检出率，早期诊断原发性肝癌的方法。

引自：《中华外科杂志》, 2000, 38(1): 128

例三：**To improve** our understanding of intratesticular hormone concentrations.

为增进对睾丸内激素浓度的了解。

引自：*J Androl*, 2010, 31(2): 138

例四：The new Systemic Lupus International Collaborating Clinics (SLICC) 2012 classification criteria aimed **to improve** the performance of systemic lupus erythematosus (SLE) classification over the American College of Rheumatology (ACR) 1997 criteria.

新的系统性红斑狼疮国际合作诊所（SLICC）2012 分类标准旨在提高系统性红斑狼疮（SLE）分类效果，以超越美国风湿病学会（ACR）1997 标准。

引自：*Arthritis Care Res (Hoboken)*, 2015, 67(8): 1180

（九）寻找/求型

寻找/求型用来表述寻找解决某种问题的证据、方法、药物、材料、物质等，常用的动词或动词词组有 search for、discover、ascertain、find、find out、explore 等，与其搭配的名词常有 evidence、material、method 等词。例如：

例一：**To search for** and validate potential molecular pathogenic machanisms in the trabecular meshwork(TM) responsible for the elevated intraocular pressure(IOP) associated with glaucoma.

寻找并验证小梁网（色素沉着）导致青光眼相关眼内压升高的潜在分子致病机制。

引自：*Investigative Opthalmology & Visual Science*,2008,49(5):1916

例二：**To discover** new candidate vaccine antigen **for** *schistosomiasis*.

为了寻找预防日本血吸虫病的候选疫苗分子。

引自：《中国人兽共患病杂志》, 2001, 17(1): 45

例三：**To explore** the association between cardiac injury and mortality in patients with COVID-19.

探索 COVID-19 患者心脏损伤与死亡率的关系。

引自: JAMA Cardiol, 2020, :e200950

例四： **To find the best** sample-collecting and template-making **methods** in malaria diagnosis with PCR.

在聚合酶链反应（PCR）检测疟疾中寻找最佳的标本采集和模板制备方法。

引自:《中华检验医学杂志》, 2001, 24(1): 21.

例五： **To find out the differences of** Creutzfeldt-Jakob disease (CJD) between patents in China and other countries.

探索中国人种克-雅病与其他国家的差异。

引自:《中华内科杂志》, 2000, 39(2): 94

例六： **To ascertain** the acquisition of cytomegalovirus infection following exchange transfusion and factors affecting such transmission in newborn infants at a tertiary care hospital in India.

为了查明在印度第三级医疗机构中新生儿输血后巨细胞病毒感染以及影响感染的因素。

引自: Indian Paediat J, 2006, 73(6): 519

（十）观察型

观察型一般用来表达对某种药物治疗后或术后的疗效，或者是对某种病理、生理现象的观察。常用的句法结构为 To observe/assess+effect/result/change of…。例如：

例一： **To observe the effectiveness of** arsenic trioxide (As_2O_3)in the **treatment of** acute promyelocytic leukemia (APL).

观察三氧化二砷对急性早幼粒细胞白血病的疗效和特点。

引自:《中华血液学杂志》, 2000, 21(1): 67。

例二： **To assess the efficacy and safety of** high-dose IVIG as a treatment option in patients with therapy-resistant chronic spontaneous urticarial (CSU).

观察大剂量免疫球蛋白静脉注射对难治性慢性自发性荨麻疹的疗效和安全性。

引自: Ann Allergy Asthma Immunol, 2010, 104(3): 253

例三： **To observe the results of the treatment for** neurogenic fecal incontinence.

观察神经源性大便失禁治疗后的排便功能。

引自:《中华小儿外科杂志》, 2000, 21(1): 32

例四： **To observe the** phenotypic **changes of** renal tubulo-interstitial cells in human glomerulonephritis.

观察人类肾小球肾炎时肾小管间质细胞发生的表型转化现象。

引自:《中华肾脏病杂志》, 2000, 16(1): 7

例五：**To assess the relationship of** tea consumption with common carotid artery intima-media thickness (CCA-IMT) and carotid plaques.

观察饮茶与颈总动脉中膜厚度（CCA-IMT）和颈动脉斑块的相关性。

引自：*Arterioscler Thromb Vasc Biol*, 2008, 28(2): 353

（十一）报告型

报告型用来表述对某项研究、实验、观察结果或进展进行的报告，常以 To report the result/evolution of...的形式出现。

例一：**To report the result of** ultrastructure observation of the cysticercus cysts in human brain with SEM.

报告用扫描电镜观察脑内寄生的猪囊胞超微结构的结果。

引自：《中国人兽共患病杂志》, 2001, 17(1): 67

例二：**To report** endothelial cell densities (ECDs) and their correlation to anterior chamber depth (ACD) after implantation of the Artisan intraocular phakic lens.

报告植入 Artisan 人工晶状体后内皮细胞密度（ECDs），及其与前房深度（ACD）的相关性。

引自：*Ophthalmology*, 2008, 115(4): 608

例三：**To report** an outbreak with linezolid and methicillin-resistant *S. aureus* (LRSA) in an intensive care department and the effective control measures taken.

报告一起重症监护病房内利奈唑胺和甲氧西林耐药金黄色葡萄球菌（LRSA）的暴发事件和采取的有效控制方法。

引自：*JAMA*, 2010, 303(22): 2260

（十二）分析型

分析型是对某种疾病的致病性、临床特征、流行特征、治疗效果等进行分析，英语表述常用 determine、analyze、evaluate 等动词，也可以其他动词不定式引导，加以 by analysis。例如：

例一：**To determine** if the expression of human copper–zinc superoxide dismutase (CuZnSOD) within the lungs of mice protects against the development of emphysema.

分析人铜锌过氧化物歧化酶在小鼠肺内表达是否能防止肺气肿。

引自：*J Respir Crit Care Med*, 2005, 172(5): 530

例二：**To analyze** the clinical and microbiological profile of patients with blood culture-negative (BCN) early prosthetic valve endocarditis (PVE) in order to define the most appropriate empiric treatment.

分析早期人工瓣膜心内膜炎（PVE）血培养阴性（BCN）患者的临床和微生物学特征，以确定最适当的治疗方案。

引自：Heart, 2010, 96(10)：743

例三：**To determine** the prevalence of adrenal insufficiency, risk factors and potential mechanisms for its development, and its association with clinically important outcomes in critically ill children.

分析肾上腺功能减退的发生率、危险因素和潜在的发病机制，及其对重症儿童患者预后的影响。

引自：Am J Respir Crit Care Med, 2010, 182(2)：246

例四：**To analyze the clinical and the pathological characteristics of** pancreatic carcinoma in diabetics (DPC) **and to explore the relationship between** diabetes mellitus and pancreatic carcinoma (PC).

分析胰腺癌合并糖尿病的临床和病理学特征，并探讨糖尿病与胰腺癌之间的关系。

引自：《中华内分泌代谢杂志》, 2000, 16(2)：91

例五：**To determine the combined influence** of leisure-time physical activity and weekly alcohol intake on the risk of subsequent fatal ischaemic heart disease (IHD) and all-cause mortality.

分析业余体育运动与每周饮酒量对致死性缺血性心脏病（IHD）和全因死亡率的复合影响。

引自：Eur Heart J, 2008, 29(1)：19

（十三）总结型

在临床研究中，有些论文的目的是对以往的资料或经验进行总结后提出观点，这类"目的"表达多用 summarize 等引导，且常与"the experience in"连用。

例一：**To summarize** the clinical characteristics of acute pandysautonomia in childhood, to gain better understanding of the diagnosis and differential diagnosis.

总结儿童急性全自主神经功能不全的临床特征、诊断及鉴别诊断。

引自：《中华儿科杂志》, 2010, 48(6)：454

例二：**To summarize** the available evidence on timing of perioperative antibiotics for cesarean delivery.

总结关于剖宫产手术期间抗生素应用时间选择的现有证据。

引自：Am J Obstet Gynecol, 2008, 199(3)：301e1

例三：**To summarize** and assess current evidence from randomized controlled trials

(RCTs) on anterior cruciate ligament injuries, with special reference to graft type and surgical technique.

根据随机临床试验（RCTs）证据，同时参照移植类型和手术方式，总结和评估前交叉韧带损伤的治疗效果。

引自：Arthroscopy, 2009, 25(10)：1139

例四：**This article summarizes** the results of studies investigating prevalence, impact on outcomes, and cessation interventions for smoking in the transplant population.

本文总结了移植人群吸烟流行率、对结果的影响和戒烟干预的结果。

引自：Am J Med, 2019, 132(4): 413

（十四）了解型

汉语的"了解"从其词义的内涵来看，该词所表述的语义较为狭窄，故不能用对等的英文词来表示这一语义关系。医学论文中的"了解"，是通过一定的深入研究来揭示某种现象，因此，其对应的常用英文用词较为宽泛，如 study、investigate、determine、clarify 等。

例一：**To characterize** differences in postoperative opioid prescribing across surgical, nonsurgical, and advanced practice providers.

了解手术、非手术和高年资医生之间术后使用阿片类药物的差异。

引自：Annals of Surgery, 2020, 271(4): 680

例二：**To investigate** the occurrence and drug resistance of extended-spectrum beta-lactamases (ESBLs)-producing strains of *Shigella* in pediatric patients, as as to provide information for clinical treatment.

了解儿科临床分离志贺菌产超广谱 β 内酰胺酶（ESBLs）的状况及耐药情况，为临床治疗提供参考。

引自：《中华儿科杂志》, 2010, 48(8): 617

例三：**To further clarify** the role of cell proliferation and apoptosis in the pathogenesis of renal tubulointerstitial fibrosis.

了解细胞增殖与凋亡在肾小管间质纤维化中的意义。

引自：《中华肾脏病杂志》, 2000, 16(1): 24

例四：**To gain more insight in** the role of the small intestine in development of obesity and insulin resistance, dietary fat-induced differential gene expression was determined along the longitudinal axis of small intestines of C57BL/6J mice.

为更多地了解小肠在肥胖和胰岛素抵抗中的作用，（我们）在 C57BL/6J 小鼠小肠纵轴检测了饮食性脂肪诱导的差异基因表达。

引自：BMC Med Genomics, 2008, 1(12): 14

（十五）调查型

汉语中的"调查"所指的语义为"为了了解情况进行考察（多指到现场）"，因此，英语常用 investigate 表示。常用句式为"To investigate+relationship、element、curative effect"等。用于表述某疾病的流行病学调查，或某疾病在某一范围内的影响因素，某菌的耐药率等。事实上，英语中对于"调查"这一概念表达，用词更为宽泛。注意比较以下例证。

例一： The aim of the present study was **to examine** the influence of childhood respiratory infections on adult respiratory health.

本研究的目的是调查幼年呼吸道感染对成年呼吸系统健康状况的影响。

引自：*Eur Respir J*, 2009, 33(2): 237

例二： **To investigate the treatment outcome in** newly diagnosed acute leukemia patients .

调查初发性急性白血病的疗效及影响因素。

引自：《中华血液学杂志》, 2000, 21(1): 17

例三： **To investigate** the group B *Streptococcus* (GBS) colonization rate **and the relationship between** vaginal colonization of GBS **and** the maternal and neonatal outcome.

调查孕妇 B 族溶血性链球菌（GBS）带菌与产科不良妊娠结局的关系。

引自：《中华妇产科杂志》, 2000, 35(1): 32

例四： The aim of this study was **to evaluate** the association between meniscal damage in knees without surgery and the development of radiographic tibiofemoral OA.

目的旨在调查膝关节半月板损伤的非手术治疗和 X 线在骨性关节炎诊断方面的进展。

引自：*Arthritis Rheum*, 2009, 60(3) : 831

（十六）其他类型(混合表达)

在某些研究中，为了将相关因素加以考虑，研究者通常在"目的"表达中采用部分并列结构，如引导词的并列，研究内容的并列等。需要注意的是，在混合表达中一定要注意动词与名词概念搭配的一致性。例如：

例一： **To explore** the predictors of prostate biopsy outcomes, and **to develop** the prediction nomogram.

探讨前列腺穿刺结果的相关预测因素，构建前列腺穿刺结果的预测列线图模型。

引自：《复旦学报(医学版)》, 2020, 47(1): 12

例二： **To study and compare** the long-term results of VVI and AAI pacing in sick sinus syndrome.

了解并比较 VVI、AAI 起搏治疗病窦综合征（病窦）的远期疗效。

引自:《中华心血管杂志》, 2000, 28(1): 45

例三： **To assess** the safety of interleukin-6 receptor inhibition and **to collect** preliminary data on the clinical and immunologic efficacy of tocilizumab in patients with systemic lupus erythematosus (SLE).

为了评估白细胞介素-6 受体抑制剂托珠单抗（tocilizumab）的安全性，并收集有关托珠单抗治疗系统性红斑狼疮（SLE）患者的临床及免疫疗效的初步资料。

引自: *Arthritis Rheum*, 2010, 62(2) : 542

例四： **To reevaluate** the current criteria for diagnosing allergic fungal sinusitis (AFS) and **determine** the incidence of AFS in patients with chronic rhinosinusitis (CRS).

重新评估过敏性真菌性鼻窦炎（AFS）当前诊断标准，并确定慢性鼻窦炎（CRS）患者过敏性真菌性鼻窦炎的发病率。

引自: *Mayo Clin Proc*, 1999, 74(9): 877

例五： **To compare** sexual problems among HIV-positive and HIV-negative women and **describe** clinical and psychosocial factors associated with these problems.

比较 HIV 阳性和 HIV 阴性妇女间的性生活问题，并描述了与这些问题有关的临床和心理因素。

引自: *J Acquir Immune Defic Syndr*, 2010, 54(4): 360

从上述实例可以发现英文中的搭配问题。在英文中，动词和名称搭配使用时，最易出现问题的是概念搭配错误。如果动词后出现的是两个不同概念，就要选择不同的动词与名词搭配。上述例三至例五，由于搭配的概念不同，所以选择了不同的动词。

三、"Objective" 句中动词形式的选择

结构式摘要在语篇结构格式和措辞等方面有别于报道性摘要和指示性摘要等，动词形式的使用也有所不同。但是，结构式摘要中，"目的"句的动词形式相对固定，即采用简略式 "To+do" 的表达形式（本章所列例句均为此类形式，故例证从简）。而在报道性摘要或指示性摘要中，由于语体上的差异，通常采用完整句陈述目的，这就涉及动词形式的变化问题。"目的"句中涉及的动词形式有两种。

（1）在介绍本文的中心意图，说明本文（研究）亟待解决的问题时，动词常用一般式，即一般现在式。

例一： The purpose of this report/paper **is** to describe the clinical presentation of 40 such patients with rupture of the spleen.

本文旨在介绍 40 例类似的脾破裂患者的临床表现。

例二：This paper **is** aimed to investigate this hypothesis on 38 patients.

本文目的旨在通过对 38 例患者进行研究，探讨这一假说（的真实性）。

（2）交代研究的目的，用-ed 动词形式，即一般过去式。英语中的时间通常融于抽象和具体之中，它不像汉语中描述的那么具体，如"昨天、今天、明天"。在很多情况下，英语动词所涉及的时间概念必须要有参照点，如"患者手术结果如何？"这句话的英文应表示成"How was the operation with the patient?"而不是"How is the operation with the patient?"，其原因为，谈论这一"结果"时，"结果"已经成了过去的状态。同样的道理，交代研究的目的，亦即表示研究过程中所做的一切已经成为过去。

例一：The purpose of this study **was to** investigate the complications of renal transplant.

本文旨在研究肾移植患者的并发症。

例二：This experiment **was done to** explore the effect of imipramine hydrochloride on blood pressure.

本实验旨在探寻盐酸丙咪嗪对血压的影响。

以上介绍了医学论文英文摘要中有关**"目的"句（Objective or Aim）**表达方式和方法。表示研究目的时，结构式摘要中英文通常采用简洁表达式："To+动词原形"，然而，国内外医学期刊还是存在一定的差异，某些期刊在结构式摘要中同样使用完整句表达"目的"，因此，作者需要注意拟投期刊的格式要求。此外，在书写"目的"句时一定要注意引导词的使用及其固定搭配，以及内容的简明性、完整性、科学性、检索性和准确性。

四、练 习

4-1　按照语境，选择适当的英语动词，将下列"目的"句译成英文

1. 探讨铅中毒对大鼠全血、粪便和尿液中微量元素铅和硒的影响。

2. 了解食管癌与贲门癌患者术后残余食管和胸腔胃的病理生理变化，为提高患者术后生活质量提供客观依据。

3. 评估肺栓塞诊断策略的似然比（likelihood ratios），并通过预测概率（pretest probability）来决定其临床应用价值。

4. 分析中国独生子女政策对人口生育率、理想子女数和出生性别比的影响。

5. 监测初级保健机构中新发直肠出血患者的结直肠癌和腺体瘤的患病风险。

6. 确定动脉粥样硬化危险因素的发生及治疗在世界许多国家是否具有可比性。

7. 研究低剂量阿司匹林治疗后男性和女性血小板反应性的差异。

8. 比较西罗莫司洗脱支架（sirolimus-eluting）和紫杉醇洗脱支架（paclitaxel-eluting）的安全性和疗效。

9. 评估 PAC（pulmonary artery catheter）对重症患者的影响。

10. 对妊娠期慢性病发病风险的证据进行总结。

11. 冠状动脉钙化（CAC）是亚临床动脉粥样硬化的标志。本研究的目的是确定 CAC 与受教育程度之间的关系，并检查心血管危险因素及其作为潜在介导因素发生的变化。

12. 测定 NP-CRNs 在一家退伍军人医院（veterans hospital）人群中的发病率，并明确其与结直肠癌的联系。

13. 系统回顾当前可利用的有关饮酒与年龄相关性黄斑变性（age-related macular degeneration）风险的资料。

14. 观察大鼠脑缺血再灌注损伤时海马神经元 NF-κB 及 ICAM-1 随再灌注时间表达的变化，探讨姜黄素脑保护的分子机制。

15. 探讨 survivin 基因在鼠急性胰腺炎中的表达及其意义。

16. 探讨胎肝基质细胞和骨髓基质细胞在诱导胚胎干细胞向血液血管干细胞分化中的作用，分析基因表达差异。

17. 探讨羟甲基戊二酸单酰辅酶 A（HMG-CoA）还原酶的抑制剂辛伐他汀（SV）联合全反式维 A 酸（ATRA）对人早幼粒细胞白血病 NB4 细胞株增殖、分化与凋亡的影响，以及肾母细胞瘤（WT1）基因/转录因子人细胞周期调节蛋白依赖性 myb 样蛋白 1（hDMPl）基因表达变化。

18. 比较多西紫杉醇与紫杉醇联合吡柔比星（THP）和环磷酰胺（CTX）的新辅助化疗方案治疗局部进展期乳腺癌的临床疗效和毒性。

19. 分析中国年轻乳腺癌的临床病理特征，并探讨年轻乳腺癌患者的预后。

20. 通过多中心调查，前瞻性研究早产儿视网膜病（ROP）发病相关危险因素。

第五章　医学论文英文摘要"Methods"写作

医学论文英文摘要"Methods"旨在提供论文的科学依据，概括研究所用原理、条件、材料、对象和方法，并说明有无对照。有助于读者了解作者的设计思想，从方法学角度评价设计的合理性和优越性。

尽管"摘要"写作对字数有一定的限制，但描述"Methods"时，仍然需要采用最具有高度概括性的语言，对正文中所使用的关键方法予以提炼。这些要素包括研究方案、如何分组、实验对象（人或实验动物，包括对照）、研究对象人口特征（年龄、性别和其他重要信息）、处置方法、数据收集及其处理方法等。

随机临床试验报告应介绍该研究的所有主要方面，包括方案（研究的人群、干预或暴露因素、结果和统计因素分析的基本原理）、干预的安排（随机方法、治疗组分布隐匿）和隐匿的方法（盲法）。

综上所述，医学论文英文摘要"Methods"的写作内容包括两大层次——研究方案和研究过程，具体包括：①研究对象，应说明研究对象是患者、健康人，还是动物（何种动物）。介绍研究对象的一般情况，如年龄、性别、诊断，是否为特别群体、特别种属及研究地点等。研究组和对照组均应说明。②研究方法：包括研究设计类型，即说明是哪一类研究，如随机分组、双盲、对照、多中心等；所用主要治疗、干预、处理方法或技术名称，如描述治疗方法时应介绍主要疗法或药名、剂量、给药途径及疗程，主要检测项目（一般不主张用缩略语）；主要终点指标或转归指标（primary or main endpoint or outcome measure），如死亡率、病死率、生存率、生存时间等。例如："**Methods** In this phase 3, double-blind trial, we randomly assigned 715 patients with hepatitis B e antigen (HBeAg)-positive chronic hepatitis B who had not previously received a nucleoside analogue to receive either 0.5 mg of entecavir or 100 mg of lamivudine once daily for a minimum of 52 weeks. The primary efficacy end point was histologic improvement (a decrease by at least two points in the Knodell necroinflammatory score, without worsening of fibrosis) at week 48. Secondary end points included a reduction in the serum HBV DNA level, HBeAg loss and seroconversion, and normalization of the alanine aminotransferase level."（*N Engl J Med*, 2006, 354：1001）。"这篇摘要"Methods"部分的字数并不多，不足 100 个词，但提供的信息很全面。首先说明了研究的设计类型，是Ⅲ期、双盲、随机临床试验。研究对象是乙型肝炎 e 抗原阳性的慢性乙型肝炎患者，他们以往未接受过核苷类似物药物治疗。作者对治疗所用的药物、

剂量和疗程都做了明确的说明。描述主要终点指标是至 48 周时组织学有改善，并且在括号内更具体地说明是指在纤维化不恶化的情况下，Knodell 坏死炎症分数至少减少 2 分，同时也说明了次要终点指标的内容。这样，读者便可清晰地了解，这项研究所采用的主要观察指标是"硬指标"，是能客观而准确地反映疗效或病情变化的指标。实验对象若为动物，英文摘要中的 Methods 既不能完全照搬正文中的方法，也不可过于简单或笼统。大体上应包含品种或品系、遗传学背景、微生物学质量控制、体重与等级、动物龄与性别、所有动物数量、处置方式。尽管英文摘要中的 Methods 和正文中的 Methods 在文字描述上有繁简之分，但摘要中的 Methods 仍然需要借助高度概括性描述，体现正文所使用的 Methods。

一、"Methods" 写作中应包含的内容

研究对象如果是患者，在"方法"句中应首先介绍研究对象数量、选择标准、剔除标准及分组情况，还应介绍清楚患者的年龄、性别、某种疾病的临床分期、分型等对研究结果有一定影响的临床特征。研究对象如果是动物，需说明动物的种系、性别、健康状况及分组情况。如有必要，影响到因变量的动物年龄、体重等影响因素，也应概括列出。大体上，Methods 中各要素描述可归纳如下。

1. 纳入标准

例一： Patients>40 years of age with documented peripheral arterial obstructive disease, intermittent claudication, and an ankle-brachial index between 0.30 and 0.80 were eligible for inclusion and were randomized to receive orally either buflomedil or placebo for 2 to 4 years.

纳入标准为年龄>40 岁的具有明确记录的外周动脉阻塞性疾病、间歇性跛行、踝臂指数在 0.30～0.80 的患者，随机化分配接受口服丁咯地尔或安慰剂应用 2～4 年。

引自：*Circulation*, 2008, 117(6): 816

例二： Inclusion criteria were (1) a previous ablation procedure of pulmonary vein (PV) encircling performed for drug-refractory persistent atrial fibrillation; (2) a "complete" intraprocedural end point, which consisted of voltage abatement inside the lesions, PV disconnection, and exit-block pacing from inside the lesions, attained in all PVs; and (3) stable sinus rhythm documented during a minimum follow-up of 2.5 years after the procedure. Twenty volunteers were selected (12 males, mean age 59±7 years) and underwent a repeat electrophysiological study.

纳入标准：①持续性 AF 药物控制失败，且曾接受过环肺静脉消融术(PV)者；②完整的术中靶点为损伤位点内电压受抑、肺静脉电隔离、所有肺静脉内损伤处传出阻滞；③术后至少有 2.5 年随访期内记录到稳定的窦

性心律。共有 20 例患者入选〔12 例男性，平均（59±7）岁〕，全部接受电生理检查。

引自：Circulation, 2008, 117(2): 136

例三： Children with standard-risk hepatoblastoma who were younger than 16 years of age were eligible for inclusion in the study.

符合本研究纳入的对象为年龄＜16 岁的标危型肝母细胞瘤患儿。

引自：N Engl J Med, 2009, 361(17): 1662

例四： Patients aged 35-85 years were eligible for enrolment if they had blood pressure more than 140/90 mm Hg despite antihypertensive treatment and were willing to self-manage their hypertension.

入选患者均符合以下条件：年龄 35～85 岁，血压均高于 140/90 mmHg（无论是否行抗高血压药治疗），且有自我管理高血压的意愿。

引自：Lancet, 2010, 376(9736): 163

2. 排除标准及观察指标

例一： Exclusion criteria included known abdominal abscess and non-steroidal anti-inflammatory drug (NSAID) use.

排除标准包括腹部脓肿及使用非甾体抗炎药者。

引自：Gastrointest Endosc, 2008, 68(2): 255

例二： Exclusion criteria included comorbid history of epilepsy, <2 PNES/month, and IQ <70. The primary outcome was seizure frequency at end of treatment and at 6-month follow-up. Secondary outcomes included 3 months of seizure freedom at 6-month follow-up.

排除标准：癫痫史，每月小于 2 次精神性非癫痫发作（PNES），智商（IQ）<70。主要观测指标为治疗结束时和 6 个月随访期的发作频率。次级指标包括 6 个月随访期中 3 个月内无癫痫发作。

引自：Neurology ,2010, 74(24): 1986

例三： Patients with a history of AF before and during hospitalization were excluded.

排除住院之前及住院期间发生心房颤动的患者。

引自：Am J Cardiol, 2010, 105(12): 1655

例四： Patients with tumors of low malignant potential and mucinous carcinomas metastatic to the ovary from other primary sites were excluded.

低度恶性潜能肿瘤患者及原发于其他部位而后转移至卵巢的患者予以排除。

引自：Obstet Gynecol, 2010, 116(2 Pt 1): 269

3. 分组标准及处置方法

例一： Twenty-four swine, treated with streptozotocin to induce diabetes and fed a high-fat diet, were allocated into early (n=12) and late (n=12) atherosclerosis groups. Intima-media thickness was assessed by intravascular ultrasound in the coronary arteries at weeks 4 and 8 in the early group and weeks 23 and 30 in the late group.

24 只猪，用链唑霉素诱导糖尿病模型，并饲以高脂饮食，随机分配至早期（n=12）和晚期（n=12）动脉粥样硬化组。早期组于建模后第 4、8 周，晚期组于建模后第 23 周和第 30 周应用血管内超声评价冠状动脉的内膜-中层厚度。

引自: Circulation, 2008, 117(8): 993

例二: Six patients with bilateral geographic retinal atrophy due to AMD (age range, 55-83 years) were recruited for the study. The visual acuities of the patients ranged from 20/76 (0.58 logMAR) to 20/360 (1.26 logMAR). An additional six younger (age range, 22-31 years) and six older (age range, 54-78 years) normally sighted individuals were recruited as control subjects. fMRI data were acquired on a 3.0-Tesla, scanner while subjects performed visually guided saccade (VGS) and smooth-pursuit (SmP) tasks.

选取 6 名因患 AMD 导致双侧地图状视网膜萎缩的患者，年龄 55～83 岁，视力 20/76（0.58 logMAR）～20/360（1.26 logMAR）。另选取视力正常的 6 名年轻者（22～31 岁）和 6 名年长者（54～78 岁）作为对照对象。功能磁共振成像仪能量设定在 3.0 特斯拉，当受试者在进行视觉引导的扫视运动（VGS）和平稳跟踪运动（SmP）时，进行扫描获取数据。

引自: Invest Ophthalmol Vis Sci, 2008, 49(4): 1728

例三: Participants were 735 older men (mean age 60 years) without a history of coronary disease or diabetes at baseline from the Normative Aging Study. Anxiety characteristics were assessed with 4 scales (psychasthenia, social introversion, phobia, and manifest anxiety) and an overall anxiety factor derived from these scales.

受试者是 735 名老年男性（平均年龄 60 岁），按标准衰老研究基线，纳入时无冠心病或糖尿病史。采用四个量表（精神衰弱、社交内向、恐惧和明显焦虑)评估焦虑特征,再对这些量表得出的总体焦虑因子进行评估。

引自: JACC, 2008, 51(2): 113

例四: Two consecutive menstrual blood loss measurements were performed in 77 healthy women aged 21-55 years, classified as midreproductive age (n=21, control group), late-reproductive age (n=17), early-menopausal transition (n=16), and late-menopausal transition (n=23). Serum hormone levels (estradiol [E2], progesterone, follicle-stimulating hormone, luteinizing hormone, and inhibins) were measured three times per week from the start of one menstrual period to the end of the subsequent menstrual period.

对 77 例 21～55 岁的健康女性连续进行两个月经周期月经失血量测定。这些对象分为生育年龄中期（$n=21$，对照组）、生育年龄后期（$n=17$）、早期绝经过渡期（$n=16$）和晚期绝经过渡期（$n=23$）。从一个月经期开始到下一个月经期结束，每周三次测量血清激素水平（雌二醇[E2]、孕激素、卵泡刺激素、促黄体激素和抑制素）。

引自：Obstet Gynecol, 2010, 115(2 Pt 1)：249

4. 研究时间

例一： A total of 1216 patients with≥37 weeks of gestation assigned as monitoring group were performed central electronic monitoring during labor from Nov.1997 to Mar.1998. A total of 1137 patients with same gestational age assigned as control group were monitored by using intermittent auscultation during labor from Nov.1996 to Mar.1997. The rate of fetal distress, neonatal asphyxia, cesarean section, and using of forceps or vacuum extractor in the 2 groups were compared.

对 1997 年 11 月至 1998 年 3 月在我院分娩的孕周≥37 周的 1216 例孕妇（监测组）进行 CEMS 监护，并与 1996 年 11 月至 1997 年 3 月在我院分娩的孕周≥37 周、未行 CEMS 监护的 1137 例孕妇（对照组）进行比较，分析两组胎儿窘迫发生率、新生儿窒息发生率、剖宫产率和阴道手术产率。

引自：《中华妇产科杂志》，2000, 35(1)：17

例二： We reviewed 6159 consecutive outpatients with chronic stable heart failure at baseline, short-term (3-month) follow-up, and long-term (6-month) follow-up between 2001 and 2006. Clinical, demographic, laboratory, and echocardiographic data were reviewed from electronic medical records. Mortality rates were determined from 6-month follow-up to end of study period.

回顾分析 2001～2006 年门诊就诊的 6159 例慢性稳定性心衰患者的基线、短期（3 个月）随访和长期（6 个月）随访资料。从电子病案中回顾临床、人口统计学、实验室检查和超声心动图资料。从 6 个月随访期到试验期结束计算死亡率。

引自：JACC, 2008, 51(5)：569

例三： Clinical data of 100 cases of TBM admitted to Peking Union Medical College Hospital from January 1982 to December 2003 were investigated retrospectively. Data were collected with regard to the clinical, laboratory and demographic characteristics of the patients as well as the results of radiological investigations and data of clinical outcome.

回顾性分析 1982 年 1 月至 2003 年 12 月间在北京协和医院确诊或临床诊断为结核性脑膜炎的 100 例住院患者的临床资料。

引自：《中华内科杂志》，2007, 46(1)：48

例四： A retrospective analysis was performed in the Department of Endocrinology, Peking Union Medical College Hospital from October 1981 to June 2019. Patients with PAI as the first symptom were enrolled. The etiology of PAI was analyzed and the clinical characteristics was also summarized.

回顾性分析北京协和医院内分泌科 1981 年 10 月至 2019 年 6 月以 PAI 为首发症状的病例资料，对病因进行分析并总结临床特点。

引自:《中华医学杂志》, 2020, 100(12): 915

5. 研究对象（人或实验动物）特征（包括性别、年龄、种族等）及样本量

例一： We assessed the association between exercise capacity and mortality in black (n=6749; age, 58±11 years) and white (n=8911; age, 60±11 years) male veterans with and without cardiovascular disease who successfully completed a treadmill exercise test at the Veterans Affairs Medical Centers in Washington, DC, and Palo Alto, Calif. Fitness categories were based on peak metabolic equivalents (METs) achieved. Subjects were followed up for all-cause mortality for 7.5±5.3 years.

对黑色人种[n=6749；（58±11）岁]和白色人种[n=8911，（60±11）岁]成年男性退伍军人的运动耐量和死亡率之间的相关性进行评价，参试者患有或无心血管疾病，在华盛顿特区、加利福尼亚州帕洛阿尔托市的退伍军人事务医疗中心成功完成了平板运动试验。以峰值代谢当量（METs）进行健康分级。随访（7.5±5.3）年，观察受试者的全因死亡率。

引自: *Circulation*, 2008, 117(5): 614

例二： Peritoneal macrophages (PM) were isolated from nine wild-type C57BL/6 male mice (wild-type group) and nine myeloid-specific Sirt1 knock-out mice (knock-out group). RNA samples were extracted from macrophages stimulated with 1 µg/ml LPS. Sequencing and the differentially expressed lncRNA were screened after the RNA was quantified. The threshold set for up-and down-regulated genes was a fold change (wild-type group/knock-out group) ≥2 and P≤0.05. Afterwards, gene ontology (GO) and pathway enrichment analysis were conducted and co-expression network map was constructed.

选取野生型 C57BL/6 雄性小鼠 9 只（野生型组）和髓系特异性敲除型小鼠 9 只（敲除型组），分离腹腔巨噬细胞，1 µg/ml 的 LPS 处理细胞，提取总 RNA 并进行质量检测，合格后进行测序实验，以差异倍数（野生型组/敲除型组）≥2 且 P≤0.05 为纳入标准，检测野生型组和敲除型组中 lncRNA 差异表达谱，并对差异 lncRNA 进行基因本体（GO）分析和信号通路分析，构建共表达网络图，从而了解 lncRNA 参与的生物学功能。

引自:《中华医学杂志》, 2020, 100(12): 893

例三：Twenty CD38$^{-/-}$ male mice (8-week-old) and 20 wild-type (WT) male C57BL/6J mice (8-week-old) were randomly selected to construct the model of approximately 25% of the total body surface area (TBSA) burn injury. The cardiomyocytes (CMs) were separated from neonatal mice (1day) to construct the H/I injury model. Ad-CD38 adenovirus was transfected into CD38$^{-/-}$ primary CMs to callback CD38 expression. Animal experiments were grouped into WT-control group, CD38$^{-/-}$-control group, WT-burn group, and CD38$^{-/-}$-burn group (10 mice in each group). Primary CMs were divided into 6 groups: WT-normoxia group, CD38$^{-/-}$-normoxia group, CD38$^{-/-}$+Ad-CD38-normoxia group, WT-H/I group, CD38$^{-/-}$-H/I group, CD38$^{-/-}$+Ad-CD38-H/I group. The release of lactic dehydrogenase (LDH) from CMs and the cell viability were measured to estimate the level of myocardial injury. Ultrastructure of cardiomyocytes was examined by electron microscope. CD38 protein level and mitochondrial apoptosis-related proteins were detected by Western blot. Flow cytometry was used to detect mitochondrial reactive oxygen species (MitoSOX) of CMs under H/I condition. Cardiac function of mice was detected by ultrasonic apparatus.

随机选取 8 周龄 CD38$^{-/-}$雄性小鼠和野生型（WT）雄性 C57BL/6J 小鼠各 20 只构建烧伤模型，动物实验分为 WT 对照组、CD38$^{-/-}$对照组、WT 烧伤组、CD38$^{-/-}$烧伤组各 10 只，烧伤 24 h 后取材进行实验。利用出生 1 d 的小鼠乳鼠培养原代心肌细胞构建细胞缺血缺氧模型。细胞实验分为 WT 常氧组、CD38$^{-/-}$常氧组、CD38$^{-/-}$+Ad-CD38 常氧组、WT 缺血缺氧组、CD38$^{-/-}$缺血缺氧组、CD38$^{-/-}$+Ad-CD38 缺血缺氧组。通过检测乳酸脱氢酶（LDH）释放及细胞活性明确心肌细胞缺血缺氧损伤程度；电镜检测心肌细胞超微结构；免疫印迹检测心肌细胞中 CD38 蛋白及线粒体凋亡相关蛋白水平；流式细胞技术检测心肌细胞线粒体活性氧（MitoSOX）水平；凋亡试剂盒检测心肌细胞凋亡情况；小动物超声仪检测小鼠心功能。

引自：《中华医学杂志》, 2020, 100(12): 904

6. "方法"分组技巧

对于"Methods"分组，许多作者通常缺乏前瞻性考虑，即使用过于复杂的分组定义。复杂的分组定义无论是对摘要还是正文中的"结果"描述会导致语言冗长，甚至杂乱、晦涩，难以理解。例如："serum uric acid test result group and non-hyperuricemia group"［血尿酸结果组非高尿酸血症组（NUA）组］，"salmeterol/fluticasone propionate versus tiotropium group and salmeterol/fluticasone propionate group"（丙酸沙美特罗/氟替卡松对噻托吡铵组和丙酸沙美特罗/氟替卡松组）。这样定义分组，由于中心词"group"前使用了过长的修饰语，使语言缺乏精练，尤其在大型研究，如果研究分组超过 3 个以上，在后续"结果"描述时，极易造成读者理解障碍。因此，我们在"methods"中将研究对象进行分组时，应前瞻性地考虑到"结果"描述是否能实现简洁、明了。

例一：**Methods**：Experimental rats were divided randomly into 6 groups (*n*=7): A saline-aspirated control (group Ⅰ), sterile saline aspirated with CUR treatment (group Ⅱ), PEG aspirated (group Ⅲ), PEG aspirated with CUR treatment (group Ⅳ), AC aspirated (group Ⅴ), and AC aspirated with CUR treatment (group Ⅵ). After aspiration, treatment groups Ⅱ, Ⅳ, and Ⅵ were given 150 mg/kg CUR intraperitoneally once a day for 7 days. After 7 days, the rats were humanely killed, and both the lungs and serum specimens from all groups were evaluated histopathologically, immunohistochemically, and biochemically.

方法：将实验大鼠随机分为 6 组（*n*=7）：生理盐水吸入对照组（Ⅰ组）、无菌生理盐水吸入+CUR 治疗组（Ⅱ组）、PEG 吸出组（Ⅲ组）、PEG 吸出+CUR 治疗组（Ⅳ组）、AC 吸出组（Ⅴ组）和 AC 吸出+CUR 治疗组（Ⅵ组）。抽吸后，Ⅱ组、Ⅳ组和Ⅵ组腹腔注射 150 mg/kg CUR，每天一次，共 7 天。7 天后，处死大鼠，并对所有组大鼠的肺和血清标本进行组织病理学、免疫组化和生物化学评价。

【析】本篇分组就是值得效仿的实例，让复杂分组定义简洁化，从而便于"结果"比较分析描述。

引自：*J Pediatr Surg*, 2012, 47(9): 1669

例二：The rats were randomized into the following groups according to the time interval and treatment to which each was subjected:

The acute phase groups:

1. Group A, the sham laparotomy group(negative control), was instilled only with 0.9% saline after preparation of the distal esophagus.

2. Group B, the untreated group(positive control), underwent caustic esophageal burn and received daily 1 ml of 0.9% saline, intraperitoneally.

3. Group C, the treatment group underwent caustic esophageal burn and received daily(each 24 h) 40 mg/kg allopurinol for 2 days, intraperitoneally.

根据每只大鼠接受治疗的时间间隔和治疗情况，将其随机分为以下几组：

急性期组：

1. A 组，假开腹组（阴性对照组），仅在远端食管准备后用生理盐水灌注。

2. B 组，未处理组（阳性对照组），采用腐蚀性食管灼伤，每日 1 ml 生理盐水，腹腔注射。

3. C 组，治疗组，腐蚀性食管灼伤治疗，每日（每 24 h）予 40 mg/kg 别嘌呤醇 2 天，腹腔注射。

The chronic phase groups:

1. Group X, the sham laparotomy group(negative control), was instilled only with 0.9% saline after preparation of the distal esophagus.

2. Group Y, the untreated group(positive control), underwent caustic esophageal burn and received daily 1 ml of 0.9% saline, intraperitoneally.

3. Group Z, the treatment group underwent caustic esophageal burn and received daily(each 24 h) 40 mg/kg allopurinol for 3 days, intraperitoneally.

慢性期组：

1. X 组，假开腹组（阴性对照组），在准备远端食管后，仅用生理盐水灌注。

2. Y 组，未治疗组（阳性对照组），腐蚀性食管灼伤，每日 1 ml 生理盐水，腹腔注射。

3. Z 组，治疗组，腐蚀性食管灼伤治疗，每日（每 24 h）予 40 mg/kg 别嘌醇 3 天，腹腔注射。

【析】这是一项大型研究，分组比较复杂。为使分组简洁明了，先定义分组，再对各组研究内容进行补充说明，这样的分组方法值得效仿。

二、"Methods" 写作中的表达方法

1. 直接（分组）表达法

此法直接说明研究对象分为几组，每一组的数量、实验内容，一般用于两组以上的表达，也有用阿拉伯数字（1 、2 、3 等）、罗马数字（Ⅰ、Ⅱ、Ⅲ等）或英文字母（A 、B 、C 等）表示，表达分组的常用句型如下所述。

（1）……被随机分成……：...be (randomly)divided /categorized into...

（2）……被随机分成……：...be randomized into...

（3）……被随机分成……：... be (randomly) separated into...

（4）……以……标准（划分）：...based on...

（5）……被随机分成……：...be (randomly) allocated (in)to...groups

（6）……被分成……：...were grouped into...

（7）……被分成……：...were stratified into...

（8）按如下（因素）分组：The groups were as follows...

这种表达方法的优点是清晰明了，读者一眼就能看出研究对象及其具体情况。

例一：Participants **were divided into 2 groups:** (1) youth-onset type 2 diabetes mellitus (onset <20 years of age) and (2) older-onset type 2 diabetes mellitus (onset 20 - <55 years of age). Events and person-years of follow-up were stratified in a time-dependent fashion by decades of age.

参试者分为两组：2 型糖尿病发病于青年期（发病年龄＜20 岁）和 2 型糖尿病发病于青壮年期（发病年龄 20～＜55 岁）。随访安排和随访人年按时间依赖方式以每 10 岁进行分层。

引自：*JAMA*, 2006, 296(4): 421

例二： Forty adult male Sprague-Dawley rats **were randomly divided into** 4 groups (n=10), namely the control group, LPS group, low-concentration sevoflurane group and high-concentration sevoflurane group. Following sevoflurane pretreatment for 30 min and a washout period for 10 min, all the rats received intraperitoneal injection of LPS or normal saline (NS) and were sacrificed 12 h later to observe the myocardial histopathology. Apoptosis of the cardiomyocytes was detected with TUNEL assay, and enzyme-linked immunosorbent assay was used to detect serum cTnI level and myocardial TNF-α level.

健康成年雄性 SD 大鼠 40 只，随机分为 4 组（n=10）：对照组（C 组）、LPS 组（L 组）、低浓度七氟醚预处理组（S_1 组）、高浓度七氟醚预处理组（S_2 组）。七氟醚预处理 30 分钟，洗脱 10 分钟后，采用腹腔注射 LPS 方法制造大鼠脓毒症模型，并于 LPS 注射后 12 h 收集大鼠心肌及血液标本，光镜下观察心肌组织常规病理形态学改变，末端标记（TUNEL）法检测细胞凋亡，ELISA 法检测大鼠血清肌钙蛋白（cTnI）含量及心肌组织肿瘤坏死因子（TNF-α）含量。

引自：南方医学大学学报, 2014, 34(11): 1680

例三： Patients **were divided into 4 groups based on** coronary angiography: No significant stenosis (n=42), 1-vessel disease (n=72), 2-vessel disease (n=64), and 3-vessel disease (n=56).

根据冠脉造影结果，将患者分为 4 组：无显著狭窄（n=42），1 支血管病变（n=72），2 支血管病变（n=64）及 3 支血管病变（n=56）。

引自：*JAMA*, 2004, 291: 1857

例四： Patients **were stratified by** prior octreotide therapy (stratum 1: everolimus 10 mg/d, n=115; stratum 2: everolimus 10 mg/d plus octreotide long-acting release ［LAR］, n=45). Tumor assessments (using Response Evaluation Criteria in Solid Tumors) were performed every 3 months. Chromogranin A (CgA) and neuron-specific enolase (NSE) were assessed monthly if elevated at baseline.

患者依据先前奥曲肽治疗的情况进行分层［第 1 层：依维莫司 10 mg/d，共 115 例；第 2 层：依维莫司 10 mg/d+奥曲肽长效缓释剂(LAR)，共 45 例］。每 3 个月进行一次肿瘤评估（采用实体肿瘤治疗疗效评价标准）。如果患者在基线时出现嗜铬粒蛋白(CgA)和神经元特异性烯醇酶（NSE）升高，则对上述两个指标每月检测一次。

引自：*J Clin Oncol*, 2010, 28(1) : 69

例五： Patients with moderate-to-severe COPD **were randomized to** double-blind indacaterol 150 or 300 μg or placebo, or open-label tiotropium 18 μg, all once daily, for 26 weeks.

中度至重度慢性阻塞性肺疾病患者随机双盲服用茚达特罗 150 μg 或 300 μg 或安慰剂，或开放标签噻托溴铵 18 μg，每天一次，共 26 周。

引自：*Am J Respir Crit Care Med*, 2010, 182(2): 155

例六： Participants **were randomized to** 1 of 4 groups for 6 months: Control （weight maintenance diet）; calorie restriction (25% calorie restriction of baseline energy requirements); calorie restriction with exercise (12.5% calorie restriction plus 12.5% increase in energy expenditure by structured exercise); very low-calorie diet (890 kcal/d until 15% weight reduction, followed by a weight maintenance diet).

参试者在 6 个月内随机分为 4 组：对照组（饮食可维持体重）；限制热量组（限制基线所需能量的 25%）；限制热量+运动组（限制 12.5% 的热量+运动增加 12.5% 的能耗）；极低热量饮食组（每日摄入 890 kcal，直至体重减少 15%，随后采用维持体重的饮食）。

引自：*JAMA*, 2006, 295: 1539

例七： Patients **were categorized into 2 groups**: The high-MPO group included patients in the third tertile of MPO levels (>75.0 microg/L; 127 patients), and the low-MPO group included patients in the first (<52.6 microg/L) and second tertiles (52.6-75.0 microg/L)of MPO levels (255 patients).

患者分为两组：高髓过氧化物酶（MPO）组，包括处于 MPO 第三级的患者(>75.0 μg/L；127 例);低 MPO 组,包括 MPO 处于第一级(<52.6μg/L) 和第二级（ 52.6～75.0 μg/L ）的患者（ 255 例 ）。

引自：*Am Heart J*, 2008, 155(2)：356

例八： Thirty non-diabetic uremic patients undergoing maintenance hemodialysis **were divided into** the following groups: (1)nifedipine group ;(2)calcitriol group;(3) placebo group. The level of PTH receptor mRNA was measured by semi-quantitative RT-PCR method at the end of 8 th week.

30 例非糖尿病常规血液透析患者随机分成硝苯地平组、罗钙全组和安慰剂组，治疗 8 周。应用逆转录-聚合酶链反应（RT-PCR）方法检测用药前后 PBMC 上 PTH 受体 mRNA 表达。

引自：《中华肾脏病杂志》, 2000，16(5): 287

例九： Patients **were randomly assigned to** treatment with combined TACE-RFA (*n* = 96), TACE alone (*n* = 95), or RFA alone (*n* = 100).

患者随机分配到肝动脉化疗栓塞术（TACE）联合射频消融（RFA）组（ *n* = 96 ）、TACE 组（ *n* = 95 ）或 RFA 组（ *n* = 100 ）。

引自：*JAMA*, 2008, 299(14): 1669

例十： Thirty asthmatic children **were divided into two groups** ,one as MP-treated group, and the other as control group. All blood samples were collected before and after treatment with MP. The serum IgE, cytokine production in the cultured supernatants of PBMC, and the cytokine mRNA expression were determined by ELISA and RT-PCR methods respectively .

将临床 30 例哮喘患儿随机分为甲泼尼龙（MP）治疗组和对照组，用 ELISA 法测外周血单个核细胞（PBMC）细胞因子及血清 IgE 水平，用逆转录-聚合酶链反应（RT-PCR）测定细胞因子 mRNA 表达。

引自:《中华微生物学和免疫学杂志》，2000, 20(6): 548

2. 间接（分组）表达法

这种表达法先说明研究的内容及主要观察变量，然后说明研究对象包括哪几组/类人群；或者先说明实验组的实验内容/方法。如果设置了对照，需要对对照组（对象），数量、纳入标准等做概括性说明。说明时，可以用独立的句子或者将说明的内容放入用括号进行插注，说明实验组和对照组的数量及相关情况。此法表达句中一般不出现"group"一词。

例一：Polymerase chain reaction (PCR) assay was employed to detect human papillomavirus (HPV)-6,11,16 and 18 DNA in 30 pregnant women in the first trimester, 42 in the second and 31 in the third (who were followed up to their puerperium),and 30 non-pregnant women asking for intrauterine device in our out-patient clinical were taken as controls.

采用聚合酶链反应（PCR）技术检测 103 例孕产妇（观察组）宫颈及阴道分泌物、外周静脉血标本中人乳头状瘤病毒 HPV-6、HPV-11、HPV-16、HPV-18 型 DNA，其中孕早期 30 例、孕中期 42 例、孕晚期 31 例，孕晚期妇女监测到产褥期；以同期门诊要求带宫内节育器妇女 30 例为对照组，同时检测孕晚期妇女分娩的新生儿咽部分泌物标本。

引自:《中华妇产科杂志》，2000, 35(9): 523

例二：Intravenous esomeprazole bolus, 80 mg, followed by 8-mg/h infusion, over 72 hours or matching placebo, each given after successful endoscopic hemostasis. Intervention was allocated by computer-generated randomization. After infusion, both groups received oral esomeprazole, 40 mg/d, for 27 days.

全部患者都成功接受了内镜止血后，由计算机随机分组，或接受大剂量静脉注射埃索美拉唑 80 mg 后，再以每小时 8 mg 输注 72 小时，或接受安慰剂治疗。输注之后，两组都口服埃索美拉唑，每天 40 mg，共 27 天。

引自: *Ann Intern Med*, 2009, 150(7) : 455

例三：Hepatitis C virus-positive patients with bridging fibrosis or cirrhosis who did not respond to peginterferon and ribavirin were randomized to groups that were given maintenance peginterferon for 3.5 years or no treatment. HCC incidence was determined by Kaplan-Meier analysis, and baseline factors associated with HCC were analyzed by Cox regression.

对聚乙二醇化干扰素和利巴韦林治疗无应答的桥接纤维化或肝硬化的丙型肝炎病毒阳性患者，随机分组，给予聚乙二醇化干扰素治疗 3.5 年或者不接受任何治疗。使用 Kaplan-Meier 分析测定肝癌发病率，Cox 回归分析与 HCC 相关的基线因素。

引自：*Gastroenterology*, 2009, 136(1): 138

例四： Demographic data (age, sex, and race) and histology from 1074 patents with cutaneous T-cell lymphoma were stratified by age of onset and race and analyzed using Chi-square test.

1074 例皮肤 T 细胞淋巴瘤患者的人口数据（年龄、性别、种族）和组织学资料，按照发病年龄和种族进行分组，进行卡方检验分析。

引自：*J Am Acad Dermatol*, 2009, 60(2): 231

例五： We randomly assigned 48 surgical patients ≥65 yr of age to receive single intranasal doses of dexmedetomidine or placebo (5:1 ratio) in four sequential dose cohorts: 0.5, 1.0, 1.5, and 2.0 μg/kg. Each dose cohort comprised two groups of six subjects: a group of subjects using β-blockers and a group not taking β-blockers. Vital signs and sedation depth (Modified Observer's Assessment of Alertness and Sedation ［MOAA/S］ and bispectral index) were measured for 2 h after administration. Blood samples were taken to determine dexmedetomidine plasma concentrations.

我们将 48 名年龄≥65 岁的外科患者随机分为 4 个连续剂量组，分别接受右美托咪定或安慰剂（5：1）的单次鼻内给药：0.5、1.0、1.5 和 2.0 μg/kg。每个剂量队列包括两组，每组六名受试者：一组受试者使用 β 受体阻滞剂，另一组不使用 β 受体阻滞剂。给药后 2 小时测量生命体征和镇静深度［修正的观察者警觉和镇静评估（MOAA/S）和脑电双频谱指数］。采集血样以测定右美托咪定的血浆浓度

引自：*BJA*, 2020, 124(4):411

例六： From 1994 to March 2006, 1545 consecutive patients with aortic stenosis underwent isolated surgical AVR at the Department of Cardiac Surgery of Heidelberg. Both additive and logistic EuroSCOREs were calculated for each patient and summed for expected 30-day mortality. Expected and observed mortalities were compared, particularly with respect to 'high-risk' status and era of operation.

从 1994 年到 2006 年 3 月，相继有 1545 名主动脉瓣狭窄患者在海德堡医院心脏外科接受了离体 AVR 手术。对每例患者的可加模型及预测性回归 EuroSCOREs 进行计算、求和，以预测 30 天的死亡率。比较预期死亡率和观察死亡率，重点对'高危'状态和手术时期进行了比较。

（注：EuroSCOREs 是一种开发用于预测冠脉手术的手术死亡率的系统）

引自：*Eur Heart J*, 2009, 30(1)：74

例七： We randomly assigned critically ill patients with acute kidney injury and failure of at least one nonrenal organ or sepsis to receive intensive or less intensive renal-replacement therapy. The primary end point was death from any cause by day 60. In both study groups, hemodynamically stable patients underwent intermittent hemodialysis, and hemodynamically unstable patients underwent continuous venovenous hemodiafiltration or sustained low-efficiency dialysis. Patients receiving the intensive treatment strategy underwent intermittent hemodialysis and sustained low-efficiency dialysis six times per week and continuous venovenous hemodiafiltration at 35 ml per kilogram of body weight per hour; for patients receiving the less-intensive treatment strategy, the corresponding treatments were provided thrice weekly and at 20 ml per kilogram per hour.

将合并有至少一个肾以外的器官衰竭或脓毒血症的急性肾损伤危重患者随机分配到强化或非强化肾替代治疗组。主要治疗终点是 60 日内任何原因引起的死亡。两个研究组中，血流动力学稳定的患者接受间断血液透析，血流动力学不稳定的患者接受持续静脉血液透析或维持性低效透析。强化治疗组患者接受间断血液透析和维持性低效透析是每周 6 次，持续静脉血液透析的速度为 35 ml/(kg·h)；非强化治疗组患者接受相应治疗分别是每周 3 次和 20 ml/(kg·h)。

引自: *N Engl J Med*, 2008, 359(1): 7

关于研究对象的数量，可以直接表述在研究对象的前面，或使用"数词+of+对象"表达，也可使用括号插注的方式间接表达，例如：

例一： Sixty coronary heart disease (CHD) and 40 normal subjects were recruited to participate the study.

60 例冠心病患者和 40 例健康人参加此项研究。

引自:《中华心血管病杂志》, 2000, 28(3): 271

例二： Consecutive CRT patients (*n*=309) followed at our institution were retrospectively studied for percentage of RA pacing and incidence of high atrial rates, as determined by regular device interrogations.

入选我中心的 309 例接受心脏再同步化治疗（CRT）患者，用标准仪器测定，研究右心房起搏比率与快速房性心率的关系。

引自: *Am Heart J*, 2008, 155(1)：94

例三： 1763 participants (829 M and 934 F; 38 to 88 years of age) of the Framingham Heart Study Offspring cohort underwent CMR of the thoracoabdominal aorta using an ECG-gated 2D T2-weighted black-blood sequence.

参加弗明翰心脏研究后代队列的 1763 人（829 名男性和 934 名女性，年龄 38～88 岁）通过心电图门控的二维 T2 加权的'黑血'扫描序列进行胸腹主动脉 CMR 扫描。

引自：Arterioscler Thromb Vasc Biol, 2008, 28(1)：155

例四： Ninety-seven RA patients who were classified by their rheumatologists as being in remission were studied. Disease activity was assessed by the DAS-28 and simplified disease activity index (SDAI). US examination was performed in mode B and power Doppler (PD) in 42 joints.

按风湿病学家分类，纳入本研究的共有 97 例处于类风湿关节炎（RA）的患者。采用 DAS-28 和简化的疾病活动指数（SDAI）对疾病的活动性进行评价。对 42 个关节进行 B 型超声和能量多普勒超声（PD）检查。

引自：Rheumatology（Oxford），2010, 49（4）：683

三、主要研究手段的表述

不同研究课题所采用的技术方法不同，如形态学研究常采用解剖法、组织切片、显微镜、电镜、组织化学和细胞化学、细胞培养、细菌培养、原虫培养等方法；机能学方面的研究常采用电生理、生化测试、同位素、免疫等方法，所有这些方法均是实验手段。在 Methods 写作中，实验手段常用下列方式来表达。

（一）用介词或介词短语 with、by 、by means of 等词语表示

例一： CIMT images were captured **by** a single ultrasonographer at 1 center and read **by** a single treatment-blinded reader using automated edge-detection technology.

在每个中心由一位超声检查操作者采集颈动脉内膜中层厚度（CIMT）影像，由一位不了解治疗分组情况的判读者应用自动边缘检测技术进行判读。

引自：JAMA, 2006, 296: 2572

例二： Extended-spectrum β-lactamases (ESBLs) producing strains in E.coli and K. pneumoniae were detected **by** double disc synergy test, inhibitor-potentiated disc diffusion test and inhibitor combined with minimum inhibitory concentrations (MIC) determination of third-generation cephalosporins. The bacterial susceptibility testing of ESBLs-producing strains was assayed by Kirby-Bauer method.

双纸片法、酶抑制剂增强纸片散法、酶抑制剂联合三代头孢菌素最低抑菌浓度（MIC）测定法和 E-试验；Kirby-Bauer（KB）法测定 ESBLs 株对抗菌药物的敏感性。

引自：《中华传染病杂志》, 2000, 18(3): 151

例三：The expression levels and localization of TGF-beta1, Smad3, and Smad7 in liver tissue were **detected by** immunohistochemistry.

采用免疫组织化学法测定肝脏转化生长因子 β1、Smad3、Smad7 的表达水平，并对其进行定位。

引自：*Hepatobiliary Pancreat Dis Int*, 2009, 8(3): 300

例四：The temporal ocular expression of the chemokine PBP before and during corneal infection over several days by *Pseudomonas aeruginosa* **was examined by** immunohistochemistry.

应用免疫组化方法检测角膜绿脓杆菌感染前及感染后数天眼部颞侧趋化因子 PBP 的表达。

引自：*Exp Eye Res*, 2009, 89(6): 1035

例五：Rotavirus was detected, **by means of** reverse-transcriptase-polymerase-chain-reaction (RT-PCR) assay, in stool specimens obtained from all three infants.

从获得的所有三名婴儿的粪便样本中通过逆转录聚合酶链反应（RT-PCR）技术检测轮状病毒。

引自：*N Engl J Med*, 2010, 362(4): 314

（二）作主语，即直接用技术方法作主语，使用被动语态

例一：**The IMPACT model was used** to synthesise data for England and Wales describing CHD patient numbers, uptake of specific treatments, trends in major cardiovascular risk factors, and the mortality benefits of these specific risk factor changes in healthy people and in CHD patients.

用 IMPACT 模型综合处理英格兰和威尔士的数据，包括冠心病患者数、采取特殊治疗情况、主要心血管危险因素的变化趋势，以及这些特定危险因素改变在减少死亡方面为健康人和冠心病患者带来的受益。

引自：*BMJ*, 2005, 331(7517): 614

例二：**High-throughput sequencing was used** to detect 65 blood tumor-related genes in 191 MDS patients and 9 secondary acute myelocytic leukemia patitents (SAML), and to analyze the characteristics of abnormal genes, mutation burden, as well as the relationship with disease subtypes, chromosome karyotypes and age.

采用高通量测序靶向检测 191 例 MDS 患者和 9 例 MDS 继发急性髓细胞白血病（SAML）患者的 65 种血液肿瘤相关基因，分析异常基因特点、突变负荷及与疾病亚型、染色体核型和患者年龄等的关系。

引自：《中华医学杂志》, 2020, 100(12): 933

例三：**Techniques including biochemistry, radioimmunoassay, fluoroassays and polymerase chain reaction (RT-PCR)** were used in this study.

采用生化法、放射免疫法、荧光分析法及逆转录-聚合酶链反应技术等进行研究。

引自:《中华肾脏病杂志》, 2000, 16(4): 251

例四： **Clinical records of 12 cases of MCTD complicated with TN diagnosed** in Peking University People's Hospital from January 2008 to October 2019 were analyzed retrospectively.

回顾性分析 2008 年 1 月至 2019 年 10 月在北京大学人民医院确诊为 MCTD 合并 TN 的 12 例患者临床资料。

引自:《中华医学杂志》, 2020, 100(12): 938

（三）用 using/by using/employing +所用方法等分词结构表示

例一： Patients were categorized as "pulmonary embolism unlikely" or "pulmonary embolism likely" **using** a dichotomized version of the Wells clinical decision rule.

采用 Wells 临床评定标准二分法将患者分为"肺栓塞可能性小"和"肺栓塞可能性大"两组。

引自: *JAMA*, 2006, 295(2): 172

例二： Diffusion of riboflavin through the cornea was assessed **by using** infrared-excited, two-photon microscopy of riboflavin autofluorescence, combined with second-harmonic generation of fibrillar collagen.

使用与原纤维胶原二次谐波相结合的自体荧光核黄素的红外线激发双光子显微术观察通过角膜的核黄素扩散。

引自: *Invest Ophthalmol Vis Sci*, 2010, 51(8) : 392

四、研究方案的表述

在 Methods 中应交代研究设计的名称，如前瞻性随机对照研究、回顾性研究。事实上，"方法"句的写作要根据研究方案而定。前瞻性研究，结果是主要内容，则方法要叙述得简练而有条理；回顾性研究，"方法"是论文的主体部分，所以"方法"要写得详细而具体。此外，在一些国际主流学术杂志中，如《英国医学杂志》(*British Medical Journal, BMJ*)、《美国医学协会杂志》(*The Journal of the American Medical Association, JAMA*)等，通常将研究方案分列为独立项目，即设计 (design)、范围 (地点)(setting)。同时，出于英语语言表达的简洁性，常采用短语或省略结构。

例一： Double blind randomised placebo controlled trial.

双盲随机安慰剂对照研究

引自: *BMJ*, 2006, 332: 1032

例二：　From 1996 to 2006, we prospectively included a total of 197 consecutive asymptomatic patients (99 men; age, 63±12 years) with very severe aortic stenosis. Patients were excluded if they had angina, syncope, exertional dyspnea, ejection fraction <0.50, significant mitral valve disease, or age >85 years. Very severe aortic stenosis was defined as a critical stenosis in the aortic valve area ≤0.75 cm^2 accompanied by a peak aortic jet velocity ≥ 4.5 m/s or a mean transaortic pressure gradient≥50 mmHg on Doppler echocardiography. The primary end point was defined as the composite of operative mortality and cardiac death during follow-up. Early surgery was performed on 102 patients, and a conventional treatment strategy was used for 95 patients.

1996～2006 年，我们采用前瞻性研究，先后纳入 197 例极其严重的无症状性主动脉瓣狭窄患者[99 例男性；年龄(63±12)岁]。排除符合如下条件的患者：患有心绞痛、晕厥、呼吸困难、射血分数<0.50、明显二尖瓣瓣膜疾病或年龄>85 岁的患者。极其严重的主动脉瓣狭窄界定为主动脉瓣区≤0.75 cm^2 并伴随主动脉喷射峰值速度≥4.5 m/s 或经主动脉的平均压力梯度≥50 mmHg（通过多普勒超声心动图显示）。主要研究终点设定为随访期间手术死亡率和心源性死亡双因素。102 例患者采用早期手术，95 例患者采用传统治疗方法。

【析】本例为前瞻性研究。试比较下述例三、例四回顾性研究在方法（研究方案）写作上的差异。

引自：*Circulation*, 2010, 121(13)：1502

例三：　This was a retrospective analysis at an academic fertility center. The stair-step protocol is performed as follows: 50 mg clomiphene for 5 days, ultrasonography on days 11-14. If unresponsive, immediately begin 100 mg clomiphene for 5 days and repeat ultrasound in 1 week. If still unresponsive, begin 150 mg clomiphene for 5 days and repeat the ultrasound in 1 week. Stair-step cycles were compared with published historical clomiphene outcomes for women who were nonresponsive.

这是在专科学院的生育中心进行的一项回顾性分析。阶梯式方案执行如下：50 mg 克罗米芬，应用 5 天，11～14 天后进行超声检查。如果没有反应，立即给予 100 mg，应用 5 天，1 周内重复进行超声波检查。如果仍然没有反应，给予 150 mg 克罗米芬，应用 5 天，1 周内重复进行超声波检查。对克罗米芬无反应的女性，将其阶梯周期内所观察的数据与已发表的克罗米芬观察结果进行比较。

引自：*Am J Obstet Gynecol*, 2009, 200(5): 510

例四：　This was a retrospective study of 615 patients who underwent curative intent surgery for primary rectal cancer. Preoperative chemoradiotherapy involving

50.4 Gy fractionated radiotherapy and concurrent chemotherapy was performed in patients with locally advanced rectal cancer (clinically T3 or T4). We explored associations between the number of lymph nodes retrieved in the pathologic specimen and patient demographics (age, gender, body mass index [BMI]), treatment (surgeon, sphincter-saving, preoperative chemoradiotherapy), and tumor-related variables (location, stage, histology). After adjustment for other factors, we compared the mean number of obtained lymph nodes between patients treated with preoperative chemoradiotherapy and those treated without preoperative chemoradiotherapy.

本文回顾性研究了 615 例患者，这些患者均接受过原发直肠癌根治术。局部晚期直肠癌患者（临床 T3 期或 T4 期）的术前放化疗包括 50.4 Gy 的分次放疗和同步化疗。同时分析病理标本中找到的淋巴结的数目与患者统计学信息［年龄，性别，体重指数（BMI）］、治疗（外科大夫，保肛手术，术前放化疗）和肿瘤相关变量（部位，分期，组织学）之间的联系。对其他因子进行调整之后，对术前行放化疗和未行术前放化疗的患者术后获得淋巴结的平均数目进行比较。

引自：*Ann Surg*, 2010, 252(2)：336

例五： We performed a case-control study within a population-based surveillance for acute viral hepatitis. The incidence of acute hepatitis B (AHB) was estimated for the time since 1991, and the association between AHB and the considered risk factors was analyzed for the period 2001-2005.

本研究基于人群监督范围内对急性病毒性肝炎进行的病例对照研究。对自 1991 年起急性乙型肝炎（AHB）发生率进行了评价，同时对 2001～2005 年 AHB 与相关危险因素关联性予以分析。

引自：*Clin Infect Dis*, 2008, 46(6)：868

例六： Individuals, now aged 50-59 yr, originally enrolled in a population-screening program for *Helicobacter pylori* (*H. pylori*) were contacted via postal questionnaire, utilizing the Manning criteria for IBS diagnosis. Baseline demographic data, quality of life, and IBS and dyspepsia symptom data were already on file. Consent to examine primary care records was sought, and data regarding IBS- and dyspepsia-related consultations were extracted.

利用肠易激综合征（IBS）Manning 标准，通过邮寄调查表联系年龄在 50～59 岁带有幽门螺杆菌（*H. pylori*），并最初被纳入群体筛查程序的患者。基线人口统计数据、生活质量、IBS 和消化不良症状资料已经存入档案。收集同意检查者的原始护理记录，并且提取有关 IBS 和消化不良相关的主诉资料。

引自：*Am J Gastroenterol*, 2008, 103(5): 1229

五、"Methods"写作中的常用动词及词组

由于 Methods 表达的是基本研究过程，无非是研究对象、研究手段、研究内容、研究方案，所以使用的动词具有一定的范围，且一般为及物动词。为了使读者更好地掌握这些常用动词的语义搭配及其在语境中的搭配意义，兹将常用动词列举如下。

1. divide into

divide into 意为"分成、分组"（to separate and group according to kind; classify），使用频率最高，通用于所有研究对象（人或动物）的分类。

例一： Total 2124 cases were eligible to be analysed and **divided into** ERAS groups and Non-ERAS group according to the different perioperative pathway protocol.

共 2124 例患者，根据围术期处理方案的不同分为 ERAS 组和非 ERAS 组。

引自:《中华医学杂志》, 2020, 100(12): 922

例二： Participants were **divided into** 2 groups: (1) youth-onset type 2 diabetes mellitus (onset <20 years of age) and (2) older-onset type 2 diabetes mellitus (onset 20 - <55 years of age). Events and person-years of follow-up were stratified in a time-dependent fashion by decades of age.

参试者分为两组：年轻发病 2 型糖尿病组（发病年龄 <20 岁）和年长发病 2 型糖尿病（发病年龄 20~<55 岁）。随访事件和人年按时间依赖方式以每 10 岁进行分层。

引自: JAMA, 2006, 296: 421

2. measure

measure 意为"测定"、"测量"（a reference standard or sample used for the quantitative comparison of properties），与此搭配的主要是各种化学与生化成分、含量及各种功能。

例一： Computer-based morphometric quantification of inflammatory cells (CD43), myofibroblasts (smooth muscle alpha-actin [alpha-SMA]) and collagen deposition (Sirius red and hydroxyproline content) were **measured**.

基于计算机的形态学测定对炎症细胞（CD43）、肌纤维母细胞[（平滑肌 α 肌动蛋白（α-SMA）]和胶原沉积（红色黏胶纤维和羟脯氨酸）进行测定。

引自: Hepatology, 2010, 51(3): 942

例二： Serum creatinine levels were **measured** at baseline and 1 and 2 days after contrast.

在造影前及造影后第 1、2 天进行了血清肌酐检测。

引自: JAMA, 2004, 291: 2328

例三：IGF-I concentration and GH peak after GHRH/GHRP-6 test were **measured**.

测定 IGF - I 的浓度和 GHRH/GHRP-6 试验后 GH 峰值。

引自：*J Clin Endocrinol Metab*, 2010, 95(5): 2266

例四：We **measured** Lp-PLA2 activity among 740 men and 777 women with confirmed diabetes enrolled in the Health Professionals Follow-Up Study (HPFS) and Nurses' Health Study (NHS).

我们对 740 名男性和 777 名女性糖尿病确诊者进行了 Lp-PLA2 活性测定，这些患者分别登记注册于健康专家随访研究（HPFS）和护士健康研究（NHS）。

引自：*Br J Anaesth*, 2010, 104(6)：761

3. analyze

analyze　意为"分析"（to separate into parts or basic principles so as to determine the nature of the whole; examine methodically; to make a chemical analysis of）。一般涉及对某些基本要素、方法校验、数据资料或化学分析。

例一：　Data of 122 patients, who underwent esophageal radioactive stent placement for advanced esophageal or gastric cardia cancer between January 2012 and September 2017 in Zhongda Hospital, were retrospectively **analyzed**.

回顾性分析 2012 年 1 月至 2017 年 9 月于东南大学附属中大医院接受食管内照射支架置入术治疗中晚期食管或贲门癌的 122 例病例资料。

引自：《中华医学杂志》, 2019, 99(47): 3687

例二：Cancer biological variables were **analyzed** from tumor tissue microarrays using immunohistochemistry or in situ hybridization.

应用免疫组织化学或原位杂交法对肿瘤的生物学特性进行肿瘤组织微矩阵分析。

引自：*JAMA*, 2004, 292: 1064

例三：Cross-sectional data from 4181 male individuals who underwent general health screening were **analyzed.**

分析了 4181 名接受健康普查的男性横截面数据。

引自：*Arterioscler Thromb Vasc Biol*, 2008, 28(1): 160

4. Perform

perform 意为"实施"、"执行"（to carry on；function）。该动词通常与其他名词连用，构成搭配意义。可以与其搭配的名词比较宽泛，如数据分析、手术方式方法、实验手段等。

例一：Linear regression was **performed** to adjust for factors potentially affecting the posttransfusion PLT count response.

进行线性回归以调整可能影响输血后血小板计数反应的因素。

引自：*Transfusion*, 2010, 50(7): 1552

例二： Landmark analyses were **performed** among patients who were event-free (no death, myocardial infarction [MI], or revascularization) at 6- and 12-month follow-up.

对随访期 6 个月、12 个月内无任何问题（无死亡、无心肌梗死发生或无需血管重建手术）的患者进行界标分析（landmark analysis）。

引自：*JAMA*, 2007, 297: 159

例三： Reverse-transcription polymerase chain reaction (RT-PCR) was **performed** using colonic biopsy tissues from patients with IBS-D and normal subjects.

使用 IBS-D 患者和正常受试者的直肠活检样本进行逆转录聚合酶链反应（RT-PCR）。

注：IBS-D 是指以腹泻为主的肠易激综合征（diarrhea-predominant irritable bowel syndrome）。

引自：*Dig Dis Sci*, 2010, 55(10): 2922

例四： Endothelial cell density measurements were **performed** preoperatively and at each follow-up examination using a noncontact specular microscope.

使用非接触镜面发射显微镜测量术前及每次随访检查时的内皮细胞密度。

引自：*Ophthalmology*, 2008, 115(4): 608

5. allocate

allocate 意为"分配、指定"（to distribute according to a plan; designate）。但要注意的是，该动词多用于"分组"，与介词 to 连用，多用于以人为研究对象的分组描述。

例一： 170 and 432 eligible men and women, who had indicated on a previous questionnaire that they would accept an invitation for screening, were randomly **allocated to** the intervention group (offered flexible sigmoidoscopy screening) or the control group (not contacted).

符合入选条件的 170 位男性和 432 位女性患者，且在此之前均接受过问卷调查并同意接受乙状结肠镜检查，随机分配到检查组（提供乙状结肠镜检查）和对照组（不提供乙状结肠镜检查）。

引自：*Lancet*, 2010, 375(9726)：1624

例二： The adjusted risk for the combined end point of cardiac death or nonfatal myocardial infarction during an extended mean 8.2-year follow-up period of the BIP trial was assessed in 3,090 patients **allocated to** the original bezafibrate (n=1,548) and placebo (n=1,542) groups of the trial.

在 BIP 试验延长随访期内（平均 8.2 年），3090 名患者接受了评价。被访者分为口服必降脂组（n=1548）和安慰剂组（n=1542），观察上述患者心脏死亡或非致死心肌梗死在合并终点校正后的风险。

引自：*JACC*, 2008, 51(4)：459

例三：1113 patients were randomly **allocated to** targeted intraoperative radiotherapy and 1119 were allocated to external beam radiotherapy.

1113 例患者被随机纳入靶向术中放疗组，1119 例患者被纳入外放射治疗组。

引自：*Lancet*, 2010, 376(9735): 91

6. detect

detect 意为 "检测"（to discover or ascertain the existence, presence, or fact of; to discern the true nature or character of）。该词表示 "检测" 时，所涉及的内容比较广泛，既包括手段的使用，又涉及受检测的内容，如物质水平，影像表现、基因及蛋白测定等。

例一：Combined corticotropic and somatotropic deficiencies were **detected** in two patients.

对 2 例患者复合促肾上腺皮质激素和复合生长激素缺乏情况进行了检测。

引自：*J Clin Endocrinol Metab*, 2010, 95(7): 3277

例二：Flow injection of system was assembled using HPLC, four groups of serum advanced glycosylation end products-peptide (AGE-P) level **were detected** .

利用高效液相色谱仪（HPLC）构建流动注射分析系统，检测不同人群血清小分子糖基化终产物-肽水平。

引自：《中华内分泌代谢杂志》, 2000, 16(4): 231

例三：Expression of Galectin-3 **was detected** by reverse transcriptase-polymerase chain reaction and Western blot analysis.

采用 RT-PCR 和 Western blot 检测 Galectin-3 表达。

引自：《复旦学报（医学版）》, 2007, 34(2): 169

例四：Totally 99 lymph nodes were **detected** by clinical examination, 53 nodes in the nonmalignant group and 46 nodes in the malignant group.

临床检查共检出淋巴结 99 个，非恶性组 53 个，恶性组 46 个。

引自：*International Journal of Dental Sciences and Research*, 2013, 1 (1): 8

7. collect

collect 意为 "收集"、"采集"（to bring together in a group or mass; gather. ）。主要用于资料/数据、标本/样本的收集。

例一：A community-based cohort study in which data were **collected** during all Framingham Heart Study examinations attended in the 1990s.

社区队列研究，数据收集于 20 世纪 90 年代进入 Framingham 心脏研究的所有患者检查结果。

引自：*JAMA*, 2005, 294(4): 466

例二：Air samples (1.5 m^3) were **collected** on liquid medium with a commercial sampler at 1-, 3-, 5-, and 8-m distances from patients' heads. Air control samples were collected away from *Pneumocystis pneumonia* patient wards and outdoors.

用从市场采购的采样器从距离患者头部1米、3米、5米和8米处采集空气样本（1.5 m³）置于液体培养基中。空气对照样品从远离肺孢子虫肺炎患者病房的地方及户外采集。

引自：*Clin Infect Dis*, 2010, 51(3)：259

例三： Data were prospectively **collected** on a consecutive series of 11,141 patients undergoing PCI without dialysis in northern New England from 2003 to 2005.

收集11 141例行PCI手术未接受透析患者（时间：2003～2005年；患者所在地：新英格兰北部）的资料。

引自：*Am Heart J*, 2008, 155(2): 260

8. determine

determine意为"检测、测定"（to establish or ascertain definitely, as after consideration, investigation, or calculation）。

例一： Risk factors with odds ratio (OR) and confidence intervals (CI) were **determined** using conditional logistic regression analyses.

通过条件logistic回归分析确定危险因素的比值比（OR）和置信区间（CI）。

引自：*J Hepatol*, 2010, 53(1)：162

例二： Multiorgan insulin sensitivity and very low-density lipoprotein(VLDL) kinetics were **determined** in 10 subjects with class obesity.

对10名Ⅰ型肥胖受试者进行了多器官胰岛素敏感性和极低密度脂蛋白（VLDL）动力学测定。

引自：*Obesity (Silver Spring)*, 2010, 18(8): 1510

例三： Lead content was **determined** by flame atomic absorption spectrophotometry.

用原子吸收分光光度法测定铅含量。

引自：*Studies of Trace Elements and Health*, 2006, 22(6): 35

例四： Differential gene expression was **determined** in mucosal scrapings using Mouse genome 430 2.0 arrays.

应用小鼠430 2.0阵列检测黏膜刮取物的差异表达基因。

引自：*BMC Med Genomics*, 2008, 1(12)：14

9. employ

employ意为"使用、利用"（to engage the services of; put to work），employ指"正式使用"，其内涵意义为"借助……来实施……"。通常用于研究手段或方法的使用。

例一： The Mantel-Haenszel random-effects model was **employed** for all analyses using odds ratio (OR) and 95% confidence interval.

采用 Mantel-Haenszel 随机效应模型分析比值比和95%置信区间。

引自: *Obstet Gynecol*, 2010, 116(1): 147

例二： Case-control method was **employed**, and the PCR-SSP technique was used to identify HLA-DRB1 alleles .

采用病例对照法，运用 PCR-SSP 技术测定 HLA-DRB1 等位基因型别。

引自:《中华流行病学杂志》, 2000, 21(3): 267

例三： A multi-comparative proteomic analysis was **employed** to identify differentially regulated SAT proteins by BS and/or the degree of insulin sensitivity.

采用多比较蛋白质组学分析方法，通过 BS 和（或）胰岛素敏感性来鉴定差异调节的 SAT 蛋白。

引自: *Obesity Surgery*, 2018, 26: 1757

10. use

use 意为"采用、使用"（apply for a purpose; employ）。在用法上，use 和 employ 没有明显区别，use 在医学英语中是使用频率最高的词。

例一： Among all patients who underwent surgical treatment, the direct end-to-side anastomosis strategy was applied in 26 patients, autologous pericardial-homograft patch and aortic flap were employed in 20 patients, and synthetic graft was **used** in 6 patients.

在所有接受手术治疗的患者中，26 例患者采用直接端-侧吻合，20 例患者采用自体心包同植片和主动脉瓣成形术，6 例患者采用合成移植物修复。

引自: *J Cardiothorac Surg*, 2019, 14: 82

例二： Linear mixed models were **used** to analyze the health-related quality of life (HRQL) outcomes.

采用线性混合模型对健康相关的生活质量（HRQL）结果进行分析。

引自: *Obesity Surgery*, 2018, 25: 2408

11. carry out

carry out 意为"实施、执行、实现"（to perform or complete; CONDUCT）。其语境意义通常指"……通过……手段或方法……实施……"。

例一： A case-control study was **carried out**.

采用病例对照研究的方法。

引自:《中华医学杂志》, 2000, 21(3): 287

例二： Analysis of implant and prosthesis movement was **carried out** using the Mann-Whitney U test, and a P value of $\leqslant 0.03$ was considered significant.

植入物及假体活动性分析采用 Mann-Whitney U 检验，且当 $P \leqslant 0.03$ 时为

差异有统计学意义。

引自: *Ophthalmology*, 2010, 117(8) : 1638

例三： A separate analysis was **carried out** for the combined end point of death, ventricular tachycardia, ventricular fibrillation, cardiac arrest, ischemic stroke, major bleeding, systemic embolism, pulmonary embolism, and myocardial infarction.

对死亡、室性心动过速、心室颤动、心脏停搏、缺血性卒中、严重出血、全身栓塞、肺栓塞和心肌梗死的复合终点进行独立分析。

引自: *Am J Cardiol*, 2010, 105(12): 1768

12. diagnose

diagnose 意为"诊断"[to distinguish or identify (a disease) by diagnosis]，指通过诊断辨别或识别（如疾病）。

例一： Clinical records of 12 cases of MCTD complicated with TN **diagnosed** in Peking University People's Hospital from January 2008 to October 2019 were analyzed retrospectively.

回顾性分析 2008 年 1 月至 2019 年 10 月在北京大学人民医院确诊为 MCTD 合并 TN 的 12 例患者临床资料。

引自:《中华医学杂志》, 2020, 100(12): 938

例二： Totally 143 HIV/ AIDS patients who were first **diagnosed** in Peking Union Medical College Hospital from January 1988 to April 2006 were enrolled in this study.

回顾性分析了 1988 年 1 月～2006 年 4 月在北京协和医院首诊发现并有完整病史资料的 143 例 HIV/AIDS 患者的临床资料。

引自:《中国医学科学院学报》, 2006, 28(5): 651

13. observe

observe 意为"观察"（to make a systematic or scientific observation of）。

例一： The renal tissue were **observed** by light microscopy and electron microscopy .
用光镜及电镜观察肾脏组织。

引自:《中华肾脏病杂志》, 2000, 16(1): 89

例二： We reviewed cutaneous adverse reactions **observed** with antiosteoporotic agents, including information from case reports, regulatory documents, and pharmacovigilance.

回顾病例报告、规范性文件及药物安全监视中所有关于抗骨质疏松药物所导致的药物不良反应。

引自: *Osteoporos Int*, 2010, 21(5): 723

14. assign

assign 意为 "分配、归属"（to ascribe；attribute）。该词常用于表示组别分类，其后与介词 to 连用。

例一： One hundred and thirty-seven rats were randomly **assigned to** three groups with different treatments .

137 只大鼠随机分成 3 组，采用不同方法治疗。

引自：《中华消化杂志》, 2000, 20(2): 171

例二： We randomly **assigned** 105 patients with ULMCA stenosis **to** percutaneous coronary intervention (PCI; 52 patients) or coronary artery bypass grafting (CABG; 53 patients).

随机分配 105 名无保护左主干冠状动脉（ULMCA）狭窄患者行经皮冠状动脉介入（PCI，52 例）或冠状动脉旁路移植术（CABG，53 例）。

引自：JACC, 2008, 51(5)：538

例三： Patients were enrolled between April 2001 and September 2003 and were randomly **assigned to** treatment group.

2001 年 4 月至 2003 年 9 月期间入组患者，并随机分配至各治疗组。

引自：J Clin Psychiatry, 2010, 71(5)：574

15. investigate

investigate 意为 "调查、分析、了解"（to observe or inquire into in detail; examine systematically）。

例一： The microsatellite polymorphism of MICA exon 5 in 175 unrelated healthy individuals were **investigated** using PCR-heteroduplex analysis.

用 PCR-异源双链分析法，对 175 名正常人无关个体的 *MICA* 基因第 5 个外显子微卫星多态性的分布进行研究。

引自：《中华医学遗传学杂志》, 2000, 17(3): 332

例二： The purpose of this study was to **investigate** the impact of age, sex, and hypertension (HTN) on aortic atherosclerotic burden using cardiovascular MRI (CMR) in a free-living longitudinally followed cohort.

通过自由生活纵向随访观察，应用心血管 MRI（CMR）研究年龄、性别和高血压对主动脉粥样硬化的不同影响。

引自：Arterioscler Thromb Vasc Biol, 2008, 28(1): 155

16. follow up

follow up 意为 "随访"（to keep under surveillance）。其内涵意义指通过跟踪手段去了解某种疾病的预后情况。注意，follow-up 用连字符连接成一个词时，为名词。此外，单独使用 follow 时，还有"随后，紧跟"之意。

例一： All patients were **followed up** for more than 10 years.

所有患者均随访 10 年以上。

引自：《中华肿瘤杂志》, 2000, 22: 321

例二： A total of 121 patients (median age 33.3 years; 59.5% male) were enrolled from 11 sites and **followed up** for a median of 3.7 years.

来自 11 个中心的共 121 例患者（中位数年龄 33.3 岁；59.5%为男性）纳入本研究，随访时间中位数为 3.7 年。

引自: *Circulation*, 2008, 21(8): 172

例三： All patients received lansoprazole. The duration of treatment was 3 months, **followed by** repeat endoscopy and biopsies.

所有患者接受兰索拉唑治疗。治疗时间为 3 个月，之后重复内镜和活检检查。

引自: *Gastroenterology*, 2010, 139(2): 418

17. include

include 意为"包括"（to take in as a part, an element, or a member）。

例一： A total of 128 patients with advanced Hodgkin's disease was **included** in this study.

本文以 128 例晚期霍奇金病人为研究对象。

引自：《中华肿瘤杂志》, 2000, 22(3): 333.

例二： We **included** 396 077 patients aged 66 years or older who had a history of cardiovascular disease or diabetes while undergoing medical treatment and who were alive on April 1, 1998.

研究共包括 396 077 例年龄≥66 岁，正在接受内科治疗，截至 1998 年 4 月 1 日仍然存活的有心脏病史或糖尿病史的患者。

引自: *JAMA*, 2004, 291: 1864

18. stratify

stratify 意为"把……分级，分层"（To separate into a sequence of graded status levels）。该词在"方法"分组时，通常侧重流行病学研究方案的描述。

例一： One thousand fifty-three patients were **stratified** (center, number of metastatic sites, prior adjuvant therapy, and measurable cancer) and randomly assigned.

对 1053 例患者进行分层（治疗中心、转移部位数目、初始辅助化疗和可测量肿瘤）和随机分配。

引自: *J Clin Oncol*, 2010, 28(9) : 1547

例二： Patients were **stratified** according to management strategies which included revascularization, primary amputation, palliative limb care, and aggressive local care without revascularization (conservative group).

患者按治疗策略分组，包括血管重建组、一期截肢组、姑息性肢体护理组和无血管重建的积极局部护理组（保守治疗组）。

引自：*Ann Vasc Surg*, 2010, 24(8): 1110

例三： Participants were **stratified** by aerobic fitness (characterized by preoperative cardiopulmonary exercise test), surgical specialty, and intended surgical approach (open or laparoscopic).

研究对象按有氧健身（以术前心肺运动试验为特征）、手术专科、拟行手术入路（开放或腹腔镜）进行分组。

引自：*Br J Anaesth*, 2015, 115(4): 578

19. categorize

categorize 意为"分类、归类"（Put things into a particular group with the same features）。该词强调的是把具有同类性质特征的事物进行归类，通常与介词"into"连用。

例一： The participants were **categorized into** groups according to injury severity (mild, moderate, or severe).

根据损伤严重程度（轻度、中度或严重）将研究对象予以分类。

引自：*Pediatric*, 2009, 124(6) : e1064

例二： Patients were **categorized into** 2 groups: The high- myeloperoxidase（MPO）group included patients in the third tertile of MPO levels (>75.0 microg/L; 127 patients), and the low-MPO group included patients in the first (<52.6 microg/L) and second tertiles (52.6-75.0 microg/L) of MPO levels (255 patients).

将患者分为 2 组：高过氧化物酶（MPO）组（MPO>75.0 μg/L; 127 例），低 MPO 组包括（MPO<52.6 μg/L）及（52.6～75.0 μg/L），共 255 例。

引自：*Am Heart J*, 2008, 155(2): 356

例三： The 34 urine specimens **were categorized** as voided urine (16 cases), bladder-catheterized urine (17 cases), and bladder-washed fluid (1 case).

34 份尿标本分为自主排出尿（16 例）、膀胱导管尿（17 例）和膀胱冲洗液（1 例）。

引自：*Diagn Cytopathol*, 2012, 40(9): 798

20. randomize

randomize 意为"随机……"（To make random in arrangement, especially in order to control the variables in an experiment.）。该词在"方法"分组中使用时，可以使语言更为

简洁，其后面可跟介词 to 或 into，或直接跟动词不定式做宾语。

例一：Patients were **randomized (1∶1) to** receive apabetalone, 100 mg orally twice daily (*n*=1215), or matching placebo (*n*=1210) in addition to standard care.

除标准护理外，患者随机（1∶1）接受阿帕贝特治疗，每日两次口服 100 mg（*n*=1215），或匹配安慰剂（*n*=1210）。

引自：*JAMA*, 2020, 323(16):1565-1573

例二：Ninety-five patients were **randomized to** either ECP and standard therapy (*n* = 48) or standard therapy alone (*n*=47).

95 例患者随机分为 ECP+标准治疗（*n*=48）或单纯标准治疗（*n*=47）。

引自：*Blood*, 2008, 112(7): 2667

除了以上所列举的词和词组的用法之外，在国内外医学期刊中，还有某些其他词或词组也较为常见，如动词 develop、design、introduce、undertake、undergo、group into……。措辞时，切勿试图完全对等，应从英语单词的内涵和外延意义两方面综合考虑词的选择。

六、"Methods" 句中动词形式的确定

无论是结构式摘要还是指示性摘要，研究方法基本上涉及研究过程、方法、方案设计。按时间关系划分，在研究论文发表时，这一时间过程中所从事的一切活动均成为历史。由此可知，使用 "V-ed" 动词形式应为方法句写作的主导选择。其次，影响动词形式确定的另一要素是时间参照点，如果一个句子中涉及两个不同时间段内发生的行为或存在的状态，尤其在以连接副词 when、as soon as、before、after、until 等词引导的时间状语从句中，为了区分行为或状态的先后顺序，先发生的行为或存在的状态应采用助动词 "had+-ed" 分词，即过去完成体表示（如下述例七、例八）。至于语态的使用，学者们的见解莫衷一是。这不仅涉及作者的写作风格，而且有各类期刊的投稿要求及写作时的语篇衔接。请注意观察下列例句。以下例句中，前四个例句均来自同一期刊 *Cardiology*，在同一语篇层面却出现了不同的语态（如下述例一、例二用的主动结构；例三、例四用的是被动结构），然而，国内期刊使用第一人称的主动结构较少，基本采用被动结构（如下述例五、例六）。

例一：In a multicenter trial, we **randomly assigned** 204 patients with acute myocardial infarction to receive an intracoronary infusion of progenitor cells derived from bone marrow (BMC) or placebo medium into the infarct artery 3 to 7 days after successful reperfusion therapy.

在一项多中心试验中，我们将 204 例急性心肌梗死患者进行随机分组，在成功灌注治疗后 3～7d，对梗死动脉行冠状动脉内注射骨髓（BMC）源性祖细胞或安慰剂治疗。

引自：*Cardiology*, 2007, 3: 15

例二： **We identified** all patients hospitalized with suspected myocardial ischemia in an urban academic hospital from 1991 to 1992. We **compared** presenting characteristics, treatment, and long-term mortality between patients with unstable angina (UA), minor myocardial damage (MMD), definite non-ST-elevation myocardial infarction(NSTEMI), and STEMI.

对 1991～1992 年在一所市级教学医院住院的所有疑似心肌缺血患者进行了确诊。比较不稳定型心绞痛（UA）、微小心肌损伤（MMD）、明确的非 ST 段抬高型心肌梗死（NSTEMI）和 STEMI 患者的临床特征、治疗方法和远期死亡率。

引自：Cardiology, 2007, 2: 21

例三： Twenty-four female BALB/c mice at 3-week-old **were randomly divided into** PBS group, RSV group, ovalbumin (OVA) group and OVA/RSV group (n=6 for each group).

将 24 只 3 周龄 BALB/c 雌性小鼠随机分为 PBS 组、RSV 组、卵清白蛋白（ovalbumin，OVA）组和 OVA/RSV 组，每组 6 只。

引自：《复旦学报(医学版) 》，2020, 47(1): 59

例四： A total of 705 patients **were randomized** to cilostazol 100 mg twice daily (n=354) versus placebo(n=351) for 6 months.

总共 705 例患者被随机入选西洛他唑组（n=354，100 mg，2 次/天）或安慰剂组（n=351）接受为期 6 个月的治疗。

引自：Cardiology, 2007, 2: 27

例五： A total of 148 gastric NENs **were divided into** type Ⅰ, type Ⅱ and type Ⅲ based on the classification of European Neuroendocrine Tumor Society (ENETS). Kaplan-Meier test and Cox regression model **were used** in univariate and multivariate survival analysis in 108 cases with pathological G3 gastric NEN.

将苏州大学附属第一医院和南京医科大学第一附属医院 148 例胃 NEN 按欧洲神经内分泌肿瘤协会（ENETS）临床分型标准分为Ⅰ型、Ⅱ型、Ⅲ型，比较各型胃 NEN 的临床、胃镜及病理特征，分别采用 Kaplan-Meier 检验、Cox 回归模型对其中 108 例病理分级为 G3 级的胃 NEN 患者进行单因素和多因素生存分析。

引自：《中华内科杂志》，2020, 59(4): 297

例六： The clinical and pathological data of 440 ICC patients who underwent curative-intent resection in 10 of Chinese hepatobiliary surgery centers from January 2010 to December 2018 **were collected**, and the deadline of follow-up **was April 30th**, 2019. Among them, **205 were males and 235 were females**, with age of (57.0±9.9) years (range:23-83 years).Eighty-five cases (19.3%) **had** intrahepatic bile duct stones, and 98 cases (22.3%) **had** chronic viral hepatitis.The Kaplan-Meier method **was used** for survival analysis. The univariate and multivariate analysis **were implemented** respectively using the Log-rank test and Cox proportional hazard model.

收集 2010 年 1 月至 2018 年 12 月中国 10 家三甲医院肝胆外科中心行意向性根治性手术治疗的 440 例 ICC 患者的临床病理学资料。其中男性 205 例，女性 235 例；年龄（57.0±9.9）岁（范围：23～83 岁）。85 例（19.3%）合并肝内胆管结石，98 例（22.3%）合并慢性病毒性肝炎。随访截至 2019 年 4 月 30 日。采用 Kaplan-Meier 法计算累积总体生存率，生存分析中单因素分析采用 Log-rank 检验，多因素分析使用 Cox 检验。

引自:《中华外科杂志》, 2020, 58(4): 295

注：为尊重原作，上述例五、例六中，英文与中文信息存在不完全对等情况，请读者酌情思考。

例七：**We used** the self-controlled case-series method to study the risk of first deep vein thrombosis (DVT) (*n*=7278) and first pulmonary embolism (PE) (*n*=3755) after acute respiratory and urinary tract infections. Data **were obtained** from records from general practices who **had registered** patients with the UK's Health Improvement Network database between 1987 and 2004.

应用自身对照病例系列研究方法，研究急性呼吸道和尿路感染后首次深静脉血栓形成（DVT）（*n*=7278）及肺栓塞（PE）（*n*=3755）的风险。所有资料来自于 1987～2004 年间英国健康促进网络数据库中注册的全科医师的病例记录。

引自: *Lancet*, 2006, 367(9516): 1075

例八：Of 72,829 women who **had never smoked**, 65,180 women **provided** information on smoking by their husbands, and 66,520 women **provided** information on exposure to tobacco smoke at work and in early life from family members.

72 829 名无吸烟史的女性中，65 180 人的配偶为吸烟者；66 520 位女性有烟草暴露史，包括工作场所及幼年期其家庭成员有吸烟者。

引自: *BMJ*, 2006, 8: 204

七、"Methods" 写作中常用 "方法、手段"

CT 灌注成像	CT perfusion imaging
CT 尿路造影	CT urography (CTU)
CT 血管造影	CT angiography
DNA 测序	DNA sequencing
MR 胆胰管造影	MR cholangiopancreatography
MR 尿路造影	MR urography (MRU)
MR 功能成像	function MR imaging

MTT 测定法	MTT assay
Northern 印迹杂交	Northern blotting
Seldinger 技术	Seldinger technique
Southern 印迹杂交	Southern blotting
X 线晶体衍射	X-ray crystallography
斑点杂交	dot blotting
病史采集	history taking
不对称 PCR	asymmetric PCR
彩色多普勒血流显像	color Doppler flow imaging
超声内镜检查	endoscopical ultrasonography(EUS)
巢式引物 PCR	nested primer PCR
磁共振波谱成像	MR spectroscopy imaging (MRSI)
单光子发射体层显像	single photon emission computed tomography(SPECT)
蛋白定性试验	Pandy's test/Pandy's reaction
蛋白多糖复合染色	proteoglycan complex staining
蛋白印迹技术	Western blotting
多中心、随机、双盲、安慰剂对照、平行组研究	multicenter, randomized, double-blind, placebo-controlled, parallel-group study
定量 PCR	quantitative PCR
定量系统综述	quantitative systematic review
定位克隆	positional cloning
定性系统综述	quantitative systematic review
动态血压监测	ambulatory blood pressure monitoring
镀银染色法	silver impregnation
队列研究	cohort study
多因素分析	multivariate analysis
多重 PCR	multiplex PCR
反向 PCR	reverse PCR
非实验研究	non-experimental study
非随机对照试验	non-randomized controlled trial
非血管介入技术	non-vascular interventional technique
分层分析	stratified analysis
粪便隐血试验	fecal occult blood test
腹腔镜胆囊切除术	laparoscopic cholecystectomy
肝功能试验	liver function test
肝脏穿刺抽脓术	liver abscess puncture
肝脏穿刺活体组织检查术	liver biopsy
功能互补试验	functional complementation assay

骨髓穿刺术	bone marrow puncture
骨髓活组织检查术	bone marrow biopsy
过碘酸-六甲四胺银染色	periodic silver methenamine
含铁血黄素试验（Rous 试验）	Rous test
红细胞渗透脆性试验	erythrocyte osmotic fragility test
环卵沉淀法	circunoval precipitin test
回顾性研究	retrospective study
回顾性队列分析	retrospective cohort analysis
基因芯片技术	gene chip
吉姆萨染色	Giemsa staining
经导管动脉内药物灌注	transcatheter arterial infusion (TAI)
经导管动脉栓塞术	transcatheter arterial embolization (TAE)
经导管溶栓术	transcatheter thrombolysis
经导管射频消融术	radiofrequency catheter ablation
经内镜鼻胆管引流术	endoscopic nasobiliary drainage (ENAD)
经内镜逆行性胆胰管造影	endoscopic retrograde cholangiopancreatography (ERCP)
经皮胆管球囊扩张术（成形术）	balloon catheter technique
经皮肺穿刺术	percutaneous lung biopsy
经皮冠状动脉介入治疗	percutaneous coronary intervention (PCI)
经皮腔内血管成形术	percutaneous transluminal angioplasty
静脉葡萄糖耐量试验	intravenous glucose tolerance test
聚合酶链式反应	polymerase chain reaction (PCR)
开放标签、随机化、非劣性研究	open-label, randomized, noninferiority study
口服葡萄糖耐量试验	oral glucose tolerance test
离子交换层析	ion-exchange chromatography
联合培养	combination culture
淋巴结穿刺术	lymph node puncture
淋巴结组织活检术	lymph node biopsy
流式细胞术	flow cytometry
锚定 PCR	anchored polymerase chain reaction
酶联免疫吸附测定（酶联免疫吸附试验）	enzyme linked immunosorbent assay(ELISA)
免疫沉淀法	immunoprecipitation
内镜下黏膜切除术	endoscopic mucosal resection (EMB)
逆行性尿路造影	retrograde urography
逆行性膀胱造影	retrograde cystography
逆行性肾盂造影	retrograde pyelography
逆转录 PCR	reverse transcription PCR

凝胶过滤层析	gel-filtration chromatography
葡萄糖耐量试验	glucose tolerance test
气管内插管	endotracheal intubation
前瞻性队列研究	prospective cohort study
前瞻性开放标签试验	prospective, open-labelled trial
前瞻性基于人口的研究	prospective population-based study
亲和层析	affinity chromatography
氰化物抗坏血酸试验	cyanide-ascorbic acid test
瑞氏染色	Wright's staining
扫描电镜观察	scanning electron microscopy (SEM)
实时 PCR	real-time PCR
束臂试验	touniguer test/capillary fragility test/capillary resistance test
数字 X 线荧光成像	digital fluorography (DF)
数字减影血管造影	digital subtraction angiography (DSA)
双盲试验	double-blind trial
双脱氧链终止法	chain termination method
试点随机，双盲，安慰剂对照， 　交叉试验	pilot randomized, double-blind, placebo-controlled, 　　crossover trial

八、练　习

5-1　将下列"方法"句译成英文，注意常用词的使用

（1）**方法**：制作小鼠睾丸组织切片，显微镜下观察，记录第Ⅶ相细精管的精原细胞数及第Ⅳ相细精管的次级精母细胞和处于减数分裂中期、后期的细胞数。

（2）**方法**：应用放射性核素胃排空、食管测压、24 h 食管 pH 监测、电子胃镜、摄像上消化道造影和 DeMeester 烧心症状评分对 92 例食管癌与 79 例贲门癌术后患者进行客观检查，并与正常人进行对比分析。

（3）**方法**：根据肾动脉造影结果将 69 例入选患者分为严重狭窄组 44 例；轻度狭窄组 25 例。记录两组肾动脉及冠状动脉（冠脉）介入的手术成功率和并发症，同时分别测定术前及术后 3 个月尿 α_1，β_2-MG 水平，并比较随访情况。

（4）**方法**：应用抑郁自评量表（SDS）、焦虑自评量表（SAS）、相关因素调查表对 77 例肺癌患者进行评定，其结果与 65 例鼻咽癌患者进行对照比较。

（5）**方法**：回顾性分析了 2001 年 9 月至 2006 年 10 月在我科行肝段下腔静脉全程显露布加综合征根治术的 60 例患者的临床资料。

（6）**方法**：在 426 例行前列腺癌根治术的患者中采用 Taqman 探针法检测 *CYP1B1* 基因 8 个标签单核苷酸多态性（single nucleotide polymorphism，SNP）的分布情况。采用 RT-PCR 法检测 127 例前列腺癌旁组织中 *CYP1B1* mRNA 的表达。采用 Cox 比例风险模型和 Kaplan-Meier 法进行关联性和生存分析。

（7）**方法**：采用扩增片段长度多态性（AFLP）分子标记技术对 10 省或自治区（云南、四川、广西、福建、湖南、湖北、江西、安徽、江苏和浙江）25 个钉螺种群基因组 DNA 进行扩增，分析钉螺种群间的遗传距离与地理距离的相关性。

（8）**方法**：将急性重症胰腺炎患者 40 例随机分为试验组和对照组，试验组早期行肠道内营养，对照组病情稳定后行肠道内营养，记录患者的感染率、病死率、血清白蛋白水平、Ⅰ级护理时间、Ⅱ级护理时间及住院时间。

（9）**方法**：2005 年 10 月至 2007 月 9 月对 1200 例患者采用一次性包皮环切吻合器进行手术，患者年龄 5～95 岁，其中包皮过长 904 例，包茎 296 例。

（10）**方法**：采用细胞外微电极记录技术，记录大鼠海马脑片 CA1 区群峰电位（PS）幅值和高频刺激诱发 LTP 后 PS 的增幅。

5-2　将下列句子中的部分汉语译成英语

1. The present prospective ＿＿＿＿＿＿＿（随机控制性）parallel study was conducted on 93 blood culture-proven Salmonella typhi children. All MDRTF cases were ＿＿＿＿＿（随机分成）treatment with ofloxacin or ceftriaxone.

2. ＿＿＿＿＿＿＿＿＿（81 例 ARF 患者的资料）were retrospectively＿＿＿＿＿＿（收集）. ＿＿＿＿＿＿＿（入选标准）: 5 to 15 years of age and diagnosis of ARF confirmed by 2 or more rheumatologists, ＿＿＿＿＿＿＿＿＿（持续 6 个月以上）and two or more visits.

3. Children of age 24-47 months were ＿＿＿＿＿＿＿＿＿＿（采用系统随机抽样法选择）. Information on socio-demographic factors and immunization status was obtained by house-to- house visit. ＿＿＿＿＿＿＿＿＿（疫苗免疫接种率）was computed and analysis of association between immunization coverage and socio-demographic factors was done.

4. This ＿＿＿＿＿＿＿＿＿＿＿＿（前瞻性分析研究）was ＿＿＿＿＿（做）among 400 cases, selected by simple sampling from neonates with late onset jaundice admitted in two referral hospitals of Isfahan during a 9-month period. The ＿＿＿＿＿（资料包括）the age, sex and feeding type, as well as the results of physical examination, treatment, radiology studies, etc were recorded. The etiology of jaundice was＿＿＿＿＿＿＿（经生化检测）. Urine analysis and urine culture were ＿＿＿＿＿＿（做）for all subjects. XZ and t-test were used for analysis of the data in- SPSS software.

5. Radiological chest examinations were performed for 88 children before and after remedial operations. Pre- and postoperative chest radiograph and CT were performed to ＿＿＿＿＿＿＿（测定）transversal chest width; sagittal left chest side depth, sagittal right chest side depth, sternovertebral distance, and vertebral body length. Derivative indices were also estimated: Vertebral index (VI), Frontosagittal index (FI), Haller index (HI)and asymmetry index. Computerized assessment of data was used. For＿＿＿＿＿＿（统计分析）, the software "Statistica 6.0" was used.

6. A ＿＿＿＿＿＿＿＿＿＿＿＿＿（单盲随机控制试验）created from the two week

placebo run-in periods for two nested trials that _____（比较）acupuncture and amitriptyline with their respective placebo controls. _____（对象比较）who remained on placebo continued beyond the run-in period_____（试验结束）.

7. Prospective study in NICU for three months. The nurses were asked to assess whether a baby is sick or not on the basis of observed_____（物理变量）. Both the nurses and the attending physician _____（做出评估）on a progress sheet separately. _____（统计学分析）to see the agreement of the nurses with the doctors in respect to the sickness assessment, treatment, _____（最终结果）and the agreement between the symptoms picked up by the nurses and the doctors.

8. _____（不同水平）inflammatory mediators were _____（测定）in the bronchoalveolar lavage（BAL）fluid and serum on days 1 and 4 after the identification of the pulmonary complication in 127 patients with different immunosuppressive conditions.

9. Amoebas _____（治疗）20% of human, bovine and swine milk, with 10% of human milk fractions (i.e., casein, proteins except casein and fat) or_____（用）1 mg/ml of human milk apo-lactoferrin, human secretory immunoglobulin type A (sIgA) and chicken egg-white lysozyme (i.e., purified proteins). Milk proteins _____（用……检测）immunoblot. Confocal microscopy was_____（用来）define the interaction of milk proteins (100 μM each) and amoebas. Experiments were _____（做）at least three times in triplicate, and mean and standard deviations were calculated.

10. _____（前瞻性随机单盲控制研究）was _____（采用）at a university-affiliated hospital in Israel. Institutional Research Ethics Board approved the study. Infants who were 0 to 2 months of age and presented to the emergency department with fever and therefore required urine collection for culture were_____（随机平均分成）into 2 sample collection groups: Suprapubic aspiration or transurethral catheterization. Patients _____（排除）when they were born prematurely or had had a previous sepsis workup or other painful procedures or an anomaly of the urogenital system or abdominal wall.

第六章 医学论文英文摘要"Results"写作

英文摘要的"Results"部分重点阐述研究中观察到的现象、发现的问题、获得的资料、确定的关系及达到的效果和效能等内容，对研究目的及其所提出的问题做出直接应答，是作者主要劳动成果的结晶。"结果"部分所涉及的内容必须是作者在实际研究中所获得的客观数据和发现，因此，"结果"部分的内容必须完整、清晰、准确、无误。无论是摘要还是正文，"Results"应避免单纯罗列大量原始资料，而应对资料进行统计学处理和科学的组织后，再按逻辑思维顺序依次列出。尽管不同论文摘要"Results"部分内容千差万别，但其写作仍有一定的规律可循，本章结合实例介绍如何撰写"Results"。

一、"Results"总体写作要求

英文摘要中的"Results"，作者必须凸显在研究工作中所观察到的客观资料和重要发现，以文字描述和（或）统计学资料体系研究发现（结果）的可信度及准确性。英文需用完整句子，谓语动词采用过去时态，研究所得资料如百分数、血压等数字采用临床病例书写形式，不必用书面英文表达。此外，撰写医学论文英文摘要"Results"部分尚需注意以下几个方面。

1. 避免使用疑问句和感叹句，注意正确使用简化字和标点符号。

2. "Results"以文字描述方式给出研究所获的资料，如果所涉及的资料较多，叙述的顺序可按重要性大小排列，如先叙述主要实验结果，接着叙述次要结果，最后给出对照组的结果；亦可先叙述对照组的结果和次要结果，然后重点描述主要结果，但一定要突出研究的关键性资料。

3. 注意使用定性和定量的词汇，而模糊资料，如 probably、possibly、approximately、about、rare 等应避免使用，另外，如"Thirteen out of 100 cases（100 例中的 13 例）"不要写成"A small portion out of 100 cases（100 例中的小部分）"。

4. 尽可能使用规范术语，对已经规范化了的人名、地名、机构名称及本专业读者能清楚理解的已经规范化了的缩略语、略称、代号（如 DNA 等），需使用通用的规范名称，其余的代号首次出现时应给出全称。注意使用法定计量单位、国际单位和国际通用符号，不用非公知公认的符号和术语，否则，会影响读者对文章内容的把握。

5. 所用的人称一般为第三人称。

6. 英文动词时态必须与事情发生时间相一致。"Results"部分主要叙述研究中所获得的客观资料及所观察到的现象，这一切均发生在作者撰写论文之前，故常采用一般过去时态。若叙述客观存在或基本规律，可用一般现在时。

7. 英文摘要中的"Results"，只能使用统计学处理后的结果数据来说明差异或某种情形的趋势变化，不可使用图表。

8. 无论是摘要还是正文中的"Results"，都是作者本人的研究结果，着重叙述客观研究发现资料，因此，不要掺杂前人或他人的探索研究工作，更不要加入个人对结果优劣性的主观评价。

让我们初步感知和熟悉结构式和非结构式摘要中的"Results"写作方法及内容描述的差异。

例一：【**Summary**】Criteria for diagnosis of Alzheimer's disease (AD) is not available in China. The international criteria is not a proper choice due to issues such as translation and lead to low diagnostic rate and high rate of missed diagnosis. The research group of Alzheimer's Disease Chinese (ADC) reviewed knowledge and techniques in neuropsychology, neuroimaging, molecular biology, and clinical neurology, and systematically studied the detection techniques such as memory, language, visuospatial, executive function, and medial temporal lobe visual scores on MRI, and their optimal threshold and diagnostic value for the diagnosis of AD. Through a systematic review and consensus meeting, a diagnostic framework for screening AD in the Chinese population was established. Among these methods, an operational standard for clinical pathology models increased the diagnostic sensitivity by 15%. The sensitivity and specificity of screening memory impairment increased by 18.1% and 11.6% , respectively. The sensitivity of screening medial temporal lobe atrophy increased by 24.5% and missed diagnosis was decreased by 34.5%. An operational standard for clinical biology models, incorporating the latest molecular imaging and molecular biology techniques, has enabled the early diagnosis of AD in China. The framework combines a principled diagnostic guideline with an operational screening protocol, which is applicable to all clinical settings and of great significance for the early detection, early diagnosis and early treatment of AD.

【提要】阿尔茨海默病诊断无中国标准，采用国际标准因语言环境等因素影响，我国痴呆诊断率低且漏诊率高。本研究小组利用神经心理学、神经影像学、分子生物学、临床神经病学等知识和技术，对阿尔茨海默病诊断涉及的记忆、语言、视空间、执行、行为和功能以及磁共振成像内侧颞叶视觉评分等检测技术及其最佳阈值和诊断价值进行了系统研究，并通过小组专家共识方式，建立了适用于中国人群的阿尔茨海默病筛查和诊断框架，改善了我国阿尔茨海默病的诊断率和准确度。其中，一个临床病理学模式的操作标准性能达到了同类技术的领先水平，使诊断敏感度提高 15%，筛查记忆损害的敏感度和特异度分别提高 18.1%和11.6%，检出内侧颞叶萎缩的敏感度提高 24.5%，漏诊率下降 34.5%；一个临床生物学模式的操作标准将诊断标准下的最新分子影像学和分子生物学诊断参数整合到框架中，推动我国阿尔茨海默病早期诊断技术迈向国际先进水平。该框架是原则性的诊断标准与操作性的诊断参数相结合的产物，适用于我国临床环境，对阿尔茨海默病早发现、早诊断、早治疗具有重要意义。

引自:《中华内科杂志》, 2019, 58(2): 91

例二：Importantly, we revealed that PDGF-CC targeting acted not only on multiple cell types important for pathological angiogenesis, such as vascular mural and endothelial cells, macrophages, choroidal fibroblasts and retinal pigment epithelial cells, but also on the expression of other important angiogenic genes, such as PDGF-BB and PDGF receptors. At a molecular level, we found that PDGF-CC regulated glycogen synthase kinase (GSK)-3beta phosphorylation and expression both *in vitro* and *in vivo*. Activation of GSK3beta impaired PDGF-CC-induced angiogenesis, and inhibition of GSK3beta abolished the antiangiogenic effect of PDGF-CC blockade.

重要的是，我们发现 PDGF-CC 靶向不仅作用于对病理性血管生成起重要作用的多种细胞（如血管壁和内皮细胞、巨噬细胞、脉络膜成纤维细胞、视网膜色素上皮细胞），而且影响其他重要的血管新生基因（如 PDGF-BB 和 PDGF 受体）的表达。我们发现 PDGF-CC 在体内和体外分子水平调控糖原合成酶激酶（GSK）-3β 磷酸化和表达。活化 GSK3β 可损伤 PDGF-CC 诱导的血管生成，抑制 GSK3β 可影响 PDGF-CC 阻断抗血管生成作用。

引自: *Proc Natl Acad Sci*, 2010, 107(27): 12216

例三：【Findings】Between June 13, 2016, and Oct 27, 2017, we enrolled and assessed 1035 women with suspected pre-eclampsia. 12 (1%) women were found to be ineligible. Of the 1023 eligible women, 576 (56%) women were assigned to the intervention (revealed testing) group, and 447 (44%) women were assigned to receive usual care with additional concealed testing (concealed testing group). Three (1%) women in the revealed testing group were lost to follow-up, so 573 (99%) women in this group were included in the analyses. One (<1%) woman in the concealed testing group withdrew consent to follow-up data collection, so 446 (>99%) women in this group were included in the analyses. The median time to pre-eclampsia diagnosis was 4.1 days with concealed testing versus 1.9 days with revealed testing (time ratio 0.36, 95% CI 0.15-0.87; $P=0.027$). Maternal severe adverse outcomes were reported in 24 (5%) of 447 women in the concealed testing group versus 22 (4%) of 573 women in the revealed testing group (adjusted odds ratio 0.32, 95% CI 0.11-0.96; $P=0.043$), but there was no evidence of a difference in perinatal adverse outcomes (15% $vs.$ 14%, 1.45, 0.73-2.90) or gestation at delivery (36.6 weeks $vs.$ 36.8 weeks; mean difference -0.52, 95% CI -0.63 to 0.73).

【结果】在 2016 年 6 月 13 日至 2017 年 10 月 27 日期间，我们纳入并评估了 1035 名疑似子痫前期妇女，其中 12 名（1%）妇女不符合纳入条件。在 1023 名符合条件的妇女中，576 名（56%）纳入干预（暴露检测）组，447 名（44%）纳入其他隐蔽试验（隐蔽检测组）常规护理组。在披露的检测组中，有 3 名（1%）妇女失访，最终有 573 名（99%）妇女被纳入本研究，但隐蔽检测组中有一名对象（<1%）在我们随访数据收集过程中主动退出，因此，最终纳入本组的实际对象为 446 人（>99%）。子痫前期诊断隐蔽试验的中位时间为 4.1 天，暴露试验为 1.9 天（时间比：0.36，95%CI 0.15～0.87；$P=0.027$）。隐蔽试验组 447 名妇女中有 24 名（5%）报告了产妇严重不良结局，而暴露试验组 573 名妇女中有 22 名（4%）报告了产妇严重不良结局（调整后的优势比 0.32，95%CI 0.11～0.96；$P=0.043$），但没有证据表明围产期（15% $vs.$ 14%，1.45，0.73～2.90）或分娩时（36.6 $vs.$ 36.8 周）存在不良结局（平均差为 -0.52，95% CI -0.63～0.73）。

引自：*Lancet*, 2019, 393: 1807

例四：【Results】The recovery time of conscious and spontaneous breathing in group D were significantly shorter than that in group C ($P<0.05$). The MAP and HR of the two groups at T_1-T_5 were significantly lower than those at T_0 ($P<0.05$). The levels of P_{peak} in group C at T_3-T_5 was significantly higher than those in group D ($P<0.05$). The SpO_2 values in the group D at T_1-T_5 were significantly higher than those in group C ($P<0.05$). The $P(A-a)O_2$ values in the group D at T_1-T_5 was significantly lower than those in group C ($P<0.05$). The levels of IL-6, IL-8 and MDA in group D at T_1-T_5 were significantly lower than those in group C ($P<0.05$). The levels of IL-10 and SOD in group D at T_1-T_5 were significantly higher than those in group C ($P<0.05$). The values of IQA, AI, and the expression of CHOP mRNA and their protein in the two groups at T_4 were significantly higher than those at T_2 ($P<0.05$). The values of IQA, AI, and the expression of CHOP mRNA and their protein in group D at T_4 were significantly lower than those in group C ($P<0.05$).

【结果】D 组患者术后清醒和自主呼吸恢复时间均显著短于 C 组（均 $P<0.05$）；两组患者 T_1～T_5 时刻 MAP、HR 水平显著低于 T_0 时刻。C 组

患者 $T_3 \sim T_5$ 时刻 P_{peak} 水平均显著高于 D 组（均 $P<0.05$）。D 组患者 $T_1 \sim$ T_5 时刻 SpO_2 均显著高于 C 组，P（A-a）O_2 水平均显著低于 C 组（均 $P<0.05$）。D 组患者 $T_1 \sim T_5$ 时 IL-6、IL-8 和 MDA 水平均显著低于 C 组，IL-10 和 SOD 水平均显著高于 C 组（均 $P<0.05$）。两组患者 T_4 时刻 IQA、AI 及 CHOP mRNA 和蛋白表达水平均显著高于 T_2 时刻（均 $P<0.05$），且 D 组 T_4 时刻 IQA、AI 及 CHOP mRNA 和蛋白表达水平显著低于 C 组（均 $P<0.05$）。

引自:《中华医学杂志》, 2020, 100(1): 37

从上述四个实例中我们可以发现，非结构式摘要和结构式摘要对"Results"的描述存在一定的差异。例一在"结果"中给出的是重点数据；例二则直接陈述重要发现；例三和例四虽然同为结构式摘要，但例三以统计学处理后的重点数据独立呈现，而例四则以同样的方式，以更为详细的数据，对研究结果进行对比，从而突出研究结果的差异。

二、"Results"写作中的常用词及短语

遣词造句是一项非常重要的基本功，通过翻阅大量医学期刊，就会发现医学论文英文摘要"Results"部分中存在一定数量使用频率相对较高的词汇和和短语，在此枚举部分，希望对提高读者的写作水平有所帮助。

（一）常用名词

（1）总结"Results"时，常需要对某些成分或指标的表达水平予以描述，多数作者会选用名词 level。

例一： Both low EF and diastolic dysfunction were independently related to higher **levels** of BNP.

EF 降低及舒张功能不全均与 BNP 水平升高独立相关。

引自: *JAMA*, 2006, 296(18): 2209

例二： The **level** of Ki-67 expression in low grade NHL was lower than that in high grade（$P<0.01$）

Ki-67 在低度恶性 NHL 组中的表达低于高度恶性组（$P<0.01$）

引自:《中华内科杂志》, 2001, 40(7): 452

（2）由于"Results"中主要转述的是客观资料，因此，常用第三人称形式表述（注：这是国内期刊普遍认可的形式，但国外期刊用第一人称复数形式较为常见，如上述一、例三：we enrolled…），如使用"the result of"或"results in"作主语引导所观察到的现象、发现的问题及获得的资料。尽管如此，对"结果"描述时，基于语境信息较为明显，在结构式摘要中应尽可能避免使用"The results of…showed that…"这种表达。因为结构

式摘要中的标题词"Results"本身就提示了"结果",所以撰写结构式摘要"Results"时,直接描述"结果"即可,此可避免冗词。当然,如何措辞不能一概而论,具体情况要根据语篇衔接的需要。

例一：**The results of** serologic tests **showed that** 7 cases were infected by hepatitis B alone and other 2 cases were superinfected with hepatitis B and hepatitis E virus.

乙型肝炎病毒感染 7 例,乙型肝炎病毒、戊型肝炎病毒重叠感染 2 例。

引自:《中华传染病杂志》,2000, 18(2): 166

例二：**Results in** situ hybridization were in conformity with that of immunohistochemistry / Western blot in our research.

原位杂交与免疫组织化学染色和（或）Western blot 结果具有一致性。

引自:《中华病理学杂志》,2000, 29(1): 85

例三：**Results revealed** significantly improved naming accuracy of treated items $(F[1,9]=5.72, P<0.040)$ after anodal tDCS compared with sham tDCS. Patients who demonstrated the most improvement were those with perilesional areas closest to the stimulation site. Crucially, this treatment effect persisted at least 1 week after treatment.

结果显示,与假 tDCS 治疗相比,正极 tDCS 对治疗项的命名准确性有显著改善（F[1,9] = 5.72, $P<0.040$）。改善最大的患者为病灶区接近刺激点的患者。重要的是,这种治疗效果最低能持续到治疗后 1 周。

注：tDCS 意为 transcranial direct-current stimulation(经颅直流刺激)。

引自: *Stroke,* 2010, 41(6): 1229

（3）"Results"句中涉及研究对象（病例）、样品及标本时,英文常用 patients、participants、subjects、case、sample、specimen 等词来表示。

例一：Among the 1856 diabetic participants, 96 had youth-onset type 2 diabetes mellitus. The age-sex–adjusted incidence of diabetic ESRD was 25.0 **cases** per 1000 person-years.

在 1856 例糖尿病参试者中,96 例为年轻发病。校正年龄及性别后,年轻发病 2 型糖尿病者终末期肾疾病（ESRD）的发生率为每 1000 人年 25.0 例。

引自: *JAMA,* 2006, 296: 421

例二：The present study included 12 **cases**, 1 males and 11 females, average age was(40±13)years.

12 例患者中男 1 例,女 11 例,平均年龄（40±13）岁。

引自:《中华医学杂志》,2020, 100(12): 938

例三：The mean (SD) age of trial **participants** was (62.9±10.7) years and increased from (62.3 ±11.2) years in 2001-2006 to (64.0±10.4) years in 2013-2018 $(P =0.01)$.

试验参与者的平均年龄（SD）为（62.9±10.7）岁，从 2001～2006 年的（62.3±11.2）岁增加至 2013～2018 年的（64.0±10.4）岁（$P=0.01$）。

引自：*JAMA Cardiol*, 2020, doi: 101001/jamacardio20200359

例四： Monospecific anti-Ro52 reactivity was found in 51 (12.7%) of the 402 **samples** tested.

402 例检测血清样本中，发现 51 例（12.7%）有单一特异性抗 Ro52 抗体。

引自：*Postgrad Med J*, 2010, 86(1012): 79

例五： E-CD was expressed in all of 10 **specimens** of normal cervical epithelia.

正常宫颈上皮组织中 E-CD 100%表达。

引自：《中华肿瘤杂志》, 2000, 22(5): 496

（4）"Results" 中描述两组或多组实验结果之间的差异，常用名词 difference。

例一： Nonfatal acute MI occurred in 321 (7.2%) and 267 (6.0%) in the 2 groups (HR, 0.83; 95% CI, 0.71-0.98; $P=0.02$), but no **differences** were seen in the 2 other components of the primary end point.

两组发生非致命性 MI 者分别为 321 例（7.2%）和 267 例（6.0%）（HR, 0.83；95%CI, 0.71～0.98；$P=0.02$）。但是另外两个一级终点指标两组未见显著性差异。

引自：*JAMA*, 2005, 294(19): 2437

例二： The **difference** between the 2 groups of patients were statistically significant.

两组患者间差异有显著性(与预防组相比)。

引自：《中华肿瘤杂志》, 2000, 22(4): 315

例三： Among the abnormal genes, the mutation frequency of U2AF1 (37.3%) and ASXL1 (41.6%) were higher, and there were significant **differences** in mutation burden among different abnormal genes ($F=91.946$, $P<0.001$). There were differences in the number of gene mutations among different subtypes of MDS, and the number of EB-2 gene mutations was the highest (2.2±1.5).

MDS 患者检出异常基因中，U2AF1（37.3%）和 ASXL1（41.6%）等突变频率较高，且不同异常基因间突变负荷间差异有统计学意义（$F=91.946$，$P<0.001$）。不同亚型 MDS 患者，基因突变个数存在差异，EB-2 型基因突变个数最多（2.2±1.5）个。

引自：《中华医学杂志》, 2020, 100(12) : 933

（5）在提到新方法、新途径时通常要与实际情况相比较，表述新方法与实际情况误差时，常用 deviation，意为 the difference、especially the absolute difference、between one number in a set and the mean of the set（误差，偏差）。

例一： The **deviation** of the software measurement was less than 4% of actual size at most in our reliability demonstration.

软件测量经初步证实其最大误差小于 4%。

引自:《中华整形外科杂志》, 2000, 16(1): 87

例二: The adjusted relative risk (95% confidence interval [CI]) of MI associated with each standard **deviation** increase in anxiety variable was 1.37 (95% CI 1.12 to 1.68) for psychasthenia...

心肌梗死相关的焦虑变量升高的标准差校正的相对危险度为 1.37（95% CI, 1.12～1.68）……

引自: *JACC*, 2008, 51(2): 113

（6）"Results"句中通常需要对分子生物学中某一因素的表达水平进行阐述,可用英文单词 expression。

例一: Our data show that MLL germline infant ALL specifies a gene **expression** pattern that is different from both MLL-rearranged infant ALL and pediatric precursor B-ALL.

数据显示,混合型白血病(MLL)种系婴儿急性淋巴母细胞白血病(ALL)所特有的一种基因表达类型,与 MLL-重排婴儿 ALL 和小儿前体 B-ALL 都有所不同。

引自: *Blood*, 2010, 115(14) : 2835

例二: The **expression** of Prrx2 decreased 91.2% in MDA-MB-231 cells and 88.7% in MCF-7 cells after transfection with interfering vectors ($P<0.05$).

转染干扰载体后 MDA-MB-231 细胞 Prrx2 表达水平下降 91.2%；MCF-7 细胞表达水平下降 88.7%, 差异均具有统计学意义（$P<0.05$）。

引自:《中华医学杂志》, 2020, 100(12): 942

例三: Immunohistochemical staining revealed that the positive rate of MMP-7 protein was 67.3% in colorectal carcinoma and 30.0% in controls ($P<0.05$); the **expression** of MVD was 41.32±6.39 in the colorectal carcinoma and 24.17±6.23 in controls ($P<0.05$).

大肠癌及对照组 MMP-7 的表达水平分别为 67.3%和 30.0%（$P<0.05$）, MVD 在大肠癌及对照组的表达分别为 41.32±6.39、24.17±6.23（$P<0.05$）。

引自:《第四军医大学学报》, 2007, 28(6): 506

（二）常用动词及其结构和用法

"Results"部分的写作常涉及对研究中所观察到的事实或所发现的现象予以陈述,或陈述数量的增减,或对研究数据予以比较等。然而,英语语言有别于汉语,如可数名词有单复数形式变化,动词不仅涉及主谓一致、动词形式变化,而且某些动词还有其特定的搭配使用要求。本节拟将"Results"写作中一些使用频率较高的动词就其意念功能和搭配归类如下。

（1）陈述研究、实验、调查所获得的结果，即所观察或所发现的事实。常涉及动词：show、find、observe、see、suggest、indicate、reveal、document、demonstrate、exhibit 等。动词形式取其过去式。针对不同的语篇衔接或篇章逻辑关联，这类动词可有主动或被动结构表达形式。动词句型如下：

1）The result(s) showed that...　　　　　结果表明……

2）The result(s) suggested that...　　　　结果表明……

3）The result(s) indicated that...　　　　结果表明……

4）The result(s) revealed that...　　　　结果表明……

5）The result(s) documented that...　　　结果表明……

6）The result(s) demonstrated that...　　结果表明……

7）We found that…　　　　　　　　　（我们）发现……

8）We observed that…　　　　　　　　（我们）观察到……

9）It was found that…　　　　　　　　（我们）发现……

10）It was seen that…　　　　　　　　（我们）观察到……

11）It was observed that…　　　　　　（我们）观察到……

12）It was found to…　　　　　　　　（我们）发现……

例一： Comparison within the cohort **showed that** mild hypothyroidism prior to T_4 therapy was associated with increased risk of mortality from ischemic heart disease *vs.* biochemical euthyroidism (HR, 2.08; 95% CI, 1.04-4.19).
队列内比较显示，与甲状腺生化检查正常者比较，T_4 治疗前轻度甲状腺功能不全与缺血性心脏病的死亡危险增加相关（HR，2.08；95% CI，1.04～4.19）。

引自：*JAMA*, 2005, 294: 71

例二： Analysis of the first 5 minutes of each resuscitation by 30-second segments **revealed that** chest compression rates were less than 90/min in 28.1% of segments.
按照 30 秒时段对每例复苏最初 5 分钟进行分析发现，在 28.1% 的时段胸外按压频率低于 90 次/分。

引自：*JAMA*, 2005, 293: 305

例三： We **found that** housekeeping genes tend to be less polymorphic than tissue-specific genes for both rare and common single-nucleotide polymorphisms SNPs.
（我们）发现，对于罕见或常见单核苷酸多态现象，持家基因少见于组织特异性基因。

引自：*Mol Biol Evol*, 2009, 21: 236

例四： Euthyroid, subfertile women with TAI undergoing IVF **demonstrated** significantly higher risk for miscarriage compared with controls (four studies-fixed effects RR:

1.99, 95% confidence interval: 1.42-2.79, $P<0.001$).

与对照组相比，甲状腺功能正常，但生育力低下且伴有甲状腺自身免疫（TAI）疾病的女性，接受体外受精（IVF）后其流产风险更高（4 项研究固定效应 RR：1.99，95%CI：1.42～2.79，$P<0.001$）。

引自：Eur J Endocrinol, 2010, 162(4): 643

例五： Similar reductions **were seen** in levels of serum apolipoprotein B, triglycerides, and Lp(a) lipoprotein.

血清载脂蛋白 B、甘油三酯、Lp（a）脂蛋白水平出现类似的下降。

引自：N Engl J Med, 2010, 362(10)：906

例六： Increased risks of all-cause and circulatory deaths *vs.* age- and period-specific mortality **were observed** in follow-up in those not requiring, or prior to, T_4 therapy.

随访发现无需 T_4 治疗或 T_4 治疗之前的患者中，与相应年龄段和时间段内死亡率相比，患者全因死亡和循环系统疾病死亡危险增加。

引自：JAMA, 2005, 294: 71

例七： This analysis **revealed that** reduced levels of C4, but not C3, were independently associated with the two-month pre-flare period.

分析结果显示，C4 水平降低（而非 C3），与发作前两个月的病程有独立的联系。

引自：Lupus, 2010, 19(11): 1272

例八： No significant association was found between intraoperative $rScO_2$ values and POCD.

未发现术中局部脑氧饱和度($rScO_2$)值和术后认知功能障碍（POCD）之间存在显著相关性。

引自：Br J Anaesth, 2019, 123(2): 196-205

例九： Stratified analyses **indicated that** smoking duration was associated with lower PD risk within fixed intensities of smoking.

分层分析提示，吸烟持续时间在固定吸烟强度时与较低帕金森病（PD）发生危险相关。

引自：Neurology, 2010, 74(11): 878

例十： At the end of the 3-month treatment period, the RSV-PLC group (*n*=71) **exhibited** significantly elevated EDN levels ($P<0.0001$).

治疗 3 个月末，与初始水平相比，RSV-PLC 组（*n*=71）患者 EDN 水平显著升高（$P<0.0001$）。

引自：J Pediatr, 2010, 156(5)：749

（2）研究结果中常需要对观测到的各种数据指标的数量变化予以描述，即数量的增减或生化/生理指标的上升或下降等。常用动词：increase、rise、raise、go up、elevate、decrease、fall、reduce、decline、drop、lower 等。与这些动词连用的主要介词为 by 或 to，但要注意 by 或 to 所表达的意义有所不同。By（to the amount or degree of）表示纯增、减净数，不包括底数在内，即实际增加或减少的数目，在句中可以省略。例如："Cell number increased by almost 50% during the first 24 h after the beginning of treatment."。又如："He is older than I by three years." 等于"He is three years older than I."。而 to（until and including）表示增加到什么数目，不是纯增减数。简单地说，包括底数。例如："Cell number increased to 1000"（1000 包括在内）。除此之外，还要注意上述动词在表达概念时其语义搭配。

1）结果写作中常见概念动词搭配（表 6-1）

表 6-1　结果写作中常见概念动词搭配

概念范畴	上升/增加	下降/减少
体温（temperature）	raise, rise, go up	decrease, drop, lower
血压（blood pressure）	elevate	drop, fall, lower
抵抗力（resistance）	strengthen, increase, build up	fall, weaken, lower
体重（body weight）	gain, put on	lose, reduce
心输出量（cardiac output）	increase	reduce, decrease
细胞数（cell count）	increase	decrease
颅内压（intracranial pressure）	elevate	lower, fall, drop
疼痛（pain/suffering）	aggravate	alleviate, ease
出生率（birth rate）	increase, rise	decline
增长率（increase rate）	increase	decline, decrease, slow
通透性（permeability）	increase	decrease
血容量（blood volume）	increase	decrease
血流（blood flow）	increase	decrease
组织灌注（tissue perfusion）	increase	decrease
炎性反应（inflammatory reaction）	exacerbate	abate
风险（系数）（risks）	increase, rise	decrease, reduce
事件（疾病）发生率（incidence）	increase, rise, rebound	decrease, fall, drop
生化指标（biochemical indicator）	ascend, increase	reduce, lower, descend
面积（area）	enlarge, extend	reduce
程度（degree）	improve, enhance	fall, reduce
基因/蛋白表达（gene/protein expression）	enhance, up-regulate	inhibit, down-regulate

2）用法例举

例一：There was a decrease in BMI in both treatment groups up to week 12, thereafter stabilizing with orlistat but **increasing** beyond baseline with placebo. At the end of the study, BMI had **decreased** by 0.55 with orlistat but **increased by** 0.31 with placebo (P=0 .001).

至 12 周时，两组 BMI 均有下降；此后，奥利司他组体重维持稳定而安慰剂组则超过基线。研究结束时，奥利司他组 BMI 下降 0.55，而安慰剂组则增加 0.31（$P=0.001$）。

引自：JAMA, 2005, 293: 2873

例二： Recipient diabetes, age, male gender, African American race, **elevated** peak panel reactive antibody and increased cold ischemia time were independent risk factors for delayed graft function.

移植受体者罹患糖尿病、年龄、男性、非洲裔美国人、群体反应性抗体峰值升高、冷凝血时间延长等是导致移植肾功能延迟恢复（DGF）的独立危险因素。

引自：Am J Transplant, 2010, 10(2)：298

例三： At 6 months, fasting insulin levels were significantly **reduced** from baseline in the intervention groups (all $P<0.01$), whereas DHEAS and glucose levels were unchanged.

6 个月时，各干预组空腹血糖水平较基线明显降低（均 $P<0.01$），而 DHEAS 和葡萄糖水平没有改变。

引自：JAMA, 2006, 295: 1539

例四： Finally, compared with control normal mice and to young preautoimmune (NZBxNZW)F1 animals, the frequency of cells secreting autoantibodies reacting with peptide 1-25 was significantly **raised** in the spleen and bone marrow.

最后，与对照正常小鼠和幼年预先自身免疫（NZBxNZW）F1 的动物相比，脾脏和骨髓中细胞分泌自身抗体（与肽 1-25 反应自身抗体）的频率显著增加。

引自：J Immunol, 2010, 184(7): 3937

例五： HRs for stroke were non-significantly **raised** for subjects with asymptomatic CHD (1.36 (0.47, 3.91)).

无症状 CHD 受试者卒中的风险率（HRs）无显著增加[1.36(0.47~3.91)]。

引自：Eur Heart J, 2008, 29(1)：327

例六： Although mortality for CABG surgery overall **declined** significantly over time (P for trend <0.0001), mortality for CS patients undergoing CABG did not change significantly during the 4-year study period ($P=0.07$).

尽管冠状动脉旁路移植术（CABG）死亡率随着时间在逐步下降（趋势 $P<0.0001$），在 4 年研究期内心源性休克（CS）患者接受 CABG 的死亡率没有显著改变（$P=0.07$）。

引自：Circulation, 2008, 117(7)：876

例七： Nicotine exposure upregulated the expression of hypoxia inducible factor 1alpha and vascular endothelial growth factor and **enhanced** angiogenesis but inhibited the expression of bone morphogenetic protein 2 and impaired bone healing.

尼古丁使缺氧诱导因子-1α和血管内皮生长因子的表达上调，并增加了血管形成，但抑制了骨形态发生蛋白2的表达，并影响骨的愈合。

引自: *J Bone Miner Res*, 2010, 25(6): 1305

（3）对研究所发现的"结果"进行比较或对比时，常用的动词有 compare。该动词常与介词 with 或 to 连用，搭配意义有所不同。"'Compare with' is often used when looking at the ways in which two things are like and unlike each other.", 即比较两件事物的异同时使用 compare with。而 "'Compare to' is often used when showing that two things are alike.", 即在表示两件事物相似的情况下常使用 compare to。

例一：**Compared with** the control group, the lead content in the rats' whole blood, faeces and urine of the poisoning group was significantly higher (*P*<0.01), selenium content in the whole blood and urine was significantly higher (*P*<0.05), while in the faeces was significantly lower (*P*<0.01).

与对照组相比，中毒组大鼠全血、粪便和尿液中铅含量均显著升高（*P*<0.01），全血和尿液中硒含量亦明显升高（*P*<0.05），粪便中硒含量明显降低（*P*<0.01）。

引自: *Studies of Trace Elements and Health,* 2006, 6: 22

例二：A significantly higher number of babies with ARF weighed less than 2500 g as **compared to** those without ARF (86.5% *vs.* 67.6%; *P*=0.008).

相对于未罹患急性肾衰竭婴儿来看，有相当数量的急性肾衰竭患儿体重普遍低于 2500 g（86.5% *vs.* 67.6%; *P*= 0.008）。

引自: *Ind J Pediatr*, 2006, 73(1): 19

例三：Patients with elevated levels of BNP at study entry and with BNP levels lower than 80 pg/ml at 4 months tended to have only modestly increased risk (HR, 1.7; 95% CI, 1.0-2.9) **compared with** patients with BNP levels lower than 80 pg/ml at both visits.

有些患者在进入研究和第4个月时 BNP 水平均小于 80 pg/ml，有些患者在进入研究时 BNP 水平有所升高。而在第4个月时 BNP 水平小于 80 pg/ml，与前者相比，后者出现死亡或新发 CHF 的危险略有增加（HR, 1.7；95%CI 1.0~2.9）。

引自: *JAMA*, 2005, 294: 2866

例四：There were 16 patients in 869 UC inpatients who were diagnosed with CRC during a period of 7548 person years and the incidence rate of UC-CRC was 1.84%. **Compared to** UC inpatients without CRC, a longer course of disease (OR=1.087, 95% CI:1.046-1.129), a lower usage rate of 5-Aminosalicylic Acid(5-ASA) (OR=0.218, 95% CI:0.052-0.915) and a higher incidence rate of intestinal stenosis (OR=16.533, 95% CI:3.824-71.478) were found in UC inpatients with CRC.

869 例 UC 患者共随访 7548 人年，其中有 16 例患者发生了结直肠癌，结直肠癌的发生率为 1.84%。与 UC 不合并结直肠癌患者相比，UC 合并结直肠癌患者病程较长（OR=1.087，95% CI：1.046～1.129）、5-氨基水杨酸（5-ASA）应用比例较低（OR=0.218，95% CI：0.052～0.915）、肠梗阻的发生率较高（OR=16.533，95% CI：3.824～71.478）。

引自:《中华医学杂志》, 2020, 100(8): 599

在结果的写作中，除了用动词之外，另一种常见表达是使用 compare 的同根名词，如 in comparison with 或 in contrast, on the contrary。

例一： **In contrast**, MGMT status determined by Q-RT-PCR and IHC showed little or no correlation with overall survival.

相比之下，由 Q-RT-PCR 和免疫组织化学决定的 MGMT 的状况与整体存活率均没有相关性或相关性不大。

引自: *J Neurooncol*, 2010, 97(3) : 311

例二： Although increase of IMT in CB region was more pronounced (+26%) than that in CCA region (+13%) in patients with pheochromocytoma **in comparison with** essential hypertensive patients, the level of statistical significance was comparable (*P*=0.003 and *P*=0.007, respectively).

虽然与原发性高血压患者相比，嗜铬细胞瘤患者 CB 区 IMT（26%）的增加比 CCA 区（13%）更明显，但统计显著性水平相当（*P*=0.003 和 *P*=0.007）。

引自: *J Hum Hypertens*, 2009, 23: 350

（4）相关性表示法：描述研究结果中的相关性时常用动词：associate、correlate、equal、match、measure、connect 等。除此之外，还有某些名词或形容词也可表达这类概念，如 consistent。这类动词、形容词、名词常构成如下搭配。

1）...be associated with... 与……相关
2）...be inversely correlated with... 与……呈负相关
3）...be consistent with... 与……相一致
4）...be in relation to... 与……有关
5）...be connected with... 与……有关联
6）There was relationship/correlation/association between...and...
……与……之间有关
7）There was a relation/correlation of...and ... ……与……之间有关

例一： A total of 556 study participants underwent echocardiography at HF diagnosis. Preserved EF (50%) was present in 308 (55%) and was **associated with**

older age, female sex, and no history of myocardial infarction (all $P<0.001$).
共有 556 例参试者在确诊 HF 时接受了超声心动图检查。其中 EF 值正常（50%）者有 308 例（55%），多见于年长、女性和既往无心肌梗死病史的患者（均 $P<0.001$）。

引自：*JAMA*, 2006, 296: 2209

例二： No **correlation** existed between negative appendectomy rate and race, health insurance status, or hospital appendiceal rupture rate.
阴性阑尾切除率与种族、健康保险状况或医院阑尾穿孔发生率没有相关性。

引自：*JAMA*, 2004, 292: 1977

例三： It **was** not **related to** histologic type, but to histologic grade of the cancer .
（bc1-2 蛋白表达）与（乳腺）癌组织学类型无关，与组织学分级呈负相关。

引自：《中华肿瘤杂志》, 2000, 22(5): 490

例四： In this investigation, 414 nurses were screened with PTSD and 303 nurses without. IES-R score was negatively **correlated with** SSRS, CD-RISC and SES ($r=-0.275$, -0.202, -0.709, all $P<0.05$).
本研究中，414 名（57.7%）PTSD 阳性，303 名 PTSD 阴性。Spearman 相关分析发现，IES-R 评分与 SSRS、CD-RISC 及 SES 评分呈显著负相关（$r=-0.275$、$r=-0.202$、$r=-0.709$，均 $P<0.05$）。

引自：《中华医学杂志》, 2020, 100(1): 32

例五： Atrial tachycardia caused an upregulation of VCAM-1 expression, which was prevented by irbesartan, **consistent with** the observed increase in plasma levels of angiotensin Ⅱ.
依贝沙坦能阻止房性心动过速导致的 VCAM-1 表达上调，与血浆中血管紧张素Ⅱ增加一致。

引自：*Circulation*, 2008, 117(6): 732

（5）差异性表示法：研究结果中需要给出统计学上的差异时，主要用动词 differ，但使用时习惯上用其同根名词 difference 或形容词 different，可用下列结构表示。

1）There was very / highly significant difference in...between...and...

……与……之间有较大差异

2）No significant /Insignificant difference was found/observed/noted in...and...

……与……之间未发现差异

3）...be different from...　　……与……之间有差异

例一： At the low serum 25-hydroxyvitamin D level (<10 ng/ml), calcium intake of less than 800 mg/d *vs.* more than 1200 mg/d was significantly associated with higher serum PTH ($P=0.04$); and at a calcium intake of more than 1200 mg/d, **there was a significant difference between** the lowest **and** highest vitamin D groups ($P=0.04$).

当血清25-羟维生素D浓度较低时（＜10 ng/ml），与钙摄入量＞1200 mg/d组相比，钙摄入量＜800 mg/d组血清PTH浓度明显升高（P=0.04）。钙摄入量超过1200 mg/d时，最低和最高维生素D组之间（血清PTH浓度）有显著性差异(P=0.04)。

引自：JAMA, 2005, 294: 2336

例二： During the period 1999-2006, age-adjusted prevalences of anti-HBc (4.7%) and HBsAg (0.27%) were not **statistically different from** what they were during 1988-1994 (5.4% and 0.38%, respectively).

1999～2006年人群样本年龄校正的抗HBc（4.7%）和HBsAg（0.27%）检出率与1988～1994年人群样本相比差异无统计学意义（分别为5.4%和0.38%）。

引自：J Infect Dis, 2010, 202(2)：192

例三： **There were no significant group differences** in age, sex, incidence of diabetes mellitus, ethnicity, or contrast volume.

两组患者在年龄、性别、糖尿病发生、种族及造影剂用量方面无显著性差异。

引自：JAMA, 2004, 291: 2328

例四： These "metabolic adaptations" (−6% more than expected based on loss of metabolic mass) **were statistically different from** controls ($P<0.05$).

上述"代谢调节"（超出预计值的-6%），与对照组相比存在显著性差异（$P<0.05$）。

引自：JAMA, 2006, 295: 1539

（三）常用介词和连词

介词，又称前置词，是英语中最活跃的词类之一，特别是一些常用介词，搭配能力特别强，可用来表示种种不同的意思。介词在句子中起着广泛的联系词语的作用。英语中的介词大致分为两类：①简单介词，如about、under、without等。②复杂介词（由两个或两个以上单字构成），如according to、due to、out of等。与介词一样，连词也是一种虚词，它不能独立担任句子成分，而起着连接词与词、短语与短语、句子与句子的作用。尽管在庞大的英语词汇家族中，介词和连词犹如沧海一粟，但其用法却相当难以把握。因此，写好一篇医学论文英文摘要，除了需要熟练使用动词、名词外，还要能够选用恰当的介词、连词，从而使英语表达简洁，逻辑关系严谨。下面结合实例介绍部分在摘要写作中常用的介词和连词。

1. in

in为最为常见的介词之一，通常用来表示范围、界限、限度及时间。表示时间时，除了介词in外，还有介词within、after和before。在表达时间概念意义时，这四个介词的主要区别在于 in 和 within 用于表示将来的时间，in 意为 after the end of…，我们要表达将来一段时间之后准备做某事，时间状语中的介词必须用 in，而不能用 after，如 "The operation may be performed in a week"（不能用 after）。Within 意为 before the end of…，如 "The operation will be performed within an hour"（不能用 before）。After 和 before 用于表示过去的时间。

例一： **In** both hypothyroidism rats and normal controls, the contents of NO, activities of NOS and nNOS mRNA gene transcription levels (corrected by GAPDH m RNA) were highest in cerebella, higher in olfactory bulbs, and lowest in hippocampuses ($P<0.05$).

无论正常组还是早减组，NO 含量、NOS 活性及 nNOS mRNA 及转录水平（经 GAPDH m RNA 纠正）均以小脑为最高，嗅脑次之，海马最低（ $P<0.05$ ）。

引自:《中华内分泌代谢杂志》, 2000, 16(2): 172

例二： Pulmonary embolism was classified as unlikely **in** 2206 patients (66.7%).

2206 例患者（66.7%）分类为肺栓塞可能性小。

引自: *JAMA*, 2006, 295: 172

2. with

with 用法繁多，意义千差万别，难于详尽分类，但在摘要中主要涉及意义：①表示原因或理由；②引导一个表示方式的状语附加语；③表示伴随的情况或事态；With 后可接名词或动词 "V-ing 形式" 表示数量的增加等自变量的变化，研究结果的变化情况；④表达做某动作的方法和技术，但要注意与介词 by 在表达这一意义时的区别。在引导方式状语时，这两个词多数情况下可以互换用于表达做某动作的方法和技术，其区别在于：with 后接有形的具体物质名词（如工具、仪器等），by 后接表示概念一类的抽象名词，该名词代表的事物看不见、摸不着。例如：

例一： The mean follow-up was 18.1±13.3 months, during which 209 (67.6%) patients had at least 1 detected high atrial rate episode consistent **with** AF. Higher percentages of RA pacing were associated **with** a greater risk of postimplant AF, **with** its incidence increasing incrementally **with** quartiles of RA pacing: 44.6%, 64.3%, 79.7%, and 81.6%, respectively ($P <0.001$).

平均随访时间为（18.1±13.3）个月，其间有 209 例（67.6%）出现至少 1 次的快速心房颤动。高右心房起搏比率与术后心房颤动发生相关，随右心房起搏四分位比率增加，心房颤动发生率分别为 44.6%、64.3%、79.7% 和 81.6%（ $P < 0.001$ ）。

引自: *Am Heart J*, 2008, 155(1): 94

例二： **With** increasing duration of diabetes, Hb-AGE was significantly increased ($P<0.01$), which was positively correlated with blood glucose concentration and HbA1c content, but more closely correlated with the latter.

随着病程的延长，Hb-AGE 水平显著增高（$P<0.01$），与血糖和 HbA1c 呈显著性正相关，但与 HbA1c 的关系更密切。

引自：《中华内分泌代谢杂志》, 2000, 16(2): 180

3. among

among 常用于多个对象，包括在所述的若干或一类事物之内。

例一： **Among** 58 cases of early gravida, the positive rates of nested-PCR and virus isolation were 8.6% and 7% respectively.

58 例早期孕妇（血液标本）中，nested-PCR 检测阳性率为 8.6%，病毒分离阳性率为 7%。

引自：《中华传染病杂志》, 2000, 18(4): 250

例二： The prevalence of anti-HBc decreased **among** persons 6-19 years of age (from 1.9% to 0.6%; $P<0.01$) and 20-49 years of age (from 5.9% to 4.6%; $P<0.01$) but not among persons 50 years of age (7.2% *vs.* 7.7%).

6～19 岁（从 1.9%至 0.6%，$P<0.01$）和 20～49 岁（从 5.9%至 4.6%，$P<0.01$）人群的抗 HBc 率下降，但 50 岁人群的抗 HBc 阳性率没有降低（7.2% *vs.*7.7%）。

引自：*J Infect Dis*, 2010, 202(2): 192

4. between

between 常用于两组对象的表述。从基本意义上来区分 among 和 between 的差异，among 表示三者或更多者之间，between 表示两者之间。但在多个事物进行比较时，要用 between 来表示这一组被比较的事物中两两的区别。

例一： There were no significant differences in progression-free survival and overall survival rates **between** the patients who underwent lymphadenectomy and those who did not.

接受淋巴结切除术的患者与未接受淋巴结切除术的患者在无进展生存率和总生存率方面没有显著性差异。

引自：*Obstet Gynecol*, 2010, 116(2 Pt 1): 269

例二： After exclusion of the eight studies that had adjusted only for age, the difference in risk **between** the sexes was substantially reduced but still highly significant.

在剔除 8 项仅根据年龄调整的研究后,两性之间危险的差异明显减小，但仍然具有极显著的统计学意义。

引自：*BMJ*, 2006, 9(3): 148

5. after

after 通常用来说明某种因素作用的前后，所研究内容的变化情况。

例一： The mortality rate within 30 days was 0.08%（95% CI, 0.01%-0.24%）; the mortality rate **after** 30 days was 0.31%（95% CI, 0.01%-0.75%）.

30 天内死亡率为 0.08%（95%CI，0.01%～0.24%），30 天后死亡率为 0.31%（95%CI，0.01%～0.75%）。

【析】After 与表示时间的"天数或小时"连用时，一定要注意 after 的位置关系，因为 after 在不同的位置，传递的信息是不一样的。试比较：①Relapse occurred in 12 patients 2 years after surgery; ②Relapse occurred in 12 patients after 2 years of surgery. 第一句指术后 2 年，12 例复发； 而第二句的意思是"手术两年后 12 例复发"。中文似乎没有多少差异，但英文暗示的意思是手术时间整整持续了两年。

引自：*JAMA Surg*, 2014, 149(3): 275

例二： **After** controlling for age, sex, race, preexisting coronary heart disease, mean arterial blood pressure, diabetes, glucose level, cholesterol level, smoking, body mass index, and study site, the presence of retinopathy was associated with a 2-fold higher risk of CHF.

校正年龄、性别、种族、已有冠心病、平均动脉压、糖尿病、血糖水平、胆固醇水平、吸烟、体重指数（BMI）和研究地点后，视网膜病发病风险随 CHF 发病会增加 2 倍。

引自：*Hypertension*, 2006, 47: 256

6. at

at 表示时间中的某一点或事物所处的状态或情况，后接具体数字或事物。

例一： The percentage of CD34$^+$ cell with the gene transduction **at** 10 ng/ml Taxol reached 38.5%.

在 10 ng/ml 紫杉醇作用下基因转导 CD34$^+$细胞的阳性率可达 38.5%。

引自：《中华血液学杂志》, 2000, 21: 234

例二： The patient relieved from abdominal pain **at** 72 hours after treatment.

经治疗后，患者腹痛于 72 小时后缓解。

引自：*N Engl J Med*, 2006, 354: 1001

例三： **At** time of surgery, 93 patients (87%) had tumors that grossly appeared to be confined to the ovary, and 14 patients (13%) had evidence of extraovarian disease. Of the 93 patients with tumors that grossly appeared to be confined to the ovary **at** surgical exploration, 51 (55%) underwent lymphadenectomy (*n*=27 pelvic and paraaortic, *n*=19 pelvic only, *n*=5 paraaortic only).

手术时，93 例患者（87%）的肿瘤大体上局限于卵巢，14 例患者（13%）

有卵巢外侵袭；93 例手术探查时肿瘤大体局限于卵巢的患者中，51 例（55%）接受了淋巴结切除术（其中 27 例在盆腔和主动脉旁，19 例仅在盆腔，5 例仅在主动脉旁）。

引自：Obstet Gynecol, 2010, 116(2 Pt 1): 269

特别提示：At 在 "结果" 及整个摘要中，还可与以下概念搭配： at baseline（在基线处）、at either the 6- or 12-month study visits（在第 6 或第 12 个月研究跟踪时）、at entry study（研究入组时）、at week 12（第 12 周时）、at the final follow-up visit（最后一次随访时）、at hospital discharge（出院时）、at initial diagnosis（首次诊断时）等。

7. of

of 是英语中最常用的介词，正因为如此，它的各种用法和意义是最难确定和分类的。摘要写作中，除了其最常见的用法之外，"of" 还可以用 "of+总体" 来叙述总体中的各个部分。

例一： **Of** the 63 young CRCs studied, forty-four (69.8%) tumors were non-mucinous carcinomas, thirty-nine (61.9%) patients were in Dukes' C or D stage.
63 例结肠直肠癌患者中，有 44 例（69.8%）为非黏液型腺癌，39 例（61.9%）肿瘤处于 Dukes C 期或 D 期。

引自：《中华病理学杂志》, 2000, 29: 412

例二： **Of** the 1983 women with unilateral invasive breast cancer, data on tumor diameter were available for 1918 women.
1983 例患单侧浸润性乳腺癌的妇女中，1918 例有肿瘤直径数据。

引自：JAMA, 2004, 292: 1064

8. out of

out of 常用于大数目中的小数目的表达，意思为 "从……当中"，如 "在××例中有××例"。

例一： Two patients with negative WB-MRI had focal and intense uptake in the ribs on BS. **Out of** 264 examined areas, bone metastases were detected in 34 (13%).
两例患者 WB-MRI 阴性而 BS 显示在肋骨有局部强烈吸收；34 例患者（13%）中，在 264 个部位发现骨转移。

引自：Radiol Med, 2008, 113(8): 1157

例二： No patient died during the perioperative period. 50 **out of** 52 patients were followed-up for 100.1 ± 70.9 months.
围手术期无死亡病例。52 例患者中有 50 例获得随访，时间为（100.1±70.9）个月。

引自：J Cardiothorac Surg, 2019, 14: 82

例三: 52 **out of** 200 (26%) neonates with sepsis had acute renal failure (ARF); only 15% of ARF was oliguric.

200 例新生儿脓毒症患儿中有 52 例（26%）并发急性肾衰竭，只有 15% 的急性肾衰竭病例并发少尿症。

引自: Ind J Pediatr, 2006, 73(1): 19

9. but

but 既可作连词，亦可作介词。But 作连词表示转折，But 作介词相当于 except，表示前后两种情况的对比。

例一: The expressions of HMGB1 and RAGE in the periodontal tissues were significantly higher in DM group than in the control group, **but** the expression of TNF-α showed no significant difference among the groups.

DM 组大鼠牙周组织中 HMGB1、RAGE 表达水平显著高于对照组，但 TNF-α 表达量与对照组比较无差异。

引自:《南方医科大学学报》, 2020, 40(1): 6

例二: The prevalence of overweight (39.8%), obesity (26.6%), and morbid obesity (3.6%) were similar in most geographic locales, **but** was highest in North America (overweight: 37.1%, obese: 36.5%, and morbidly obese: 5.8%; $P<0.001$ *vs.* other regions).

超重（39.8%）、肥胖（26.6%）及病态肥胖（3.6%）的发生率在大部分地区相似，但以北美最高（超重: 37.1%，肥胖: 36.5%，病态肥胖: 5.8%；与其他地区比较 $P<0.001$）。

引自: JAMA, 2006, 295: 180

10. while

while 作为连词使用时意义较多，摘要中主要涉及其表示转折的意义（如下述例一），即等同于 whereas，表示转折意义时可以互换使用，相当于汉语转折"然而；而；而且"。此外，while 还常用来表达让步关系（如下述例二）。

例一: TP53 mutation was associated with abnormal karyotype ($r=0.177$, $P=0.019$), especially with complex karyotype ($r=0.440$, $P<0.001$), **while** NPM1 mutation is associated with normal karyotype ($r=0.173$, $P=0.024$).

TP53 突变与异常核型相关（$r=0.177$, $P=0.019$），特别与复杂核型相关（$r=0.440$, $P<0.001$），而 NPM1 突变与正常染色体核型相关（$r=0.173$, $P=0.024$）。

引自:《中华医学杂志》, 2020, 100(12): 933

例二: These data thus demonstrate that **while** PB lin-/AP+ cells express a number of osteoblastic genes and are capable of mineralization, they are a relatively quiescent cell population, both in terms of cell proliferation and matrix synthesis.

这些数据表明，尽管外周血 lin-/AP+细胞大量表达成骨细胞基因并能够矿化，但就细胞增殖和基质合成而言，它们是相对静止的细胞群。

引自: *Bone*, 2010, 47(1): 83

例三： BS revealed focal metastatic uptake in 72%, **whereas** WB-MRI was positive in 89%.

BS 显示局部转移性吸收的占 72%，而 WB-MRI 在 89%的患者中呈阳性。

引自: *Radiol Med*, 2008, 113(8): 1157

例四： Prevalence of hypertension and drug treatment increased with advancing age, **whereas** control rates were markedly lower in older women (systolic <140 and diastolic <90 mm Hg).

高血压的患病率和药物治疗率随着年龄增加而升高，但是在老年女性控制率（收缩压<140 mmHg，舒张压<90 mmHg）呈显著性降低。

引自: *JAMA*, 2005, 294: 466

11. and

and 不仅可以表示并列关系，即意义增补，还可以表示动作的先后、意义的转折或让步，以及对比关系等。

例一： In rats of model group, glomerulosclerosis, tubular atrophy **and** interstitial mononuclear cells infiltration **and** fibrosis emerged, **and** apoptotic cells in glomeruli **and** tubuli significantly increased at the 20th week **and** the 28th week.

模型组大鼠出现肾小球硬化、肾小管萎缩、间质单核细胞浸润和纤维化，20 周和 28 周肾小球和肾小管凋亡细胞明显增多。

引自:《中华儿科杂志》, 2000, 38(5): 285

例二： Bone metastases were detected in 18 patients (55%). In 15/33 patients, WB-MRI **and** BS were concordantly negative.

发现骨转移 18 例（55%）。在 15/33 例患者中 WB-MRI 和 BS 都显示阴性。

引自: *Radiol Med*, 2008, 113(8): 1157

12. both

both 常与 and 连用，构成连词短语：both…and…，是对 and 意义的强化。此外，both 也可作为限定词单独使用。

例一： **Both** PDGF **and** EGF enabled to stimulate the proliferation of HSC in a dose-dependent manner, and the effect of the former was stronger .

PDGF、EGF 均可呈剂量依赖性地刺激肝星状细胞增殖，前者作用更强。

引自:《中华病理学杂志》, 2000, 29: 27

例二：**Both** low EF **and** diastolic dysfunction were independently related to higher levels of BNP.

EF 降低及舒张功能不全均与 BNP 水平升高独立相关。

引自：*JAMA*,2006, 296: 2209

例三：Bariatric surgery (BS) caused comparable weight reductions and improved glucose homeostasis in **both** groups.

减肥手术（BS）在这两组中都导致了类似的体重减轻和葡萄糖稳态的改善。

引自：*Obesity Surgery*, 2016, 26: 1757

13. yet

yet 在摘要写作中常用来表示的意义有"另外；除此以外（besides，in addition）；更，甚至（still more，even）；然而（nevertheless）；尽管如此，虽然（and despite this，nevertheless）"。

例一：We found half of the infants had partial features to their seizures, **yet** evidence for primary generalized seizures was rare.

我们发现，有半数的病例出现局限性发作，而全身性发作则较为罕见。

引自：*Neurology*, 2010, 74(2)：150

例二：Adjustable gastric banding had lower mortality and complication rates; **yet**, the reoperation rate was higher and weight loss was less substantial than gastric bypass.

可调节胃束带术死亡率和并发症发生率低，但再手术率较高，体重减轻方面小于胃旁路术。

引自：*JAMA Surg*, 2014, 149(3): 275

14. although/though

although/though 均表示"regardless of the fact that、even though，虽然；即使不管事实上如何；即使"之意。两词可以互换使用。

例一：Duration of noninvasive ventilation, length of stay, 28-day mortality, complications and adverse events were similar, **although** serious adverse events tended to be lower with helium (10.8% *vs.* 19.6%, *P*=0.08).

各组间在动脉血气、呼吸困难程度、呼吸速率方面没有明显差异，无创通气持续时间、住院时间、28 天死亡率，并发症、不良事件发生率均相似。然而，使用氦气以后严重的不良反应较少（10.8% *vs.* 19.6%，*P*=0.08）。

引自：*Crit Care Med*, 2010, 38(1)：145

例二：**Although** serum CEA levels were associated with metabolic syndrome, association between serum CEA and carotid plaque was significant in individuals without metabolic syndrome.

尽管 CEA 水平与代谢综合征相关，对于没有代谢综合征者，CEA 水平

仍与颈动脉斑块相关。

引自: *Arterioscler Thromb Vasc Bio*, 2008, 28(1): 160

（四） "结果"中常用的高频形容词和副词

描述"results"时，常需要对"结果"进行比较，独立或集中描述，因此，在这一部分常需要借助形容词或副词来凸显观察发现。根据概念属性关系，这类词语可包括：①程度形容词及其副词，常用的有 significant（significantly）、marked（markedly）、obvious（obviously）、considerable（considerably）、striking（strikingly）、extreme（extremely）、notable（notably）、intensive（intensively）、strong（strongly）、distinct（distinctly）、extensive（extensively）、noticeable （noticeably）、substantial（substantially）、unusual （unusually）、remarkable （remarkably）、evident（evidently）（说明：这组词都含有"明显的/地；显著的/地；典型的/地"等意义）；②表示相关性的形容词及其副词：negative （negatively）、positive（positively）；③统计结果描述的形容词及其副词：different（differently）、respective（respectively）、statistical（statistically）等。以下通过实例，就其中一些难用的常用形容词或副词进行分析说明。

1. respectively

当表达两者或两者以上的人或事物各具有不同的性质、数量时，句末需用 respectively 表示 Singly in the order designated or mentioned（分别）的含义。从逻辑关系来看，句中谓语前后的内容存在着一一对应关系，该词之前通常用逗号隔开，也有不用逗号而直接置于句中。另一个与该词意义比较接近的词是 separately。Separately 意为"existing as an independent entity"（单独，分开，即单独的作为一个独立的个体存在），句中的前后内容不存在一一对应关系。例如：

例一： The sensitivity and specificity of LIF for diagnosis of colorectal cancer was 83.3% and 94.4%, **respectively.**

LIF（激光诱发荧光光谱分析）诊断大肠癌的敏感度和特异度分别为 83.3%和 94.4%。

引自:《中华肿瘤杂志》, 2000, 22(7): 398

例二： The risk of death and recurrent congestive heart failure combined was higher in patients prescribed NSAIDs or rofecoxib than in those prescribed celecoxib (hazard ratio 1.26 and 1.27, 95% confidence interval 1.00 to 1.57, 1.09 to 1.49, **respectively**).

服用非甾体抗炎药或罗非昔布患者发生死亡和复发性充血性心力衰竭的危险性高于服用塞来昔布的患者 （危险比分别为 1.26 和 1.27, 95%CI 分别为 1.00～1.57, 1.09～1.49 ）。

引自: *BMJ*, 2005, 330: 1370

例三： Fitting the same model **separately** to all cause death, myocardial infarction, and stroke gave similar results.

把这个模型分别应用于任何原因所致的死亡、心肌梗死和卒中进行预测评估，所得的结果相似。

引自：*BMJ*, 2005, 2: 330

例四： The findings were similar when the outcomes were assessed **separately.**

三种结局分别评估，结果基本相似。

引自：*BMJ*, 2005, 330: 1370

2. statistically

在医学论文摘要"结果"的表达中，通常需要将若干研究结果进行比较，指出其是否具有统计学差异，因而 statistically 的使用频率也很高。

例一： There were no **statistically** significant differences in mean pain and physical function scores.

平均疼痛及躯体功能评分在统计学上无显著性差异。

引自：*Eur Spine J*, 2010, 19(8)：1262

例二： The hospital mortality rate was **statistically** greater among patients receiving inappropriate initial antimicrobial therapy (IIAT) compared to those initially treated with an appropriate antibiotic regimen(51.7% versus 36.4%; $P<0.001$).

接受不恰当初始抗菌治疗（IIAT）患者的医院死亡率明显高于那些接受恰当初始抗菌治疗的患者，二者相比，差异有统计学意义（51.7% *vs.* 36.4%；$P<0.001$）。

引自：*Antimicrob Agents Chemother*, 2010, 54(5): 1742

3. significant 和 significantly

significant 和 significantly 表示"值得注目地，重大的（Having or likely to have a major effect; important）"之意。前者是形容词，常修饰 difference 等名词；后者是副词，常修饰 different 及形容词比较级（如 higher，larger）等。两者都是表示差异具有显著性。

例一： MBC-11 also **significantly** decreased bone tumor burden compared to PBS-or zoledronate-treated mice ($P=0.021$, $P=0.017$, respectively).

与 PBS 或唑来膦酸治疗组小鼠相比，MBC-11 也能明显减少骨肿瘤负荷（分别为 $P=0.021$ 和 $P=0.017$）。

引自：*Bone*, 2010, 47(1)：12

例二： There were no **significant differences** in duration or severity of symptoms.

各组之间的症状持续时间或严重程度都没有明显差异。

引自：*BMJ*, 2010, 340(2): c199

例三： And gene mutations were found in 9 SAML patients, the number of mutations was **significantly higher** than that in MDS patients (χ^2=11.911, P=0.018).

9 例 SAML 患者均发现基因突变，突变个数显著高于 MDS 患者（χ^2=11.911，P=0.018）。

引自:《中华医学杂志》, 2020, 100(12): 933

例四： Twenty-one days after transplantation, laser doppler analysis demonstrated **significantly increased** blood perfusion in the human smooth muscle cell(SMC) group.

移植后 21 天，多普勒分析显示在 SMC 组血液灌注显著增加。

引自: *Arterioscler Thromb Vasc Biol*, 2008, 17: 97

4. markedly

表示程度时，markedly 与 significantly 可以互用。与 markedly 意义接近的另一个副词是 evidently。这两个副词均表示 "明显地，显著地" 意思。

例一： Treatment of people with PsA resulted in considerable financial costs and these costs varied markedly by disease severity.

银屑病关节炎(PsA)患者的治疗花费巨大，同时，治疗因疾病严重程度而有显著性差异。

引自: *Rheumatology (Oxford)*,2010, 49:1949

例二： Prevalence of hypertension and drug treatment increased with advancing age, whereas control rates were **markedly** lower in older women (systolic <140 and diastolic <90 mmHg).

高血压的患病率和药物治疗率随着年龄增加而升高，但是在老年女性中控制率（收缩压<140 mmHg，舒张压<90 mmHg）呈显著降低。

引自: *JAMA*, 2005, 294(4): 466

5. negative 与 positive

negative 意为 "Not indicating the presence of microorganisms, disease, or a specific condition（阴性的）"。Positive 意为 "Indicating the presence of a particular disease, condition, or organism（阳性的）"。这两个词在结果表达中十分常见，但容易造成用法上的错误，即语义错误。当表达 "……患者某项检查结果为'阴性'或'阳性'" 时，不能表达为 "...patient was positive/negative."，而只能表达为 "...patient's specimen was positive/negative."，但可以表达为 "HBeAg-positive" 或 "HBeAg-negative women". 注意：我们不能说某种物质是 "阳性" 或 "阴性" 的，但可以说某种反应或检查是 "阳性" 或 "阴性" 的。例如，汉语中说患者的某种抗体呈阳性，英文就不能写成 "...antibody was positive"，而应是 "Of 400 patients, 10 were positive for anti-delta antibody." 或 "...anti-delta antibody test/reaction was positive in 10."。positive/positively，negative/negatively 还可表示 "正相关或负相关"。

例一： PB lin–/AP+ cells were smaller than their BM counterparts, and both were **negative** for the pan-hematopoietic marker, CD45.

外周血 lin–/AP+细胞较骨髓中 lin–/AP+细胞小，但均不表达全血细胞标志物 CD45。

引自：*Bone*, 2010, 47(1)：83

例二： CD15 was **positive** in 43% of cases(10/23).

43%的患者（10/23）CD15 阳性。

引自：*Am J Surg Pathol*, 2010, 34(3)：405

例三： Viable counts of Enterobacteriaceae were reduced and correlated **positively** with colitis severity, while DAI was **negatively** correlated with several CAs, e.g. butyric acid.

肠杆菌的活菌数降低，并与大肠炎的严重程度呈正相关性，而 DAI 与数个 CAs 呈负相关性，如酪酸。

引自：*Scand J Gastroenterol*, 2009, 44(10)：1213

例四： Triglycerides and remnant cholesterol in early pregnancy were **positively** associated with preeclampsia.

妊娠早期甘油三酯和残余胆固醇与子痫前期呈正相关。

引自：*Am J Obstet Gynecol*, 2019, 221(2):150.

例五： Twin analyses showed a **positive** association between and vessel densities in all regions.

成对分析显示所有区域的血管密度之间存在正相关。

引自：*Br J Ophthalmol*, 2020, 104(2):157

三、"Results" 写作中的难点和重点

（一）"差异" 的英文表述

在 "Methods" 部分中，我们提到医学上应用较多的科研设计方法是组间比较设计，对于不同组别的研究结果只有进行比较，才可分出优劣。因而将两种结果进行比较分析是医学论文英文摘要 "Results" 部分写作的重点内容之一，亦是难点之一。两种结果之间的比较可以是定性比较，也可以通过直接比较精确的资料来说明不同方法、途径所导致的不同结果。

1. 直接给出不同组别的实验资料，通过资料的直接比较来阐述组间差异。

例一： Fast blood glucose, fast blood insulin and ISI were (4.2±0.7) mmol/L *vs.* (3.8±0.7) mmol/L,(107.8±48.8)pmol/L *vs.* (50.4±40.5) pmol/L, and–3.25±0.27 *vs.*–2.58±0.66 in PIH group and normal group,respectively (*P*<0.05).

妊高征患者空腹血糖为（4.2±0.7）mmol/L，空腹胰岛素为（107.8±48.8）pmol/L，胰岛素敏感性指数为−3.25±0.27。血压正常的孕妇空腹血糖为（3.8±0.7）mmol/L，空腹胰岛素为（50.4±40.5）pmol/L，胰岛素敏感性指数为−2.58±0.66。

引自：《中华妇产科杂志》, 2000, 35(10): 597

例二: Overall CAC prevalence in this sample was 9.3%. After adjusting for age, race, and sex, the odds rations (ORs) for having CAC were 4.14 (95% confidence interval[CI], 2.33-7.35) for less than high school education, 1.89(95 CI, 1.23-2.91) for high school graduate, 1.47(95%CI, 0.99-2.19) for some college, and 1.24 (95% CI, 0.84-1.85) for college graduate compared with those participants with more than a college education (*P* for trend <0.001). This was also consistent within each of the 4 race-sex groups.

总体 CAC 患病率为 9.3%。校正年龄、种族、性别后，与大学以上教育程度组相比其他各组发生 CAC 的 OR 如下：高中以下组为 4.14（95%CI：2.33～7.35），高中毕业组为 1.89（95%CI：1.23～2.91），大学组为 1.47（95%CI：0.99～2.19），大学毕业组为 1.24（95%CI：0.84～1.85）（趋势 *P*<0.001）。在 4 个种族-性别组之间上述发生 CAC 的 OR 随受教育程度变化而改变的情况一致。

引自：*JAMA*, 2006, 295(15): 1793

例三: Compared to the 2011 survey, both numbers more than doubled. We obtained detailed clinical information of 1474 AIP patients. The male-to-female sex ratio was 2.94, the mean age was 68.1, and mean age at diagnosis was 64.8. At diagnosis, 63% patients were symptomatic and nearly half of them presented jaundice. Pancreatic cysts were found in 9% of the patients and calcifications in 6%. Histopathological examination was performed in 64%, mainly by endoscopic ultrasonography-guided fine needle aspiration. Extra-pancreatic lesions were detected in 60% of the patients. 84 % patients received the initial steroid therapy, and 85% received maintenance steroid therapy. Kaplan-Meier analysis revealed that the relapsed survival was 14% at 3 years, 25% at 5 years, 40% at 10 years, and 50% at 15 years. Mortality was favorable, but pancreatic cancer accounted for death in one quarter of fatal cases.

与 2011 年的调查相比，这两个数字都增加了一倍多。我们获得了 1474 例急性肺损伤患者的详细临床资料。男女性别比为 2.94，平均年龄为 68.1 岁，平均诊断年龄为 64.8 岁。诊断时，63% 的患者有症状，其中近一半出现黄疸。胰腺囊肿占 9%，钙化占 6%。64% 的患者通过超声内镜引导下的细针抽吸进行了组织病理学检查，60% 的患者发现胰腺外病变。84% 的患者接受了初始类固醇治疗，85% 的患者接受了维持类固醇治疗。Kaplan-Meier 分析显示复发生存率在 3 年时为 14%，5 年时为 25%，

10 年时为 40%，15 年时为 50%。死亡率有效降低，但是胰腺癌占死亡病例的 1/4。

引自：*J Gastroenterol*, 2020, 55: 462

2. 使用定性形容词或动词（如 higher、lower、worse、thicker、decrease）来描述两种结果的差异，通过对不同结果的比较，直接体现出它们的区别。

例一： At baseline, 379 case subjects with depression were identified. The risk of incident diabetes mellitus was **higher** among subjects with depression when compared with nondepressed subjects, and the association remained significant after controlling for potential confounders, including diabetes risk factors.

研究伊始（基线），共有 379 名受试者被诊断为抑郁症。这部分人群糖尿病患病风险高于无抑郁症状的受试者，而且对包括糖尿病危险因素在内的诸多的潜在混杂因素进行平衡之后，这一差异仍然存在。

引自：*Am J Psychiatry*, 2010, 167(5)：580

例二： Only age, International Prognostic Index, and *MYC* rearrangement retained prognostic significance in the final model. OS was significantly **worse** for patients with rearrangement of *MYC* (survival probability at 2 years = 0.35 in 0.61 in the nonrearranged group).

最终模型中，仅年龄、国际预后指数（IPI）和 *MYC* 基因重排仍对预后有显著性意义。有 *MYC* 基因重排的患者总体生存率（OS）显著较低（2 年生存率为 0.35，而无重排组为 0.61）。

引自：*J Clin Oncol*, 2010, 28(20)：3360

例三： In the primary per protocol analysis, progression in disability was **worse** than that predicted and worse than that in the untreated comparator dataset ("deviation score" of 113%; excess in mean disability status scale 0.28).

对最初每一治疗方案结果分析发现，参试患者的残疾进展情况与未治疗患者结果相比，较预计结果要糟糕得多（偏差分数为 113%；超过平均残疾状况评分 0.28）。

引自：*BMJ*, 2009, 339: b4677

（二）省略

省略就是避免重复，突出新信息，并使上下文紧密连接的一种语法手段。英语修辞手段之一就是节约用词、避免重复。一般说来，只要不会损害结构或引起歧义，能省略的地方就应省略。"Results"写作中，为了避免不必要的重复，有些句子成分可以省略，省略后的句子结构会显得更加紧凑，简明扼要，从而使读者在有限的文字描述中获取更多的信息。

例一： *C-19 IgH* gene rearrangements were found in 9 patients, and *TCR δ* gene rearrangements in 5 patients.

9 例发生 *C-19 IgH* 基因重排，5 例出现 *TCRδ* 基因重排。

【析】这是一个并列句，*TCR δ* gene rearrangements 后省略了谓语动词 "were found"。

引自：《中华血液学杂志》, 2000, 21(5): 253

例二： If we consider 'remission' to be the absence of joints with PD signal, no differences were found by DAS-28 between patients in remission and those not in remission, although differences were present by SDAI.

如果我们将关节的 PD 信号缺失确定为疾病的恢复，则通过 SDAI 检测发现处于恢复期和非恢复期的患者之间存在差别，而 DSA-28 检测没有发现有区别。

【析】"…and those not in remission…" 的完整形式应为 "…and those were not found in remission…"，本例中省略了谓语 "were not found"。

引自: *Rheumatology (Oxford)*, 2010, 49(4): 683

例三： Immunohischemiscal study showed positive results in 15 of 16 patients and 11 of the 42 patients.

免疫组化检测显示 16 名患者中，15 名为阳性；42 名患者中，11 名为阳性。

【析】and 在句中连接两个并列宾语，在 and 后面省略了宾语的一部分 "positive results in"。

引自：《中华外科杂志》, 2001, 39(9): 702

例四： Good results were noted in 24 patients (85.7%), fair in 2, and poor in 1.

（出院时）优良者 24 例（85.7%），轻残 2 例、重残 1 例。

【析】在 fair 和 poor 之后分别省略了部分主谓语 "results were noted"。

引自：《中华外科杂志》, 2000, 38(6): 360

例五： ①The risk of DVT and PE were significantly raised, and were highest in the first two weeks, after urinary tract infection. ②The incidence ratio for DVT was 2.10 (95% CI: 1.56-2.82), and that for PE 2.11 (1.38-3.23). The risk gradually fell over the subsequent months, returning to the baseline value after 1 year. ③The risk of DVT was also higher after respiratory tract infection, but possible diagnostic misclassification precluded a reliable estimate of the risk of PE after respiratory infection.

①尿路感染后 DVT 和 PE 的风险显著升高，且在前两周为最高。②DVT 发病率比为 2.10（95%CI:1.56～2.82），PE 为 2.11（1.38～3.23）。在随后的数月里风险逐渐下降，一年后回复到基线水平。③呼吸道感染后 DVT 的风险也较高，但是可能存在的误诊影响对呼吸道感染后 PE 风险的可靠评估。

【析】本例第一句的第二个分句中 and 连接的是两个并列主语关系，为了避免重复，在语境信息十分明显的情况下，第二个分句省略了主语 "The risk of DVT and PE"；而第二句的第二个分句却应用的是省略加替代。由于第二句中涉及 3 个名词：incidence, ratio 和 DVT，为了避免产生歧义，在省略谓语 was 的同时，增加了 that 指代 ratio。

引自：Lancet, 2006, 367: 9516

（三）动词的语态和时态的选择

"Results" 部分的动词基本使用的是过去时，如若描述的某一行为或状态发生于"结果"之前，则用过去完成时，以区分句子中不同动词的时间先后关系。至于语态，摘要中 "Results" 所代表的为客观资料或观察发现，动词基本使用被动式。但欧美出版的医学刊物，虽然在"目的"与"方法"及"结论"中使用主动式比较多见，但在 "Results" 中也不乏使用第一人称复数形式的主动结构，而我们中文医学刊物基本使用第三人称主动式，但被动式比较多见。

例一： We found that employee job-specific satisfaction does not correlate with patient outcomes, whereas higher satisfaction with the organization is associated with improved patient safety.

我们发现，医生特定工作的满意度与患者的满意度无关，而对医疗机构的更高满意度与改善患者的安全有关。

【析】用第一人称主动式描述结果。

引自：Am J Med, 2019, 132(4): 530

例二： Of the four patients who completed neoadjuvant chemotherapy, two had trastuzumab; all showed a partial pathologic response. We identified two cases in which there appeared to be clinical misinterpretation of the HER2 results.

在完成新辅助化疗的 4 例患者中，有 2 例患者使用的是曲妥珠单抗；所有患者均表现出部分病理反应，同时，我们还发现了两个病例中人表皮生长因子受体 2（HER2）检测结果不符合临床发现。

【析】用第一人称主动式描述结果。

引自：Am J Clin Pathol, 2019, 152(1):7-16.

例三： A total of 440 patients **underwent** curative-intent resection and lymphadenectomy. R0 resection **were** achieved in 424 cases (96.4%) and R1 resection **were** in 16 cases (3.6%). The results of postoperative pathological examination showed that high, moderate and poor differentiation **was** 4.2% (18/426), 60.6% (258/426) and 35.2%(150/426), respectively.

440 例患者均接受意向性根治性切除治疗，其中 R0 切除 424 例（96.4%），R1 切除 16 例（3.6%）。术后病理学检查结果显示，高分化比例为 4.2%

（18/426），中分化比例为60.6%（258/426），低分化比例为35.2%（150/426）。

引自:《中华外科杂志》, 2020, 58(4): 295

例四： At the end of the study, BMI **had decreased** by 0.55 with orlistat but increased by 0.31 with placebo ($P =0.001$).

研究结束时，奥利司他组 BMI 下降 0.55。而安慰剂组则增加 0.31（$P=0.001$）。

引自: JAMA, 2005, 293: 2873

例五： In almost all of these patients, the abnormal results of liver function tests **had been noted** early after the initiation of TPN of these patients.

几乎所有的患者在开始接受全胃肠外营养后不久及在做出胆道疾病诊断之前，都有肝功能检验结果异常。

引自: Am J Dig Dis，2006, 29: 92

（四）出现大于、小于或等于号分类条件时，常用 "具体数值+or+less/lower/greater" 来表达

例一： As maternal HBsAg, HBeAg titers elevated,her infant's risk of vaccine failure also increased. When maternal HBV-DNA was 125 pg/ml or greater, HBsAg titer is 1∶1000 and HBeAg titer is 1∶100 **or greater**, the vaccine failure incidence were 33.7%, 26.3% and 31.4% respectively.

随着母亲血清 HBsAg、HBeAg 滴度的升高，其新生儿发生免疫失败的危险度升高，当孕妇血清 HBsAg 滴度≥1∶1000、HBeAg 滴度≥1∶100 时或者更高时，分别有33.7%、26.3%、31.4%的新生儿发生乙肝疫苗免疫失败，与当孕妇血清 HBV DNA 浓度≥125 pg/ml 相比,新生儿发生免疫失败的危险性相当。

引自:《中华传染病杂志》, 2000, 18(4): 232

例二： Breast cancer diagnosis by mammography screening was an independent prognostic variable reducing the relative HR for distant recurrence. This effect was equal to **or greater** than the effect of 1 cm decrease in tumor diameter (HR, 1.20; 95% confidence interval, 1.10-1.31).

通过乳腺 X 线筛查确诊乳腺癌是降低远期复发相对 HR 的独立预后变量。这种作用相当于甚至超过肿瘤直径减少 1 cm 的作用（HR, 1.20; 95%CI：1.10～1.31）。

引自: JAMA, 2004, 292: 1064

例三： Median prostate specific antigen in black and white men was 0.7 ng/ml at age 50 years **or less.**

50 岁左右的白色人种和黑色人种患者的前列腺特异性抗原中位值为 0.7 ng/ml。

引自: J Urol, 2010, 183(3): 946

（五）相关因素渐进影响（曲线）的描述

对"结果"描述时，常有些影响因素对"结果"的影响并不是简单的呈正相关或负相关，而是呈曲线关系，一种结果随另一因素的变化而变化，例如：

例一： The relative inhibitory rate of PDT for the cells **elevated along with the increase** in the concentration of sensitizer and dose of light. Under the low photodynamic dose, it **increased rapidly**, and **gradually slowed down** to reach the plateau. Under the same photodynamic dose, significant difference in the inhibitory rate between the two lines was observed ($P<0.01$), and the LD90 was also different.

随光敏剂浓度的升高和照光剂量的增加，光动力作用对细胞的相对抑制率逐渐增大，在低光动力剂量下明显上升，随后上升渐趋缓慢达平台期；相同光动力剂量下，PDT 对 2 株细胞的相对抑制率存在明显差异（$P<0.01$），LD90 剂量条件亦不同。

引自：《中华外科杂志》，2000, 38(3): 204

例二： Patients with elevated levels of BNP at study entry and with BNP levels lower than 80 pg/ml at 4 months **tended to have only modestly increased risk** (HR, 1.7; 95% CI, 1.0-2.9) compared with patients with BNP levels lower than 80 pg/ml at both visits.

有些患者在进入研究和第 4 个月时 BNP 水平均小于 80 pg/ml，有些患者在进入研究时 BNP 水平有所升高，而在第 4 个月时 BNP 水平小于 80 pg/ml，与前者相比，后者出现死亡或新发 CHF 的危险略有增加（HR，1.7；95%CI，1.0～2.9）。

引自：*JAMA*, 2005, 294: 2866

例三： RA risk was lowest among women 1 to 5 years from their last birth (RR 0.29) with risk reduction **progressively lessening** with increasing time (5-15 years, 0.51 and >15 years, 0.76), compared to nulliparous women ($P=0.007$ for trend).

与未产妇（$P=0.007$ 趋势）比较，最后一次生育后的妇女中，其 1～5 年内 RA 风险最低（RR: 0.29），随着时间逐渐延长风险下降逐渐变缓（5～15 岁，0.51 和大于 15 年，0.76）。

引自：*Arthritis Rheum*, 2010, 62(7): 1842

例四： Of the 186 patients, 114 underwent RR and 72 underwent RP. The angle of exodeviation **steadily increased over time** in both groups after surgery.

在 186 例患者中，114 例接受了直肌切除术（RR），72 例接受了直肌折叠术（RP）。两组手术后外斜视的角度随着时间的推移稳定增加。

引自：*Br J Ophthalmol*, 2020, 104(3):350-356

四、多个实验结果的英文表述

（一）两个实验结果的英文表述

两组研究对象实验结果之间有无差异，两个因素是否存在相关性，两种实验方法的比较，两种药物疗效的比较等，均有不同的英文表述方法。

1. 两组研究对象实验结果差异无显著性的表达

例一： **No significant differences between** cyclic users and continuous users in terms of endometrioma recurrence were demonstrated.

就子宫内膜异位症复发而言，周期性用药和持续用药患者未见显著性差异。

引自：*Fertil Steril*, 2010, 93(1)：52

例二： Secondary outcome analyses (modified Rankin Scale, Barthel Index, Short Form 36, and clinical vasospasm) also showed **no significant differences between the 2 groups**.

次级指标分析（改良 Rankin 量表，Barthel 指数，短表 36，临床血管痉挛）也显示两组之间无显著性差异。

引自：*Stroke*, 2010, 41(5)：921

2. 两因素相关的表达

例一： **The higher** the pathologic grade of tumor, **the lower** the expression of E-CD was.

肿瘤病理分级越高，E-CD 表达越低。

引自：《中华肿瘤杂志》, 2000, 22：496

例二： Overall, 12% of participants had a restrictive spirometric pattern at enrolment. They were less likely to be male, to smoke and to have asthma, and had lower IgE levels than subjects in the obstructive group.

总体上，12%的参与者在登记时有限制性肺功能模式。与阻塞性模式组对象相比，患者中男性比例较少，有吸烟史和哮喘史的比例亦少，并且 IgE 水平较低。

引自：*Thorax*, 2010, 65(6)：499

例三： Postoperative PT flow volume was significantly reduced ($P<0.01$), and the reduction was closely related to preoperative SV flow volume ($r=0.65$, $P<0.001$)

断流术后 PT 流量显著减少（$P<0.01$），减少幅度与术前 SV 流量显著相关（$r=0.65$, $P<0.001$）。

引自：《中华实用外科杂志》, 2001, 21(3): 149

例四: We uncovered that in CFTRDeltaF508 cells, the extracellular glutathione levels are decreased, leading to a greater sensitivity to reactive oxygen species, providing an explanation for the hyperactivation of the p38 and ERK MAPKs and increased IL-6 synthesis.

我们发现,CFTRDeltaF508 细胞外谷胱甘肽水平下降,导致其对活性氧簇的敏感性增加,这说明了 p38 和 ERK MAPKs 过度活化及 IL-6 合成增加的原因。

引自: *J Biol Chem*, 2010, 285(29): 22299

3. 对照组与实验组结果分开表达

例一: The mean (SD) age of participants was 10.7 (3.17) years. The mean (SD) FEV_1 at baseline and 168 days were 2.13 (0.85) L and 2.22 (0.86) L for the azithromycin group and 2.12 (0.85) L and 2.20 (0.88) L for the placebo group. The difference in the change in FEV_1 between the azithromycin and placebo groups was 0.02 L (95% confidence interval [CI], −0.05 to 0.08; $P=0.61$). None of the exploratory pulmonary function end points were statistically significant. Pulmonary exacerbations occurred in 21% of the azithromycin group and 39% of the placebo group. Participants in the azithromycin group had a 50% reduction in exacerbations (95% CI, 31%-79%) and an increase in body weight of 0.58 kg (95% CI, 0.14-1.02) compared with placebo participants. There were no significant differences between groups in height, use of intravenous or inhaled antibiotics, or hospitalizations. Participants in the azithromycin group had no increased risk of adverse events, but had less cough (−23% treatment difference; 95% CI, −33% to −11%) and less productive cough (−11% treatment difference; 95% CI,−19% to−3%) compared with placebo participants.

患者平均年龄为 10.7 岁,标准差为 3.17 岁。实验开始和 168 天后,阿奇霉素组平均 FEV_1 值分别为 2.13 L 和 2.22 L,标准差分别为 0.85 和 0.86;安慰剂组平均 FEV_1 值分别为 2.12 L 和 2.20 L,标准差分别为 0.85 和 0.88. 实验结束时两组 FEV_1 值的差值为 0.02 L(95%CI, −0.05~0.08, P=0.61)。所检测的肺功能观察指标均无显著性差异。21%的阿奇霉素组患者和 39%的安慰剂组患者发生了呼吸窘迫。与安慰剂组相比,阿奇霉素组呼吸窘迫降低 50%(95%CI, 31%~79%),体重增长了 0.58 kg(95%CI, 0.14~1.02)。两组在体重、静脉或吸入阿奇霉素及住院治疗方面无明显区别。与安慰剂组相比,阿奇霉素组发生不良事件的风险无增加,但咳嗽减少了(−23%, 95%CI, −33%~−11%),排痰性咳嗽减少了(−11%, 95%CI, −19%~−3%)。

引自: *JAMA*, 2010, 303(17): 1707

例二：**In study group,** sIL-6R was (196.7±12.9) μg/L; and sgp130 was (379.4±79.3) μg/L. **In control group** Ⅰ, sIL-6R was (174.8±46.2) μg/L; and sgp130 was (254.4±34.7) μg/L.

妊高征组血清 sIL-6R 浓度为（196.7±12.9）μg/L，sgp130 浓度为（379.4±79.3）μg/L；对照组血清 sIL-6R 浓度为（174.8±46.2）μg/L，sgp130 浓度为（254.4±34.7）μg/L。

引自：《中华妇产科杂志》，2001, 36(1): 18

例三： We measured the percentage of patients screened and treated after 12 months of follow-up. **In the alerting group,** 65% of the patients requiring screening were screened (relative risk versus control=1.76; 95% confidence interval, 1.41 to 2.20) compared with 35% of patients **in the on-demand group** (relative risk versus control=1.28; 95% confidence interval, 0.98 to 1.68) and 25% of patients **in the control group. In the alerting group**, 66% of patients requiring treatment were treated (relative risk versus control=1.40; 95% confidence interval, 1.15 to 1.70) compared with 40% of patients (relative risk versus control=1.19; 95% confidence interval, 0.94 to 1.50) **in the on-demand group** and 36% of patients **in the control group**.

随访 12 个月后，我们计算筛选或治疗的患者的百分比，在电子警报组，65%需要筛选的患者被筛选出来（相对于对照组的相对危险度为 1.76；95%CI，1.41～2.20），在按需决定支持组为 35%（相对于对照组的相对危险度为 1.28；95%CI，0.98～1.68），对照组为 25%。电子警报组，66%需要治疗的患者接受治疗（相对于对照组的相对危险度为 1.40；95%CI，1.15～1.70），按需决定支持组为 40%（相对于对照组的相对危险度为 1.19；95%CI，0.94～1.50），对照组为 36%。

引自：*Circulation*, 2008, 17(2): 205

（二）多个实验结果的表述

1. 多组研究对象的实验结果用 and 连接起来充当句子的并列主语、表语或宾语等成分。

例一： Overall, 7.1% of cases and 2.5% of controls had asthma (6.0% and 2.4% had LRA whereas 1.1% and 0.1% had HRA, respectively).

总体而言，7.1%的病例和 2.5%的对照者出现哮喘（6.0%和 2.4%出现 LRA，而 1.1%和 0.1%出现 HRA）。

引自：*Thorax*, 2010, 65(8): 698

例二： The major etiology and associated diagnosis consisted of 35.9% (56/156) of non-immune anemia, 9.6%(15/156) of cardiac abnormalities, 7.1% (11/156) of intrauterine infection, 6.4% (10/156) of twin problems, 5.8% (9/156) of meconium peritonitis, 5.1% (8/156) of thoracic-lung disease, 4.5% (7/156) of chromosomal abnormalities, 1.9%(3/156) of immune anemia.

主要病因分析显示，非免疫性疾病中贫血占 35.9%（56/156）、心血管系统异常占 9.6%（15/156）、宫内感染占 7.1%（11/156）、异常双胎妊娠占 6.4%（10/156）、胎粪性腹膜炎占 5.8%（9/156）、呼吸系统疾病占 5.1%（8/156）、染色体异常占 4.5%（7/156）、免疫性贫血占 1.9%（3/156）。

引自:《中华妇产科杂志》, 2011, 12(12): 905

2. 直接用①、②、③或 A、B、C 或 I 、II 、III 等分类表达。

例一：①This method can be used to quantitatively analyze HBV genome directly from serum samples with the detectable range from 20pg to 20ng per milliliter; ② Probes used in our system would not bind to non-specific genes; ③ Whole process of quantification can be finished within about 5 hours.

①方法可直接从血清标本中对 HBV 定量，可定量范围为 20 pg/ml～20 ng/ml；②不与人类基因组及其他病毒或细菌基因组非特异杂交；③定量分析全程 5 小时左右。

引自:《中华传染病杂志》, 2000, 18(1): 40

例二：Many features increased the probability of heart failure, with the best feature for each category being the presence of (1) past history of heart failure (positive LR=5.8; 95% confidence interval [CI], 4.1-8.0); (2) the symptom of paroxysmal nocturnal dyspnea (positive LR=2.6; 95%CI, 1.5-4.5); (3) the sign of the third heart sound (S3) gallop (positive LR=11; 95%CI, 4.9-25.0); (4) the chest radiograph showing pulmonary venous congestion (positive LR=12.0; 95%CI, 6.8-21.0); and (5) electrocardiogram showing atrial fibrillation (positive LR=3.8; 95%CI, 1.7-8.8). The features that best decreased the probability of heart failure were the absence of (1) past history of heart failure (negative LR=0.45; 95% CI, 0.38-0.53); (2) the symptom of dyspnea on exertion (negative LR=0.48; 95% CI, 0.35-0.67); (3) rales (negative LR=0.51; 95%CI, 0.37-0.70); (4) the chest radiograph showing cardiomegaly (negative LR=0.33; 95%CI, 0.23-0.48); and (5) any electrocardiogram abnormality (negative LR=0.64; 95% CI, 0.47-0.88). A low serum BNP proved to be the most useful test (serum B-type natriuretic peptide <100 pg/ml; negative LR=0.11; 95% CI, 0.07-0.16).

许多临床特点可增加心力衰竭的可能性，其中最突出的特点是：①具有心力衰竭既往史（阳性 LR=5.8；95% CI，4.1～8.0）；②夜间出现阵发性呼吸困难（阳性 LR=2.6；95%CI，1.5～4.5）；③听诊闻及第三心音（S3）

奔马率（阳性 LR=11；95%CI，4.9～25.0）；④胸部 X 线片示肺静脉淤血（阳性 LR=12.0；95%CI，6.8～21.0）；⑤心电图示心房颤动（阳性 LR=3.8；95% CI，1.7～8.8）。也有一些临床特点可显著降低心力衰竭的可能性，包括：①无心力衰竭既往史（阴性 LR=0.45；95%CI，0.38～0.53）；②活动时不出现呼吸困难症状（阴性 LR=0.48；95%CI，0.35～0.67）；③肺部未闻及啰音（阴性 LR=0.51；95%CI，0.37～0.70）；④胸部 X 线片未见心脏扩大（阴性 LR=0.33；95%CI，0.23～0.48）；⑤心电图未见任何异常表现（阴性 LR=0.64；95%CI，0.47～0.88）。经证实，血清 BNP 水平低下是最有价值的检查结果（血清 BNP<100 pg/ml；阴性 LR=0.11；95% CI，0.07～0.16）。

引自：*JAMA*，2005，294：1944

3. 不同年龄组（两个年龄组间）实验结果的表达

例一：**In those aged over 35 years**, trisomy 21 was detected in 5 of 92(5.4%), and **in the age under 35 years**, it was 4 out of 208 (1.9%), *P*=0.26.

高龄孕妇（年龄>35 岁）21 三体儿的检出率为 5.4%（5/92），非高龄孕妇 21 三体儿的检出率为 1.9%（4/208），*P*=0.26。

引自：《中华医学遗传学杂志》，2000，17(1)：16

例二：HPV prevalence peaked at 75% in the HIV-positive women aged 25-34 years and then declined with age to 37.5% in those≥55 years old (*P* trend<0.001).

HPV 感染率在年龄为 25～34 岁的 HIV 阳性妇女中最高，感染率为 75%，并随着年龄增加而下降，年龄≥55 岁的妇女 HPV 感染率为 37.5%（*P* 趋势<0.001）。

引自：*J Infect Dis*，2009，199(12)：1851

4. 多种影响实验结果的因素

某实验对象、方法受诸多因素的影响，"主要影响因素"可译成"the main risk factors"或"The most common risk factors"，充作句子的主语，具体的因素——罗列用 and 连接，在句子中充作并列表语、宾语等成分。

例一：Arterial catheter and central venous catheter catheter-related infection rates were 0.68% (1.0/1000 catheter-days) and 0.94% (1.09/1000 catheter-days), respectively. The daily hazard rate for colonization increased steadily over time for arterial catheters (*P*=0.008) but remained stable for central venous catheters. **Independent risk factors** for arterial catheter colonization were respiratory failure and femoral insertion. **Independent risk factors** for central venous catheter colonization were trauma or absence of septic shock at intensive care unit admission, femoral or jugular insertion, and absence of antibiotic treatment at central venous catheter insertion.

动脉导管和中心静脉导管所引起的导管相关感染率分别为 0.68%（1.0/1000 导管留置天数）和 0.94%（1.09/1000 导管留置天数）。动脉导管植入所致日感染率随时间延长而增加（$P = 0.008$），但中心静脉导管植入所致日感染概率保持稳定。动脉导管植入感染的独立危险因素为呼吸衰竭和股动脉穿刺。中心静脉导管植入感染的独立危险因素为创伤，在重症监护病房有无发生感染性休克、股静脉或颈静脉穿刺，以及中心静脉穿刺时缺乏抗生素治疗等。

引自：Crit Care Med, 2010, 38(4)：1030

例二： **The most common risk factors** were prolonged immobilization (26.2%), surgery (23.3%), hyperlipemia(21.4%), hypertension (19.4%), malignancy (13.6%), hyperhemoglobinemia (13.6%), heart disease (12.6%), trauma (9.7%) and femoral venous puncture (9.7%).

最常见的危险因素为长期卧床（26.2%）、手术（23.3%）、高脂血症（21.4%）、高血压（19.4%）、恶性肿瘤（13.6%）、血红蛋白增多（13.6%）、心脏病（12.6%）、外伤（9.7%）和股静脉穿刺（9.7%）。

引自：《中华内科杂志》, 2000, 39(8): 513

例三： **The strongest risk factors** for anal incontinence after vaginal delivery were high maternal age, high birthweight of the child, and instrumental delivery. The only risk factor for anal incontinence after caesarean delivery was maternal age.

阴道分娩后肛门失禁的最大危险因素是高龄产妇、高体重出生婴儿和器械辅助分娩。剖宫产后肛门失禁的唯一危险因素是母亲年龄。

引自：Lancet, 2019, 393(10177): 1233

五、"Results" 写作中的一些常见错误

医学论文英文摘要 "Results" 写作中常出现以下错误，特别是对于刚刚从事科研者来说更应该避免以下可能出现的问题。

1. 使用图片、表格、化学结构式、数学公式等。

2. 在 "Results" 中加入了未经证实的作者自己的主观推断、推论和解释等。

3. 重复论文文题。例如，论文题目为 "300 例肝穿刺活检并发症分析"（Analysis of the complications of liver biopsy in 300 cases），摘要里写到 "分析了我院 300 例肝穿刺活检的并发症"（The complications of 300 cases of liver biopsy in our hospital were analyzed.），这些写法都是不可取的。

4. 过多地给出次要或无用信息，忽视了主要资料或主要信息。

5. 将 "Conclusion" 内容写入 "Results"。例如：有效控制医院获得性肺炎的危险因

素是降低 HAP 行之有效的措施（Management of these risks should be effective measures to reduce the incidence of HAP.）"。

6. 语篇逻辑混乱，缺乏对应关系。描述"结果"时，整个语篇应该与"方法"形成时空对应（chronological/event sequence），即："方法"中先后做了什么，对应的就是"结果"发现或观察到了什么。

7. 缺乏精练，完全照搬正文"结果"，形似流水账，这是国内作者的通病。如下列"结果"（注：中文内容为作者的原始文本，选自本书作者审稿手记，英文为审稿人根据内容归纳综合修改）：

1）【结果】A 组 21 例病人中 18 例病人置管有效，3 例病人在置管后接受再手术治疗。平均置管时间为（17.62±9.32）d，平均住院时间为（43.14±14.97）d。B 组 17 例病人中 12 例病人置管有效，5 例病人在置管后接受再手术治疗。平均置管时间为（31.71±15.30）d，平均住院时间为（57.41±26.88）d。

Results: For group A, the effective catheterization was in 18 of the 21 patients, and 3 required second operation. The average catheter maintenance was (17.62±9.32) days, and average hospital stay(43.14±14.97) days; For group B, catheterization was effective in 12 of 17 cases, and another 5 needed reoperation. The average catheter maintenance was (31.71±15.30) days and average hospital stay(57.41±26.88) days.

2）【结果】观察组患者有效率（94.00%）与对照组（76.00%）比较，差异具有统计学意义（$P<0.05$）；观察组和对照组患者治疗后 PLI、PD、SBI 与治疗前比较，差异具有统计学意义（$P<0.05$）；观察组患者治疗后 PLI、PD、SBI 与对照组比较，差异具有统计学意义（$P<0.05$）；观察组和对照组患者治疗后 TNF-α、CRP 与治疗前比较，差异具有统计学意义（$P<0.05$）；观察组患者治疗后 TNF-α、CRP 与对照组比较，差异具有统计学意义（$P<0.05$）。

Results: The effective rate was 94.00% for observational group and 76.00% for the control group ($P<0.05$). Plaque index (PLI), probing depth (PD) and sulcus bleeding index (SBI) were different in both groups from pre-and post-treatment ($P<0.05$), and these indicators were also different between groups ($P<0.05$). TNF-α and CRP levels were different in group and between groups before and after treatment ($P<0.05$).

六、练　习

6-1　将下列句子译成英语

1. 在 190 例过去未经治疗的患者中，有 18 例死于原发性肺癌。

2. 86 例患者中 24 例症状缓解时间不长。

3. 1063 例患者发生任何原因死亡或者持久性心肌梗死或者致残性卒中。

4. 200 例脓毒症新生儿中有 52 例发生了急性肾衰竭。

5. 在进入研究时（出院前）有 4266 例患者提供了 BNP 结果，在第 4 个月时有 3618

例患者提供了 BNP 结果，在第 12 个月时有 2966 例患者提供了 BNP 结果。

6. 被抗体包裹的细菌与临床综合征的关系是无症状菌尿 15%（27/178），膀胱炎 8%（6/75）；急性出血性膀胱炎 67%（4/6）；前列腺炎 67%（2/3）；急性肾盂肾炎 62%（16/26）。

7. 在这类人群中，两根血管病变与三根血管病变的患者年死亡率平均各为 7%及 10%。

8. 21 例患者中伤口一期愈合 17 例，二期愈合 4 例（脂肪液化 4 例，合并血肿 1 例），无感染及乳头和乳晕坏死病例。

9. 除对照组 2 例出现肺部感染外，其余患者均未发生严重并发症。术后第 7 天与术前相比，实验 B 组患者血浆 GSH 浓度明显上升。

10. 最常见的共病是高血压（74.5%）、糖尿病（40.2%）、慢性肾衰竭（14.9%）和充血性心力衰竭（26.7%）；80%的患者有至少两个卒中危险因素。

6-2　仔细阅读下列 results 段落，根据篇章结构和语境在空格处填入适当的词或词组

The study was conducted _____1_____ April 1, 2004, _____2_____ April 30, 2005. Fifty-eight infants were recruited; 29 were_____3_____ to suprapubic aspiration, and 29 were randomly assigned to transurethral catheterization. Seven infants were _____4_____ because of consent withdrawal (3 patients), _____5_____ technical difficulties during videotaping (3 patients), or because the child voided during the procedure (1 patient). Twenty-seven infants _____6_____ the suprapubic aspiration group and 24 in the transurethral catheterization group completed the study. All male infants were circumcised. An adequate urine sample was obtained in 18 (66%) _____7_____ 27 patients in the suprapubic aspiration group and in 20 (83.3%) of 24 in the transurethral catheterization group. The mean Douleur Aigue du Nouveaune score was _____8_____ higher in patients who were randomly assigned to suprapubic aspiration _____9_____ patients who were randomly assigned to transurethral catheterization (7 and 4.5, _____10_____). The _____11_____ in Douleur Aigue du Nouveaune score also were significant in a subgroup analysis of boys and girls. Mean visual analogue scale scores by parents was _____12_____ in the suprapubic aspiration group compared with transurethral catheterization (63 ± 27 mm *vs.* 46 ± 26, respectively). Similarly, mean visual analogue scale scores by nurses was higher in the suprapubic aspiration group compared with transurethral catheterization (3 ± 18 mm *vs.* 43 ± 25 mm, respectively).

6-3　找出下列结果句中的词法或句法错误并改正

1. We enrolled 740 patients in 28 ICUs in Canada and the United States. There was no significantly difference in the primary outcome (28-day mortality rate) between the bronchoalveolar-lavage group and the endotracheal-aspiration group (18.9% and 18.4%, respectively; $P=0.94$).

2. The bronchoalveolar-lavage group and the endotracheal-aspiration group also have similar rates of targeted therapy (74.2% and 74.6%, separately; $P=0.90$), days alive without

antibiotics (10.4±7.5 and 10.6±7.9, *P*=0.86), and maximum organ-dysfunction scores (mean , 8.3±3.6 and 8.6±4.0; *P*=0.26). The two groups did not difference significantly from the length of stay in the ICU or hospital.

3. The nystagmus results from an imbalance in tonic activity among the two vestibular nerves.

4. Although in patients the walls of LN arterioles were significant thicker than in controls, definite stenosis was not observed. Arteriolar lumina in the LN were not only significantly larger than in the WM, which most lacunar infarcts in CADASIL occur, but also larger than in cortical GM, where infarcts virtually never exist.

5. There were 11 (55%) men, and the common age was 72 years (range, 53 to 84 years). All patients had risk factors consistent with severe atherosclerotic disease. All symptomatic carotid stenoses had inflammation, as evaluated by USPIO-enhanced imaging. On the contralateral sides, inflammatory activity was found in 19 (95%) patients. Contralaterally, there were 163 quadrants (57%) with a signal loss after USPIO when comparing to 217 quadrants (71%) on the symptomatic side (*P*=0.007).

6. Over the 6-year follow-up period, 20 ischemic strokes were registered. After adjustment for confounding factors, cases with severe obstructive sleep apnea hypopnea (defined as apnea-hypopnea index 30) at baseline had an increased risk of developing a stroke.

7. The IMR correlated significantly to the peak creatinine kinase (CK) (R = 0.61, *P*= 0.0005) while the other measures of microvascular dysfunction did not. In patients with an IMR great than the median value of 32 U, the peak CK was significantly higher compared to those having values <or=32 U (3,128 ± 1,634 ng/ml *vs.* 1,201 ± 911 ng/ml,*P* = 0.002). The IMR correlated significantly with 3 month echocardiographic wall motion score (WMS) (R = 0.59,*P* = 0.002) while the other measures of microvascular function did not.

8. Alcohol consumption patterns (i.e., the mean number of drinks per drinking day and week) was not differ significant between preconception and pre-pregnancy recognition periods but did significantly drop after pregnancy recognition.

第七章　医学论文英文摘要
"Conclusion"写作

　　结论（Conclusion）是论文最后的总体归纳和结语。所谓"结论"是指从一定的前提推论得到的结果或对事物做出的总结性判断。为了能让读者掌握论文的主要概况，摘要内容应该包含有与论文等量的主要信息。要把实验结果和讨论分析后的认识，以简明的结论形式表达出来，回答科研构思或科学假说所提出的问题，概括地传递给读者该研究工作的主要内容和结果。因而，结论是在实验结果观察和广泛论证的基础上，经过严密的分析推理，对结果和讨论做出严肃的、高度概括的论断，是论文的最后归宿，在整篇论文中起着画龙点睛的作用，是医学论文摘要的重要组成部分。

　　Conclusion 主要内容包括对结果的分析、研究、比较、评价和应用，本课题存在的问题，与本课题有关的建议和设想，以及说明创新或新发现的学术及应用价值，可否推广应用，高度概括和集中了论文的学术见解，体现了作者学术思想的深度和广度。

　　总体上，Conclusion 应写得简明扼要、精练完整、逻辑严谨、表达准确、条理清晰。概括出的"结论"应限制在"结果"所支持的范围，"结论"概括得过窄或过浅，有失材料的真实性。正文"讨论"部分的材料只能作为支持结论的旁证，不能把它作为"结论"的直接根据。"结论"要与正文的"引言"中所提出的命题相呼应，写"结论"时应注意：

　　（1）突出重点，观点鲜明地提出一点或几点见解。

　　（2）用词准确，切忌言过其实。下结论必须注意恰如其分，不能明确回答或没把握下结论时，不要勉强下结论。这部分与"结果"部分相反，这里允许用、且常用"可能、印象、看来、似乎、提示"等字眼，以便留有余地，关于类似的表达将在后续相关内容详细举例。

　　（3）文字力求精练，忌重复。一般用 1～3 个句子组成，很多摘要只用一句话表示结论。例如："**Conclusions** Exercise capacity is a more powerful predictor of mortality among men than other established risk factors for cardiovascular disease. (*N Engl J Med*, 2002; 346: 793)"。

　　（4）遵循"就事论事"（Matter-of-fact）的原则，不应夸大其辞，避免对研究本身做出评论或褒奖（这种言语在国内期刊中常有出现。例如："This paper reported application of the new technique in China for the first time."；"The present study provides theoretical and experimental basis for pathogenesis of the syndrome."）。至于研究本身的价值或意义，自有

他人来评判。

（5）忌"画蛇添足"。结论的描述应紧紧围绕或针对研究的目的和所发现的结果进行叙述，不要添加如"The possible mechanisms of the therapy were also discussed"这类话语，因为这是正文"讨论"部分的内容。

（6）标题词"Conclusion"单复数的确定。一般情况下，研究论文基本上都是针对某一特定问题所进行的研究，理论上应该用单数形式，但是，任何事物之间必然有着千丝万缕的关联，因此，使用复数形式的标题词十分常见，尤其在国外文献中更是如此（国内文献多使用单数形式）。单复数形式的取舍决定于结论部分所涉及内容的层次。

试比较：

例一：**Conclusions**　The majority of patients with mild, persistent asthma had a low sputum eosinophil level and had no significant difference in their response to either mometasone or tiotropium as compared with placebo. These data provide equipoise for a clinically directive trial to compare an inhaled glucocorticoid with other treatments in patients with a low eosinophil level.

结论　大多数轻度持续性哮喘患者的痰液嗜酸性粒细胞水平较低，与安慰剂组相比，他们对莫米松或噻托溴铵的反应没有显著性差异。这些数据为临床指导试验提供了平衡，以比较吸入糖皮质激素与其他治疗对低嗜酸性粒细胞水平患者的影响。

引自：*N Engl J Med*, 2019, 380(21):2009

例二：**Conclusion**　In this cohort, approximately two-thirds of patients with glaucoma died within 20 years of diagnosis. In most older patients with glaucoma, the overall goal of preventing visual handicap and blindness is achievable 20 years after diagnosis.

结论　该队列中，约 2/3 的青光眼患者在诊断后 20 年内死亡。在大多数老年青光眼患者中，预防视力障碍和失明的总体目标在诊断后 20 年内是可以实现的。

引自：*Br J Ophthalmol*, 2018, 102(12): 311

当一篇论文呈现在读者面前，读者考虑是否有阅读价值时，常是在读完摘要（主要为结果和结论）后才做出决定的。因此，结论写得如何对一篇论文的传播关系重大，应尽最大力量去写好。

一、"Conclusion"写作内容

"Conclusion"主要是对研究结果的分析、比较、评价、应用，提出问题、假设、建议、预测等。以下将从对实验结果的分析，对作用机制的分析，对实验结果的评价（包括疗效评价，检验方法的评价等），对结果的比较，以及提出建议几个方面加以分类，从语言表达及措辞手段等举例说明。

（一）对结果进行分析

直接总结研究所发现的结果，用陈述句表明观点或说明情况。

例一： Percutaneous microwave ablation has a good effect on colorectal cancer liver metastases and has a similar survival prognosis as surgery. For livers with color ≥ 3 cm in colorectal cancer, the long-term survival rate of the surgery-only group is greater than that of the microwave-only group.

超声引导下经皮微波消融对结直肠癌肝转移灶效果好，且与手术治疗有着相似的生存预后。但对于直径≥3 cm 结直肠癌肝转移灶，手术治疗远期效果优于超声引导下经皮微波消融。

引自:《中华医学杂志》, 2020, 100(9): 696

例二： Vortioxetine improves the behaviors of mice with depression possibly by affecting the cAMP/CREB/BDNF signal pathway.

沃替西汀产生抗抑郁作用机制可能与影响 cAMP/CREB/BDNF 信号转导通路有关。

引自:《南方医科大学学报》, 2017, 37(1): 107

例三： One in 10 patients aged 45 or more with new onset rectal bleeding had colonic neoplasia, so investigation of the bowel should be offered to all such patients, whether or not they have other symptoms.

年龄≥45 岁的新发直肠出血患者中 1/10 有结肠肿瘤，因此，无论是否伴随其他症状，都应对所有此类患者进行肠道检查。

引自: *BMJ*, 2006, 333(7558): 69

例四： Together these data suggest that C4 activation is critical for initiating renal flare while C3 activation is involved in the actual tissue damage, and that these effects are influenced by genetic variability in complement activation and regulation.

这些数据显示，C4 的激活对肾炎发作起重要作用，而 C3 的活化则导致组织损伤。这些作用都受到了补体激活与调节的遗传变异的影响。

引自: *Lupus*, 2010, 19(11): 1272

例五： These results indicate that bilateral nephrectomy upregulates the AVP-eGFP synthesis. Further studies are needed to identify the neural and/or humoral factors that activate AVP synthesis and regulate neuronal circuits during acute kidney dysfunction.

这些结果表明双侧肾切除术上调了 AVP-eGFP 合成，但需要进一步研究来确定在急性肾功能不全期间激活 AVP 合成和调节神经元回路的神经和（或）体液因子

引自: *J Physiol Sci*, 2019, 69(3): 531

（二）对作用机制分析

解释某种结果产生的原因，证明所提出的假设。

1. "作用" 的表达法

表达作用常见句型如下：
1）...play an important role in...
2）the effects of...on...were achieved by...
3）...contribute to...
4）...have (definite) effect on...
5）...play a central role in...
6）...play key role in...
7）...help to...

例一： Retinopathy is an independent predictor of CHF, even in persons without preexisting coronary heart disease, diabetes, or hypertension. This suggests that microvascular disease may **play an important role in** the development of heart failure in the general population. Some asymptomatic persons with retinopathy on an ophthalmologic examination may benefit from further assessment of CHF risk.

即使是在没有冠心病、糖尿病或高血压的人群，视网膜病仍然是 CHF 的独立危险预测因素。这提示，微血管疾病可能对普通人群心力衰竭的发病具有重要影响。某些眼科检查发现无症状视网膜病的患者，可从进一步的 CHF 危险评估中受益。

引自：*JAMA*, 2005, 293(1): 63

例二： These facts indicate that the endogenous retrovirus genes may be the important genetic factor of IDDM and **play key role in** the structure and physical function of chromosome and the pathogenesis of genetic-related disease.

人内源型逆转录病毒基因在人染色体的结构和生理功能中具有重要作用，它们的变异可能是 1 型糖尿病及其他自身免疫病和癌症等疾病的遗传因素。

引自：《中华实验和临床病毒学杂志》, 2000, 14: 105

例三： Risedronate reduces bone marrow fat in postmenopausal women. These findings are the first demonstration of an effect of bisphosphonates on marrow fat in humans *in vivo*. By regulating the amount of fat within the bone marrow, this effect **may contribute to** the beneficial effect of bisphosphonates on bone mass.

双膦酸盐能降低绝经后妇女骨髓内的脂肪含量。这些发现首次表明了双膦酸盐类药物在体内有降低骨髓内脂肪含量的作用。这可能是双膦酸盐类药物通过调节骨髓内的脂肪含量对成骨产生有利作用。

引自：*Osteoporos Int*, 2011, 22(5): 1547

例四： Intermittent ischemia **is beneficial to** recover the decreased tissue ATP lever caused by ischemia during a short period and alleviate cell injury. The ATP level of the kidney which suffered from ischemia for a long time will be hard to recover.

间断缺血有利于在短期内恢复因组织缺血造成的 ATP 水平的下降，从而减轻细胞损伤。而肾脏长时间缺血后同期内其细胞 ATP 水平将难以恢复。

引自：《中华实验外科杂志》, 2000, 17(3): 219

例五： These findings suggest that pesticides **may contribute to** atopic asthma, but not nonatopic asthma, among farm women.

这些发现表明，杀虫剂可能导致农场妇女的特应性哮喘，而非变应性哮喘。

引自：*Am J RespCri Car Med*, 2008, 177: 11

2. "机制"的表达法

"机制"在生物医学上指的是 "the involuntary and consistent response of an organism to a given stimulus"，即生物体对所受到的刺激做出的连贯反应。常可用 "be an (one) (important) of the mechanisms of..." "be related to the pathogenesis of…"

例一： PPI use does not appear to be associated with either the presence of osteoporosis or accelerated BMD loss. The association between PPI use and hip fracture is probably related to factors independent of osteoporosis.

质子泵抑制剂的使用与骨质疏松症发生和加速骨矿物质丢失无关，但使用质子泵抑制剂与髋关节骨折有关，其可能源于骨质疏松之外的其他因素。

引自：*Gastroenterology*, 2010, 138(3): 896

例二： Inducing apoptosis is an important mechanisms of killing leukemic cells by chemotherapeutic drugs.

诱导凋亡是临床治疗相关剂量的化疗药物杀伤白血病细胞的重要机制。

引自：《中华儿科杂志》, 2000, 38(3): 223

例三： In the case of comorbidity anxiety, sleep disorder is still an independent risk factor for depressive disorder, and the relationship between depressive symptoms and sleep disorder indicators of different dimensions suggests that sleep disorder plays a comprehensive role in the pathogenesis of depressive disorder.

无论是否伴有焦虑，睡眠障碍都是抑郁障碍的独立危险因素。抑郁状况与不同维度的睡眠障碍指标的关系提示睡眠障碍在抑郁障碍的发病过程中起综合性的作用。

引自:《上海交通大学学报(医学版) 》, 2020, 40(3): 333

例四: Down-regulation of CC16 expression plays a critical role in the pathogenesis of acute lung injury induced by endotoximia. The application of GH can deteriorate the lung injury induced by endotoximia through down-regulating the expression of CC16.

CC16 表达变化在内毒素血症致急性肺损伤的发病中有重要作用，生长激素可通过下调肺源性抗炎因子 CC16 的表达而加剧内毒素血症所致的急性肺损伤。

引自:《中国免疫学杂志》, 2007, 23(3): 220

（三）对实验结果做出评价

综合实验结果发现，直接给出结论，必要时可从理论上做出解释说明。

1. 疗效评价

例一: Treatment with hyperbaric oxygen possibly reduces mortality and neurological sequelae in term neonates with hypoxic-ischaemic encephalopathy. Because of the poor quality of reporting in all trials and the possibility of publication bias, an adequately powered, high quality randomised controled trial is needed to investigate these findings. The Chinese medical literature may be a rich source of evidence to inform clinical practice and other systematic reviews.

高压氧治疗可能会减少足月新生儿缺氧缺血性脑病死亡率和神经系统后遗症的发生。由于所有试验研究的质量均较差，同时可能存在发表带来的偏倚，因此需要进行有足够说服力的、高质量的随机对照研究来证实这些发现。中国的医学文献可能是影响临床实践和进行其他系统性综述的丰富的证据来源。

引自: *BMJ,* 2006, 4: 212

例二: Silencing Prrx2 expression can effectively inhibit the proliferation and growth of breast cancer, suggesting that Prrx2 may become a new target for the treatment of breast cancer.

沉默 Prrx2 表达可有效抑制乳腺癌的增殖和肿瘤生长能力，Prrx2 可能成为治疗乳腺癌的新靶点。

引自:《中华医学杂志》, 2020, 100(12): 942

例三: The clinical efficacy of Everolimus was better than Axitinib.The adverse reactions of Axitinib was similar with Everolimus. Everolimus may be a better option in the second line treatment of mRCC.

依维莫司治疗 mRCC 在疗效上优于阿昔替尼，不良反应上两者相当，故在二线治疗 mRCC 上依维莫司比阿昔替尼有优势。

引自:《复旦学报(医学版)》, 2020, 47(1): 37

例四： Monthly intermittent preventive treatment with dihydroartemisinin–piperaquine was safe but did not lead to significant improvements in birth outcomes compared with sulfadoxine-pyrimethamine.

与磺胺多辛-乙胺嘧啶相比，双氢青蒿素-哌喹每月间歇预防性治疗是安全的，但并未导致出生结局的显著改善。

引自: *Lancet*, 2019, 393(10179): 1428

2. 检验方法评价

例一： HpSA test as a non-invasive test is a highly accurate method to diagnose *H. pylori* infection in children and teenagers.

粪便抗原检测儿童及青少年 *H. pylori* 感染的方法准确度更高。

引自:《世界华人消化杂志》, 2009, 17(4): 405

例二： Joint detection of serum IgM and IgG antibodies to 2019-nCoV is an effective screening and diagnostic indicators for 2019-nCoV infection, and an effective complement to the false negative results to nucleic acid test.

血清 2019-nCoV IgM 和 IgG 联合检测可作为新型冠状病毒感染的有效筛查和诊断指标，是新型冠状病毒肺炎核酸检测假阴性的有效互补。

(注：新型冠状病毒肺炎英文名称现修订为 "COVID-19")。

引自:《中华检验医学杂志》, 2020, 43(3): 230

例三： HLA antibody screening by phenotype bead assay may prospectively identify at-risk patients for the development of alloPR. However, clinical trials are needed to validate these findings.

通过结合珠蛋白表型测定筛查人类白细胞抗原抗体，可以前瞻性地鉴别出发生异源性血小板减少症的高危患者。然而，这些结果需要临床试验来验证。

引自: *Am J Clin Pathol*, 2019, 152(2):146-154

3. 其他实验结果的评价

例一： Calcium supplements (without coadministered vitamin D) are associated with an increased risk of myocardial infarction. As calcium supplements are widely used these modest increases in risk of cardiovascular disease might translate into a large burden of disease in the population. A reassessment of the role of calcium supplements in the management of osteoporosis is warranted.

补充钙剂（不加入维生素 D）与增加心肌梗死的风险相关。钙剂应用较广泛，心血管疾病风险会随之增加，可能导致人类疾病的重大负担。骨质疏松疾病的治疗中应正确评估钙剂的作用。

引自: *BMJ*, 2010, 341 : c3691

例二：HER2 testing may be performed on biopsy specimens with a relatively high concordance rate with resection specimens, and if multiple samples are analyzed from a single patient, the HER2-positive rate increases over twofold.

人表皮生长因子受体2（HER2）检测可在活检标本上进行，活检标本与切除标本的符合率相对较高，如果从单例患者中分析多个样本，HER2阳性率会增加两倍以上。

引自：*Am J Clin Pathol*, 2019, 151(5): 461

例三：Positioning of the heart during off-pump coronary artery bypass grafting leads to a decrease in regional cerebral oxygen saturation. This decrease is associated with changes in cardiac output, haemoglobin concentration, arterial CO_2 partial pressure, and central venous pressure.

非体外循环下冠状动脉旁路移植术期间心脏定位导致局部脑氧饱和度下降，此下降与心输出量、血红蛋白浓度、动脉血二氧化碳分压和中央静脉的压力中的变化相关。

引自：*Eur J Anaesthesiol*, 2010, 27(6): 542

例四：Lung COVID-19 lesions can be shown by the initial chest HRCT, which is the preferred imaging method. Thoracic HRCT scans play an important role in the early diagnosis of COVID-19.

COVID-19患者首次胸部HRCT检查能发现肺部病灶，是首选的影像学检查方法，胸部HRCT扫描检查在COVID-19的早期诊断中有重要作用。

引自：《中华放射学杂志》, 2020, 54(4): 292

例五：MPS is demonstrated to be significantly superior to conventional macroscopic diagnosis in both detection of function of fundic varices and evaluation of efficacy of endoscopic therapy. It appears to be a safe valuable technique which should be widely accepted for routine application.

小探头超声检查无论对胃底静脉曲张的诊断还是判断其内镜治疗疗效显著优于常规内镜下肉眼诊断，是临床一种安全性好且很有价值的检查手段。

引自：《中华消化杂志》, 2000, 20(2): 114

（四）对结果进行比较

例一：Sirolimus-eluting stents result in superior clinical and angiographic outcomes compared with vascular brachytherapy for the treatment of restenosis within a bare-metal stent.

与血管近距离放射治疗金属裸支架内再狭窄比较，西罗莫司洗脱支架具有更好的临床及血管造影效果。

引自：*JAMA*, 2006, 295(11): 1264

例二：No fall-off in gains was observed for either treatment modality after treatment discontinuation. SSRIs were associated with adverse events. Gains produced by CBT were slower to emerge than those produced by CBT+SSRI and SSRI, but CBT ended sooner.

治疗结束后，每种治疗方法均未显示临床疗效下降。选择性 5-羟色胺再摄取抑制剂（SSRIs）可导致不良事件发生。认知行为治疗（CBT）所产生的效果迟现于 CBT+SSRI 和 SSRI 所产生的临床疗效，而且 CBT 疗效维持更短。

引自：J Clin Psychiatry, 2010, 71(5)：574

例三： Ethosuximide and valproic acid are more effective than lamotrigine in the treatment of childhood absence epilepsy. Ethosuximide is associated with fewer adverse attentional effects.

与拉莫三嗪相比，乙琥胺与丙戊酸在儿童失神癫痫治疗中更为有效。乙琥胺与药物不良反应相对较小有关。

引自：N Engl J Med, 2010, 362(9)：790

例四： Compared with the placebo, captopril is not only effect in lowering blood pressure, as has been established, but also effective in improving the quality of life (QQL) in hypertensives.

与安慰剂相比，卡托普利不仅能有效地降低血压，而且能提高高血压患者的生活质量。

引自：《中华心血管杂志》，2000, 28(5): 357

（五）提出建议

基于本研究所得出的结论，提出作者的观点或见解。

例一： Cardiorespiratory fitness in young adulthood and a PRS are modestly associated with midlife BMI, although future BMI is associated with BMI in young adulthood. Fitness has a comparable association with future BMI as does the PRS. Caution should be exercised in the widespread use of polygenic risk for obesity prevention in adults, and close clinical surveillance and fitness may have prime roles in limiting the adverse consequences of elevated BMI on health.

尽管青壮年人群后期 BMI 会影响其健康，但青壮年人群的心肺健康和 PRS 与中年 BMI 适度相关，且 BMI 与 PRS 同样有关，因此广泛使用多基因预防成人肥胖会存在一定的风险，应谨慎行事，密切临床监测和健身可在限制 BMI 升高对健康的不利后果方面起主要作用。

引自：JAMA Cardiol, 2020, 5(3): 40

例二： These results suggest an increased risk of myocardial infarction associated with current use of rofecoxib, diclofenac, and ibuprofen despite adjustment for many potential confounders. No evidence was found to support a reduction in risk of myocardial infarction associated with current use of naproxen. This is an observational study and may be subject to residual confounding that cannot be fully corrected for. However, enough concerns may exist to warrant a reconsideration of the cardiovascular safety of all NSAIDs.

尽管对多种可能的混杂因素进行校正,这些研究结果提示服用罗非昔布、双氯芬酸和布洛芬可以增加发生心肌梗死的危险。无证据表明服用萘普生可以降低心肌梗死发生率。这是一项观察研究,可能会受到无法完全纠正的残余混杂因素的影响,然而,必须充分意识到,我们应该对所有NSAIDs的心血管安全性重新评价。

引自: *BMJ*, 2005, 330: 1366

例三: LA epsilon analysis is a new tool that can be used to evaluate LA function. Further studies are warranted to determine the utility of LA epsilon in disease states.

LAε值分析是一种能用于评估左心房功能的新工具,有必要进行进一步研究来确定在疾病状态下LAε值研究的有效性。

引自: *J Am Soc Echocardiogr*, 2010, 23(2): 172

例四: The incidence of large intragenic mismatch repair(*MMR*) genes deletions is relatively higher in Chinese families, and *hMSH2* deletions may be more common. It is necessary to detect the large intragenic *MMR* genes deletions in the molecular detection of HNPCC.

中国人HNPCC错配修复(*MMR*)基因大片段缺失发生率较高,*hMSH2*基因缺失可能更为常见。在分子遗传学检测中有必要开展*MMR*基因大片段缺失的检测。

引自:《中国医学科学院学报》, 2006, 28(6): 837

例五: Surgical closure of isolated VSD is a safe, effective therapy. Risk of death, complete heart block, and reoperation is minimal. As new technologies for VSD closure evolve, results such as these should be considered when evaluating patients, choosing therapeutic options, and counseling families.

单纯性室间隔缺损手术修补是安全有效的疗法,发生死亡、完全性心脏传导阻滞,以及再次手术的风险较低。随着室间隔缺损修补新技术的发展,评估患者状况、选择治疗方式及进行家庭咨询时,应该对这些结果加以考虑。

引自: *Ann Thorac Surg*, 2010, 89(2): 544

例六: These prospective findings suggest that consumption of a Western dietary pattern, meat, and fried foods promotes the incidence of MetSyn, whereas dairy consumption provides some protection. The diet soda association was not hypothesized and deserves further study.

这些前瞻性发现提示，西方饮食模式的消耗量、肉食和油煎食物促进代谢综合征的发生，而每日消耗量可提供一些保护。代谢综合征与饮食中苏打摄入是否有关，值得进一步研究。

注：MetSyn: metabolic syndrome（代谢性综合征）

引自: *Circulation*, 2008, 117(6): 754

二、"Conclusion" 句与语篇连接

语篇通常指一系列连续的语段或句子构成的语言整体，不论是一则对话或一篇文章，它们都不是互不相干的句子的简单堆积，而是一些意义相关的句子为达到一定的交际目的并通过一定连接手段而实现的有机结合。语篇无论以何种形式出现，都必须合乎语法，并且语义连贯，包括与外界在语义上和语用上的连贯，也包括语篇内部在语言上的连贯。一般说来，语篇既有句法上的组织性又有交际上的独立性。一个连贯的语篇必须具有衔接成分，而且必须符合语义、语用和认知原则，句与句之间在概念上必须有联系，句与句的排列应该符合逻辑。

语篇上的衔接体现在两个方面：有形网络和无形网络。有形网络体现在表层结构上的黏着性，即结构上的衔接，主要通过语法手段（如照应、替代、省略等）和词汇手段（如复现关系、同现关系）的使用；无形网络则是语篇中语义的关联，连贯存在于语篇的底层，通过逻辑推理来达到语义连接。

结构式摘要写作，虽然 Objective、Methods、Results 和 Conclusion 自成一体，但又存在内在的语义和逻辑上的关联。例如：

Background: Rate control is often the therapy of choice for **atrial fibrillation**. Guidelines recommend strict rate control, but **this** is not based on clinical evidence. We hypothesized that lenient rate control is not inferior to strict **rate control** for preventing cardiovascular morbidity and mortality in patients with permanent atrial fibrillation. **Methods:** We randomly assigned 614 patients with permanent atrial fibrillation to undergo a lenient rate-control strategy (resting heart rate <110 beats per minute) or a strict **rate-control** strategy (resting heart rate <80 beats per minute and heart rate during moderate exercise <110 beats per minute). The primary outcome was a composite of death from cardiovascular causes, hospitalization for heart failure, and stroke, systemic embolism, bleeding, and life-threatening arrhythmic events. The duration of follow-up was at least 2 years, with a maximum of 3 years. **Results:** The estimated cumulative incidence of the **primary outcome** at 3 years was 12.9% in the **lenient-control group** and 14.9% in the **strict-control group**, with an absolute difference with respect to the **lenient-control group** of −2.0

percentage points (90% confidence interval,−7.6 to 3.5; *P*<0.001 for the prespecified noninferiority margin). **The frequencies** of the components of the **primary outcome** were similar in the two groups. More patients in the lenient-control group met the heart-rate target or targets (304 ［97.7%］, *vs.* 203 ［67.0%］ in the strict-control group; *P*<0.001) with fewer total visits (75 ［median, 0］, *vs.* 684 ［median, 2］; *P*<0.001). **The frequencies** of symptoms and adverse events were similar in the **two groups**. **Conclusions:** In patients with permanent **atrial fibrillation**, **lenient rate control** is as effective as strict rate control and is easier to achieve.

背景：治疗心房颤动通常选择控制心率。尽管治疗指南强调严格心率控制，但这一指导方针并非完全基于临床病例。我们认为，对于持续性心房颤动患者，为降低其心血管病发病率和死亡率，非严格地控制心率的疗效并不比严格心率控制的疗效逊色。方法：将 614 例持续性心房颤动患者随机分组。静息心率<110 次/分患者采用非严格心率控制，静息心率<80 次/分，中等运动强度时心率<110 次/分的患者接受严格心率控制治疗。初期观察结果包括心血管疾病因素所致的死亡，住院治疗心力衰竭，卒中，全身性栓塞，出血性疾病和致死性心律失常发生率。随访期限最低 2 年，最长 3 年。结果：3 年随访结果表明，接受非严格心率控制的患者累计发病率（主要终点）为 12.9%，严格心率控制患者累计发病率为 14.9%。就非严格心率控制看，具有−2 个百分点的绝对差异（90%CI，−7.6～3.5，*P*<0.001，未指定的非劣效性检验界限值）。两组的初期结果构成频数无明显差异。在非严格控制组有更多的患者达到了靶心率（非严格控制组 304 人，占 97.7%；严格控制组 203 人，占 67.0%，*P*<0.001），为数不多的患者获得全程随访［非严格控制组 75 人（中位数为 0），严格控制组 684 人（中位数 2），*P*<0.001］。两组中症状和副作用出现频率无明显差异。结论：治疗永久性心房颤动，非严格心率控制和严格心率控制疗效相差无几，而且前者更容易实现。

引自：*N Engl J Med*, 2010, 362(5): 1363

　　该结构性摘要中，中心词：rate control、atrial fibrillation 始终贯穿于 background、methods、results 和 conclusions 中。在 background 中，借助篇章指示照应词 this 指代中心词：rate control。在 methods 中首次提到本研究的主要观察指标，随后在 results 中通过词汇手段衔接方法之一的复现关系，即重复短语 primary outcome。最后在 conclusions 中再次重复中心词 artial fibrillation 与 rate control 之间的关联，从而使得"Conclusion"句与整个语篇既相对独立，又互为关联。

　　"结论"亦即"评论"，是作者对研究结果或实验结果予以综合，正确解释某种现象产生的原因，所解决的问题，突出本研究的创新之处，说明本研究的理论和实践意义及有待解决的问题或今后的研究方向等。虽然"结论"的表达要求简洁明了，通常用一两句话即可，但又不能孤立于整个语篇之外。缺乏逻辑关联的语篇必将难以有效传递信息。如何写好"Conclusion"句？本节拟从语篇衔接手段方面举例说明。

（一）语法手段（照应、替代、省略）

例一： This risk score is an objective aid in deciding on further management of patients with stable angina with the aim of reducing serious outcome events. The score can also be used in planning future trials.

该危险评分在客观上有助于确定稳定型心绞痛患者的进一步治疗措施，从而减少严重复发后果。该危险评分同样可以用于后期试验设计。

【析】英语中指示照应通常可以用指示代词（this/these, that/those）或者相应的限定词 ［this/these infectious disease(s)，that/those infectious disease(s)］来表示。本例中，就是利用限定词 this 起到衔接作用的。

引自：*BMJ*, 2005, 331(7521): 869

例二： Compared with secondary prevention, primary prevention achieved a fourfold larger reduction in deaths. Future CHD policies should prioritise population-wide tobacco control and healthier diet.

一级预防降低死亡的效果是二级预防的 4 倍。未来的冠心病防治策略应优先考虑控烟的人群及更健康的饮食。

【析】这是利用语义范畴上的比较照应来实现语篇连接的。很明显，这是一个对比研究，作者为了突出其中一个手段的重要性，即作者的结论。采用这一连接手段避免了不必要的重复，从而使语言表达简洁明了，中心突出。

引自：*BMJ*, 2005, 331(7517): 614

例三： An association between physical activity and myopia was observed, suggesting a protective effect of physical activity on the development and progression of myopia in university students. **The results** confirm that intensive studying is a risk factor of myopia and that myopic progression or development is more likely in medical students in their early 20 s than in their late 20 s.

身体锻炼和近视之间存在着联系，提示身体锻炼对大学生近视眼的发生和发展具有保护效应。该研究结果证实高强度学习是近视的一种危险因素，但在二十岁前，医学生更容易发生近视问题。

【析】本例采用的是替代照应连接手段，利用词的上下义关系实现语篇照应。

引自：*Invest Ophthalmol Vis Sci*, 2008, 49(4): 1322

例四： Patients with AF undergoing PCI with stenting represent a high-risk population because of age, comorbidities, and presence of stroke risk factors. These patients have a high mortality and MACE rate, **which** is reduced by anticoagulation therapy.

接受经皮冠脉支架植入术的房颤患者因其年龄，合并症和卒中危险因素而成为高危人群。这些患者的死亡率和 MACE 发生率很高，但抗凝治疗可以降低这些不良事件发生率。

注：MACE 意指 major adverse cardiac events（主要心脏不良事件）

【析】利用关系代词 which 指代前文中的 MACE rate，不仅使得语篇内容达到逻辑连贯，同时还避免了重复。

引自：*JACC*, 2008, 51(8)：818

（二）词汇手段

避免重复是一个重要的修辞手段，但是，在不引起累赘的前提下，可恰当地利用词汇重复，从而实现语篇衔接。

例一：**Results**... Major bleeding occurred in one patient (0.2%) in each group. At the end of follow-up, 14 patients in the **fondaparinux** group (3.3%) and 25 in the placebo group (6.0%) had died. **Conclusion Fondaparinux** is effective in the prevention of asymptomatic and symptomatic venous thromboembolic events in older acute medical patients. The frequency of major bleeding was similar for both fondaparinux and placebo treated patiens.

【结果】各组中各有一位患者（0.2%）发生大出血。随访结束时，安慰剂组、fondaparinus 治疗组分别死亡 25 例（6.0%）、14 例（3.3%）患者。

结论：fondaparinux 可有效预防急性内科老年患者无症状性及有症状的静脉血栓。严重出血概率两组相似。

【析】在语篇衔接照应中，常使用指示照应词，但是，如果指向性缺乏明显对应时，使用指示照应词不仅起不到连接语篇的作用，反而会导致语义模糊。此时，利用词汇重复关系这一衔接手段，就能更好地达到语篇上的衔接，如本例中就是重复 fondaparinux 一词来实现的。这种衔接手段在结果句写作中较为常见。

引自：*BMJ*, 2006, 332: 1032

例二：**A diagnostic management strategy using a simple clinical decision rule, D-dimer testing, and CT** is effective in the evaluation and management of patients with clinically suspected pulmonary embolism. **Its use** is associated with low risk for subsequent fatal and nonfatal VTE.

使用简化的临床评估标准、D-二聚体检测及 CT 检查可有效评估和处理临床肺栓塞疑似患者。这种方案的使用可降低后期发生致死性和非致死性静脉血栓栓塞风险。

【析】利用词汇 its use 照应。

引自：*JAMA*, 2006, 295: 172

例三：Baseline health-related quality of life (HRQL) was similar in patients with and without obesity-related disease prior to gastric bypass. After surgery, patients with no comorbidity had similar positive changes in HRQL as patients with one or several comorbidities. **These findings** indicate that other factors than obesity-related disease are at least as important for severely obese patients' impaired HRQL.

基线健康相关生活质量（HRQL）在胃旁路手术之前的评分，与有肥胖相关疾病的患者和没有肥胖相关疾病的患者基本接近。手术后，无共患病的患者在 HRQL 中的评分变化与有一种或多种共病的患者相似。这些发现表明，肥胖相关疾病以外的其他因素对于严重肥胖患者的 HRQL 受损至少同样重要。

【析】"结论"中用了 These findings 照应前文内容。

引自：*Obesity Surgery*, 2015, 25: 2408

（三）常用结构

"Conclusion"句写作常见结构如下：

（1）The /Our results/findings/study (ies)/data/observation/analysis/experiment (s)/investigation show (s) /showed that…

结果（发现、研究、数据、观察、分析、实验、调查）表明……

（2）The /Our results/findings/study (ies)/data/observation/analysis/experiment (s)/investigation suggest (s)/suggested that…

结果（发现、研究、数据、观察、分析、实验、调查）表明……

（3）The /Our results/findings/study (ies)/data/observation/analysis/experiment (s)/investigation confirm (s)/confirmed that…

结果（发现、研究、数据、观察、分析、实验、调查）证实……

（4）The /Our results/findings/study (ies)/data/observation/analysis/experiment (s)/investigation indicate (s)/indicated that…

结果（发现、研究、数据、观察、分析、实验、调查）提示……

（5）The /Our results/findings/study (ies)/data/observation/analysis/experiment (s)/investigation demonstrate (s) / demonstrated that…

结果（发现、研究、数据、观察、分析、实验、调查）表明……

（6）The /Our results/findings/study (ies)/data/observation/analysis/experiment (s)/investigation support (s)/supported that…

结果（发现、研究、数据、观察、分析、实验、调查）证明……

（7）The /Our results/findings/study (ies)/data/observation/analysis/experiment (s)/investigation accord (s)/accorded with…

结果（发现、研究、数据、观察、分析、实验、调查）与……一致

（8）The /Our results/findings/study (ies)/data/observation/analysis/experiment (s)/investigation agree (s)/agreed well with…

结果（发现、研究、数据、观察、分析、实验、调查）与……（非常/相当）一致

（9）The /Our results/findings/study (ies)/data/observation/analysis/experiment (s)/investigation illustrate (s) /illustrated that...

结果（发现、研究、数据、观察、分析、实验、调查）表明……

（10）The /Our results/findings/study (ies)/data/observation/analysis/experiment (s)/investigation provide (s)/provided evidence that...

结果（发现、研究、数据、观察、分析、实验、调查）提供了……证据

（11）The /Our results/findings/study (ies)/data/observation/analysis/experiment (s)/investigation point (s) /pointed out that...

结果（发现、研究、数据、观察、分析、实验、调查）表明……

（12）The /Our results/findings/study (ies)/data/observation/analysis/experiment (s)/investigation reveal (s)/revealed that...

结果（发现、研究、数据、观察、分析、实验、调查）揭示……

（13）The /Our results/findings/study (ies)/data/observation/analysis/experiment (s)/investigation supply a basis for...

结果（发现、研究、数据、观察、分析、实验、调查）提供……的基础

（14）The /Our results/findings/study (ies)/data/observation/analysis/experiment (s)/investigation is (are) consistent/ in accord/with the theory/ hypothesis/previous studies/ that...

结果（发现、研究、数据、观察、分析、实验、调查）与……理论（假说、以前的研究）相一致

（15）Results are contrasted with/different from...

结果与……相反（不同）

（16）In summary/conclusion, ...

总之，……

（17）It is concluded that...

结论是……

（18）Further analysis/experiments/study will be necessary/needed to confirm...

有必要做进一步的分析（实验、研究）以证实……

例一：This retrospective study suggested that preventive coagulation of visible vessels in the resection area after ESD may lead to a lower bleeding rate.

该回顾性研究提示内镜黏膜下层剥离术后对暴露出的血管予以预防性凝固可降低出血率。

引自：*Endoscopy*, 2008, 40(3): 179

例二：Our findings suggest that in HL, hepcidin is upregulated by IL-6. Elevated hepcidin levels result in iron restriction and signs of anemia of chronic inflammation, although hepcidin-independent mechanisms contribute to development of anemia in HL.

我们的研究表明，霍奇金淋巴瘤患者体内 IL-6 介导了铁调素的表达上

调。虽然铁调素非依赖的机制也参与了霍奇金淋巴瘤患者贫血的发生，但增高的铁调素限制了铁的利用，从而导致慢性炎症性贫血。

引自：*J Clin Oncol*, 2010, 28(15)：2538

例三：The results of this preliminary study suggest the potential application of MB-photodynamic inactivation of plasma virus is an useful approach in clinical practice.

初步证明，亚蓝/光化学法可高效灭活血浆中的模型病毒，与此同时，几种凝血因子的活性也受到了不同程度的影响。

引自：《中华实验和临床病毒学杂志》, 2000, 14(1): 52

例四：The current study demonstrates that CRT reverses LV remodelling in heart failure patients with chronic RV pacing in a similar way as in primary CRT recipients, even after very long periods of RV pacing. Our data, therefore, may have important implications for the treatment of pacemaker-dependent patients with heart failure, and support the use of CRT in this setting.

这项研究表明，与 CRT 植入治疗相似，即使在右心室起搏很长一段时间后，CRT 也能有效逆转慢性 RV 起搏心力衰竭患者的 LV 重塑。因此，本研究对需依赖起搏器的心力衰竭患者治疗具有重要意义，且支持在此情况下应用 CRT。

引自：*Eur Heart J*, 2010, 31(12)：1477

例五：Our results suggest that oral sildenafil is a safe and effective alternate for persistent pulmonary hypertension following congenital heart surgery in children.

研究结果表明，口服昔多芬是治疗患儿先天性心脏病术后出现的持续性肺动脉高压的一种安全而且有效的替代疗法。

引自：*Eur J Cardiothorac Surg*, 2010, 38(1)：71

例六：In conclusion, these data indicate that LV pressure in patients with CCTGA affects the degree of TR and that septal shift caused by changes in LV and RV pressure is an important mechanism.

总之，该研究数据表明患有先天矫正型大动脉转位症（CCTGA）的患者中左心室压力可以影响三尖瓣反流（TR）的程度，并且由于左右心室压力的变化所导致的室间隔移位是一个重要的发病机制。

引自：*Am J Cardiol*, 2010, 105(5)：735

例七：Our results are similar to those observed with probiotic strains and suggest that indole could be important in the intestinal epithelial cells response to gastrointestinal tract pathogens.

我们的研究结果与对益生菌菌株的研究结果类似，这表明吲哚在肠道上皮细胞对胃肠道病原体的反应中可能起着重要的作用。

引自：*Proc Natl Acad Sci U S A*, 2010, 107(1)：228

三、功能篇："可能性"表示法

"Conclusion"作为研究结果的终极性总结，从严格意义上说，所得出的"结论"不应含糊其辞。对此，有不少学者坚持认为，既然结论源于结果，即是由具体"结果"抽象演绎出的一般性原理，结论应是肯定的。事实上，随着科学研究的进展、创新和新发现，这就意味着没有终极性的结论。其次，任何一项研究一定是研究者新思想的体现，研究者可能限于目前的研究技术手段或现有硬件设备的技术支持，但本着严谨的科学态度，某些"结论"就不会那么肯定，这与不成熟的研究是大相径庭的。显然，这些"结论"可能会起到抛砖引玉的作用。用英文写作和汉语写作在措辞方面存在较大的差异，对某些功能意念的表达就不可能完全对等。本节就这一问题从语义、语用方面对"可能性"表示法做分析对比，以期提高读者的措辞能力。

人们对事物的看法或某一结果的判断，通常涉及对"可能程度"（degrees of likelihood）的估计。对"可能程度"的不同看法都带有主观判断的成分。主观判断有别于臆断，它是建立在客观事实的基础上所得出的某种结论，是一种理性上的分析判断。

（一）完全可能

"完全可能"是指对所陈述的内容有百分之百或接近百分之百的把握，汉语中可用"必定、肯定、一定"等词语来表示，在英语中常用的表达：①用形容词 sure 或 certain；②用副词 surely、definitely、certainly、undoubtedly；③习惯用语"There's no doubt(that)... "；④情态动词 must。此外，若做否定判断，可与否定词 not 或 no 连用。但要注意的是，must 不可与 not 或 no 连用。

例一： Undoubtedly, the laboratory markers **must be** the criteria for diagnosis of ARF.

毫无疑问，该生化指标完全可以作为急性肾衰竭的诊断标准。

引自：*Lancet*,2010,376(9736):163

例二： Therefore, research efforts **must be** continued to focus on oral agents with chances of high cure rate.

因此，今后的研究工作应继续注重在具有高治愈率的口服药物上。

引自：*J Health Popul Nutr*, 2000, 18: 33

例三： This new knowledge would **undoubtedly** translate into a more efficient prevention and treatment of this common post-operative complication that is associated with a major health and economic burden.

毫无疑问，这种新认知必会促进对此类常见术后并发症进行更有效的预防和治疗，而这种常见术后并发症与健康和经济负担密切相关。

引自：*JACC*, 2008, 51(8): 793

例四： We found no evidence that etomidate is associated with worse outcome than thiopental or propofol in patients undergoing emergency laparotomy, but we **cannot be certain** that etomidate is well tolerated in this group of patients. More data are required to address this issue **definitively**.

在急诊剖腹探查手术中，与使用硫喷妥钠或丙泊酚诱导麻醉相比，没有证据表明在预后方面，使用依托咪酯诱导会更差，但我们无法确定本组患者是否对依托咪酯有较好的耐受性，该结论还需要更多的数据来证明。

引自：*Eur J Anaesthesiol*, 2010, 27(5)：481

（二）很可能

"很可能"是对所陈述的内容有相当大的把握，如70%～90%的把握，但还没有达到完全的把握，相当于汉语口语中的"多半"。英语中表达"很可能"有下列几种表示法：①用 probable（adj.）、likely（adj.）、probably（adv.）等；②用情态动词 will、should、ought to 等。Will 表示"可能性"时，含有"根据其固有特点和规律很可能……"，should 和 ought to 含有"按道理，按常规或按已知情况等很可能会……"的意思。Should 和 ought to 的本意是"应该"，在句中有时有"可能性"和"理应"两种意思兼备；③用 may 或 might。要注意的是，从情态动词在语境中所反应的"确定性"与"不确定性"意义看，ought to 和 might 暗示"最不确定性"，"Conclusion"句中应慎用这两个词。

例一：Breast cancer estrogen-receptor (ER) status **may** also help predict which patients benefit from advances in adjuvant chemotherapy.

雌激素受体状态有助于预测哪些乳腺癌患者可从新型辅助化疗中获益。

引自：*JAMA*, 2006, 295: 1658

例二：These data revealed, for the first time, that DBZ promoted multiple key steps of angiogenesis, at least in part through Akt and MAPK signalling pathways, and suggest it **may** be potentially developed further for treating myocardial infarction and other cardiovascular diseases.

这些数据首次揭示，丹参素冰片酯（DBZ）至少部分通过 Akt 和 MAPK 信号通路促进血管生成的多个关键过程，并提示 DBZ 可能被进一步开发用于治疗心肌梗死和其他心血管疾病的药物。

引自：*Br J Pharmacol*, 2019, 176(17): 3143-3160

例三：The rate of appendiceal rupture in school-aged children was associated with race and health insurance status and not with negative appendectomy rate and therefore is more **likely** to be associated with prehospitalization factors such as access to care, quality of care, and patient or physician education.

学龄儿童的阑尾穿孔发生率与种族和健康保险状况相关，而与阴性阑尾切除率无关，因此更可能与某些入院前因素有关，如是否能得到治疗、治疗的质量及患者或医生受教育的情况等。

引自：*JAMA*, 2004, 292: 1977

例四：Given uncertainties about the balance between the risks and benefits of bariatric surgery in the long term, the decision to undergo surgery **should** be based on a high quality shared decision making process.

从长远看，鉴于减肥手术的风险和收益之间的平衡存在不确定性，是否采用手术治疗应取决于有效的共同决策过程。

引自：*BMJ*, 2014, 349: 3961

例五：The results suggest that neostigmine **might be** safer than sugammadex when assessing only the incidence of anaphylaxis.

结果表明，仅就过敏反应发生率而言，新斯的明可能比 sugammadex 更安全。

引自：*BJA*, 2020, 124(2): 154

（三）可能

"可能"常用的表达方法：possible(*adj.*)、possibly、perhaps、maybe(*adv.*)、possibility(*n.*)等词汇。

例一：BMD loss is greater in hip and slower at spine in DM women during menopausal transition. Women with DM have a higher risk of fractures, **perhaps** because of their earlier menopause.

在绝经过渡期，糖尿病（DM）妇女的髋关节骨密度（BMD）流失较快，而脊柱骨密度流失较慢。糖尿病妇女骨折风险较高可能与更年期提前有关。

引自：*Osteoporos Int*, 2011, 22(5): 1367

例二：In addition, **it is possible that** even moderate calorie restriction may be harmful in specific patient populations, such as lean persons who have minimal amounts of body fat.

除此之外，对于某些特定人群，一定程度上限制热量摄入可能是有害的，如偏瘦体格者。

引自：*JAMA*, 2007, 297: 986

例三：We conclude that long-term use of coumarins is associated with enhanced extracoronary vascular calcification, **possibly** through the inhibition of MGP carboxylation.

我们推断长期使用香豆素与外周动脉钙化的增加有关，这可能是因为香豆素抑制了 Gla 基质蛋白（MGP）的羧化。

引自：*Blood*, 2010, 115(24)：5121

四、"Conclusion"句中几个常用动词特殊用法及其结构

在本章中，我们已经给出了"Conclusion"句写作常见表达方式，除此之外，医学

论文英文摘要结论写作常涉及动词 suggest、propose、recommend、show、conclude、indicate、illustrate、confirm 等，同时，为了语言表达多元性，这些动词除了使用常见的动词句型结构外，还可以使用其同根名词。常用结构如下所述。

1. suggest

suggest 在 "Conclusion" 句中的意思为 to give signs of、make clear、indicate（暗示，表明），其后由连接代词 that 引起的从句中，谓语动词由于陈述的是真实条件，因此，that 从句中谓语动词通常用一般式。如果所表达的结论，在作者看来有必要做进一步论证时，其后 that 从句中的谓语动词可接非真实条件结构。

（1）...suggest(s) that...：……的研究结果表明……。
（2）It is suggested that...：本研究/实验等表明……。

例一： Current vaccination strategies prioritizing elderly persons may be less effective than believed at reducing serious morbidity and mortality in this population, which **suggests that** supplementary strategies may be necessary.
目前优先考虑老年人的疫苗接种战略在降低这一人群的严重发病率和死亡率方面可能还不是想象中的那么有效，但至少表明疫苗接种可能是一种补救措施。

引自：*Ann Intern Med*, 2020, 172(7): 445

例二： Positive HPHIS are positively associated with DM and IGT independently. **It is suggested that** the population with positive HPHIS may be an important risk factor for development of DM.
高血压家族史（HPHIS）阳性与糖尿病、IGT 的发生呈独立正相关，提示 HPHIS 阳性是糖尿病的重要发病危险因素之一。

引自：《中华内科杂志》, 2000, 39(6): 395

特别提示："It is suggested that..." 属于无主结构，使用时应考虑到句子与句子之间的一致性，即句子与句子之间的逻辑关联。因此，上述例二应修改为 "Positive HPHIS are positively associated with DM and IGT independently, **suggesting that/which suggests that** the population with positive HPHIS may be an important risk factor for development of DM."。

例三： **Results suggest that** malignant hypertension **is** yet another disease related to cigarette smoking.
本研究表明，恶性高血压是另一种与吸烟有关的疾病。

引自：*Stroke*, 2003, 34: 2285

例四： **These results suggest that** treatment with tolterodine ER plus tamsulosin for 12 weeks **provides** benefit for men with moderate to severe lower urinary tract symptoms including overactive bladder.

上述结果提示，托特罗定缓释片+坦索罗辛联合治疗（12 周）对有中、重度下尿路症状（包括膀胱过度活动症）的男性患者有益。

引自：JAMA, 2006, 296: 2319

2. conclude

1）We conclude that…：我们的结论是……。

2）It is concluded that…：结论是……。

3）Our conclusion is that…：我们的结论是……。

4）It can be concluded that…：可以得出……结论。

5）Conclusion can be reached/drawn that…：可以得出……结论。

例一：**We conclude that** both gain and loss of homeobox genes were important for the evolutionary change of phenotypic characters in bilateral animals.

我们的结论是同源异形基因的得失对于两侧对称动物表型特征的进化都十分重要。

引自：Mol Biol Evol, 2005, 21: 236

例二：**Conclusion can be reached that** the pancreas is sometimes permanently damaged during infectious hepatitis.

由此可见，在传染性肝炎患病期间胰腺有时会受到永久性损害。

引自：Nucleic Acids Res, 2006, 24: 3875

特别提示：conclusion 作名词使用时，与之搭配的动词可以是 reach 或 draw。

例三：We concluded that including etoposide in the initial treatment of EBV-HLH patients can improve their prognosis, especially adult patients. This may be because that adult patients are recognized as "higher risk" patients.

我们的结论是，早期使用依托泊苷治疗 EBV-HLH 患者，可以改善其预后，尤其是成年患者。这可能是因为成年患者被认为是"高风险"患者。

引自：Br J Haematol, 2019, 186(5):717-723

3. propose

通常情况下，propose 后的从句应用非真实条件结构，但如果表示"提出"（To put forward for consideration, discussion,or adoption）、"认为"（To make known as one's intention）等含义时，其后由 that 引起的从句中谓语动词则用真实条件结构。

1）The authors propose that…：作者建议……。

2）It is proposed that…：建议……。

例一：Endovascular treatment may thus be **proposed** as an alternative to surgical clipping at this location. Nevertheless, a longer follow-up period is necessary to determine its efficacy, particularly in cases of unruptured aneurysms.

血管内治疗方法很有可能替代该部位的外科夹闭手术治疗，但需要较长时间的随访期来确定该治疗的有效性，尤其是在治疗未破裂的动脉瘤时更需要注意。

引自：J Neurosurg, 2010, 112(4)：703

例二： The authors **propose that** supportive management must remain the mainstay of therapy even in severely intoxicated patients.

作者认为，即使对于重度中毒患者，支持疗法应为首选治疗方法。

引自：Biochem Pharmacol, 2000, 59: 847

例三： We **propose that** SHP functions as a novel tumor suppressor in the development of HCC. These findings provide new insight into the molecular mechanisms leading to this common cancer and may have both diagnostic and therapeutic applications.

研究者提出 SHP 可能是肝细胞癌发展过程中一个新肿瘤抑制基因，有可能成为肝细胞分子机制新的研究方向，并且有望运用于诊断和治疗。

引自：Gastroenterology, 2008, 134(3)：793

4. recommend

recommend 后接 that 引起的从句中谓语动词要用非真实条件结构。

1）The authors recommend that…：我们建议……。

2）It is recommended that…：建议……。

例一： A two-tablet increase in L-T(4) initiated at confirmation of pregnancy significantly reduces the risk of maternal hypothyroidism during the first trimester and mimics normal physiology. Monitoring TSH every 4 wk through midgestation **is recommended**.

研究证明，妊娠初期增加左旋甲状腺素 2 片可明显降低孕妇妊娠前 3 个月甲状腺功能减退的风险，且母体呈现正常生理功能，但建议妊娠中期每 4 周一次监测 TSH 水平。

引自：J Clin Endocrinol Metab, 2010, 95(7): 3234

例二： Furthermore, as anti-Ro52 reactivity is more prevalent than anti-Ro60 reactivity in certain autoimmune conditions, specific testing for their distinction in clinical practice **is recommended**.

而且，在某些特定自身免疫状态下，抗 Ro52 抗体活性比抗 Ro60 抗体活性更为常见。为区别上述抗体在临床应用中的特点，有必要对其进行特异性试验。

引自：Postgrad Med J, 2010, 86(1012)：79

例三： In high-risk patients, remission induction regimens must be improved, and allogeneic SCT **should be recommended** in patients achieving second complete remission.

在高危患者中，必须改善诱导缓解治疗方案，达到第二次完全缓解患者，推荐接受异体干细胞移植治疗。

引自：*J Clin Oncol*, 2010, 28(14)：2339

五、其他常用表达法

（一）"影响因素"的表达

1）…be associated with…：……与……有关。

2）…be affected by…：……受……影响。

3）… be an important risk factor for…：……对……是高危因素。

4）…be closely related to…：……与……密切相关。

5）…be involved in…：……与……有关。

6）There are some relationship between…：……与……有关。

7）…be one of the primary causes for…：……重要原因之一。

8）There is some association between…：……与……有关。

9）…may lead to/result in/account for…：……可能导致……（是……的原因）。

10）…is related /due/attributed to…：……与……有关（由于……，归因于……）。

例一： Episodes of AHFS **are associated with** transient increases in markers of myocyte injury and ECM turnover that may reflect an acceleration of pathological myocardial remodeling during AHFS.

急性心衰综合征（AHFS）发作与反映急性心衰综合征期间病理性心肌重构加速的心肌细胞损伤标志物瞬间升高和细胞外基质（ECM）代谢有关。

引自：*Circ Heart Fail*, 2010, 3(1)：44

例二： Systemic inflammation in the decompensated heart failure **may contribute to** RVF after LVAD implant left ventricular assist device right ventricular failure.

失代偿性心力衰竭所致的全身性炎症可能导致左心室辅助装置（LVAD）植入后发生右心室衰竭（RVF）。

引自：*J Cardiothorac Surg*, 2019, 14: 80

例三： Pericardial fat **is correlated with** multiple measures of adiposity and cardiovascular disease risk factors, but VAT is a stronger correlate of most metabolic risk factors. However, intrathoracic and pericardial fat **are associated with** vascular calcification, which suggests that these fat depots may exert local toxic effects on the vasculature.

心包脂肪与不同肥胖程度和心血管病危险因素相关，但VAT与绝大多数代谢性危险因素相关性更强，然而，胸内和心包脂肪与血管钙化相关，从而提示脂肪沉积可能对血管造成毒性影响。

引自: Circulation, 2008, 117(5): 605

例四: Increased serum total bilirubin level **is associated with** reduced PAD prevalence.
血清总胆红素升高与降低 PAD 发病率相关。

引自: Arterioscler Thromb Vasc Biol, 2008, 28(1): 166

例五: Continuing annual breast cancer screening past age 75 years **did not result in** substantial reductions in 8-year breast cancer mortality compared with stopping screening.
与不做任何筛查相比，每年对 75 岁以上人群进行乳腺癌筛查并不能使 8 年乳腺癌死亡率大幅下降。

引自: Ann Intern Med, 2020, 172(6): 381

（二）"标志"的表示法

1）...be as an indicator of...: ······作为······的标志。

2）...be used as an objective indicator in...: ······作为······的客观标志。

3）...be regarded as an important judgement line in...:
······作为······的重要判断指标。

4）...become an indicator for...: ······是······的指标。

例一: Examination of VEGF expression can help to select the patients who need chemotherapy and radiotherapy, and may **be as an indicator** of prognosis.
检测 VEGF（血管内皮生长因子）表达可作为胃癌的预后指标，有助于对术后病人放化疗的选择提供依据。

引自:《中华试验外科杂志》, 2000, 17(1): 42

例二: PreS1 is more sensitive than HBeAg when as a serological index of HBV infection and reproduction. Determination of PreS1 has a great application value in diagnosis and treatment of hepatitis B. PreS1 could be taken as **a new serological indicator for** infectivity and replication of HBV.
PreS1 抗原作为乙肝感染和复制的血清学指标敏感性高于 HBeAg，对提示乙肝患者的病情发展和转归有重要临床意义。PreS1 可以作为一项新的乙肝病毒复制的传染性指标。

引自:《第四军医大学学报》, 2007, 28(5): 442

例三: Hence, identification of SLE patients who cannot dismantle NETs might be a useful **indicator of** renal involvement. Moreover, NETs might represent a therapeutic target in SLE.
因此，系统性红斑狼疮（SLE）患者体内的 NETs 降解程度可能是评估其肾脏受累的一个有用指标。不仅如此，NETs 还可能是 SLE 的一个新的治疗靶点。

引自：*Proc Natl Acad Sci U S A*, 2010, 107(21): 9813

（三）有待解决的问题和对未来的展望表示法

在"结论"句中，作者如果认为在一次性研究中难以解决诸多问题或研究中产生了新的相关问题时，应做出客观评价。同时也是为从事同类研究的同行提供研究信息。另外，在结论的结尾句中，也可以对本研究的应用方向提供线索，即本研究的前景。写作时可用下列句式表达。

1）Whether...remains to be determined：是否……有待确定。

2）Whether...is yet to be determined：是否……有待确定。

3）Further analysis/experiments will be necessary：有必要做进一步的分析（实验）。

4）It is necessary to make/carry out (a) further study on...：有必要对……做更深入研究。

5）There are some/several limitations to...：……存在（一些）不足之处。

6）... should be further explored/investigated...：……应进一步探讨（研究）。

7）...will be required：……需要……。

例一：Treatment of peanut-allergic children with epicutaneous immunotherapy **remains to be determined**.

治疗儿童花生过敏症的疗效有待进一步验证。

引自：*JAMA*, 2019, 321(10): 946

例二：The use of acid-suppressive therapy, particularly proton pump inhibitors, is associated with an increased risk of community-acquired *C. difficile*. The unexpected increase in risk with nonsteroidal anti-inflammatory drug use should **be investigated further.**

抑酸治疗（特别是质子泵抑制剂的使用）与社区获得性艰难梭状芽孢杆菌感染的危险增加有关。非甾体抗炎药的使用也增加这一危险，对于这一意外结果尚需开展进一步研究。

引自：*JAMA*, 2005, 294: 2989

例三：This study provides longitudinal biochemical evidence that lactation duration is independently associated with lower incidence of diabetes. **Further investigation is required** to elucidate mechanisms that may explain this relationship.

这项研究提供了纵向生化证据，表明哺乳时间与较低的糖尿病发病率独立相关，但这两种之间的关系机制需要进一步研究论证。

引自：*JAMA Intern Med*, 2018, 178(3): 328

例四：Our data demonstrated that higher levels of cystatin C are associated with an increased risk of HF and that such association may be limited to hypertensive individuals. **Additional studies are warranted to further examine** the relationship between hypertension and cystatin C on the risk of HF.

我们的数据表明，较高水平的胱抑素 C 与心力衰竭风险增加相关，这种相关性可能仅限于高血压个体。还需要更多的研究来进一步验证高血压和胱抑素 C 在心力衰竭风险中的关系。

引自：*American Heart Journal*, 2008, 155(1): 82

例五： The authors found no evidence that the clinical presentation associated with an ICA occlusion was related to patency of other extra or intracranial arteries to act as collateral pathways. **Further work is required to investigate** what determines the clinical effects of ICA occlusion.

研究未发现ICA阻塞的临床症状与其他开放的颈外或颅内动脉形成的侧支循环相关，尚需进一步的研究探寻何种因素决定了 ICA 阻塞的临床症状。

引自：*J Neurol Neurosurg Psychiatry*, 2006, 77(6): 7291

例六： In clinical settings, however, the limitations of such a simple measure of predominant symptom dimensions should be borne in mind and further work on their validity and utility is needed.

然而，在临床环境中，我们需要重视的是，主要症状维度的简易测量方法仍存在一定的局限性，对此，还需要对其有效性和实用性进行进一步的研究。

引自：*Psychiatry Res*, 2010, 18(1): 25

六、"Conclusion"句中动词形式的确定和语态

在结构式摘要中，撰写"Conclusion"句时英语动词常涉及下述三种形式。

（一）动词的一般式，即一般现在时

这是"Conclusion"句中最常用的动词形式。"Conclusion"句中如果作者认为其结论具有普遍性，可用一般现在时。

例一： For individuals with no cardiovascular risk factors as well as for those with 1 or more risk factors, those who **are** obese in middle age have a higher risk of hospitalization and mortality from CHD, cardiovascular disease, and diabetes in older age than those who **are** normal weight.

对没有心血管危险因素的人群和有1个或1个以上危险因素的人群而言，中年时肥胖者老年后因 CHD、心血管疾病或糖尿病住院和死亡的风险高于中年时体重正常者。

引自：*JAMA*, 2006, 295: 190

例二：This method **is rapid, accurate, simple, and economical** for detecting *E.coli*.

本法是一种快速、准确、简易和廉价的检测大肠埃希菌的方法。

引自：《中华检验医学杂志》, 2000, 24(3): 168

例三：Extubation and NIV **are feasible** in patients who stabilize during ECLS therapy.

临时体外生命支持（ECLS）治疗期间稳定的患者中，拔管和无创通气（NIV）是可行的。

引自：*J Intensive Care Med*, 2020, doi: 101177/0885066620918171

（二）动词的过去式，即一般过去时

若作者认为该结论为研究结束时的结论，而该结论并不具备普遍性，则用过去式；如果"结论"句陈述的是前期观察发现，动词应用过去式（提示：国外医学期刊在"结论"句中动词用过去式比较多见，国内某些期刊则较少使用过去式动词）。

例一：These results suggest an increased risk of myocardial infarction associated with current use of rofecoxib, diclofenac, and ibuprofen despite adjustment for many potential confounders. No evidence **was found** to support a reduction in risk of myocardial infarction associated with current use of naproxen.

尽管对多种可能的混杂因素进行校正，但这些研究结果提示服用罗非昔布、双氯芬酸和布洛芬可以增加发生心肌梗死的危险。没有发现支持服用蔡普生可以降低心肌梗死发生率的证据。

引自：*BMJ*, 2005, 330: 1366

例二：Among patients with stable coronary disease and moderate or severe ischemia, we **did not find** evidence that an initial invasive strategy, as compared with an initial conservative strategy, **reduced** the risk of ischemic cardiovascular events or death from any cause over a median of 3.2 years.

在稳定的冠状动脉疾病和中度或重度缺血的患者中，我们未发现证据证明与最初的保守治疗策略相比，初始侵入性治疗（中位数 3.2 年）可降低缺血性心血管疾病或任何原因导致的死亡风险。

引自：*N Engl J Med*, 2020, 382: 1395

例三：Habitual vigorous activity **was not associated with** increased risk of subsequent MI in subjects with established CHD, but additional data for stroke would be useful.

冠心病患者日常剧烈体力活动与心肌梗死风险增高无关，但与卒中的相关性还有待进一步研究。

引自：*Eur Heart J*, 2008, 29(3): 355

例四： The metabolic syndrome **was associated with** increased risk of AF. The metabolic derangements of the syndrome may be important in the pathogenesis of AF.

代谢综合征和 AF 发生危险的增加相关，提示代谢失调在 AF 的发生过程中可能十分重要。

引自：*Circulation*, 2008, 117(10)：1255

例五： In this 12-week trial, the thyroid hormone analogue eprotirome **was associated with** decreases in levels of atherogenic lipoproteins in patients receiving treatment with statins.

为期 12 周的研究显示，在接受他汀治疗的患者中，甲状腺激素类似物 Eprotirome 能降低致动脉粥样硬化脂蛋白的水平。

引自：*N Engl J Med*, 2010, 362(10)：906

（三）表示未来时间的动词形式

这一动词形式可用来表达作者对本研究的预期效果或展望。英语中表示未发生的行为可以借助多种动词形式，如一般现在时，情态助动词 will、be+to do 等形式。按传统英语语法概念，或称之为一般将来时。如若表达作者客观、委婉的看法或建议时，可用情态助动词 "should+动词原形" 来表达。

例一： One in 10 patients aged 45 or more with new onset rectal bleeding had colonic neoplasia, so investigation of the bowel **should be** offered to all such patients, whether or not they have other symptoms.

年龄≥45 岁的新发直肠出血患者中 1/10 有结肠肿瘤，因此，无论是否伴随其他症状，对所有此类患者都应进行肠道检查。

引自：*BMJ*, 2006, 4: 273

例二： Evidence suggests that more intensive lowering of low-density lipoprotein cholesterol (LDL-C) than is commonly applied clinically **will provide** further benefit in stable coronary artery disease.

证据显示，与临床常规降脂比较，对稳定性冠状动脉疾病患者施行强化降脂降低低密度脂蛋白胆固醇可进一步获益。

引自：*JAMA*, 2005, 294: 2437

例三： There were no significant differences in short-term clinical success and technical success between octogenarians and non-octogenarians. However, octogenarians showed a significantly higher incidence of perioperative adverse events, particularly in major adverse events and non-technical adverse events. Peroral endoscopic myotomy for octogenarians **should be** carefully applied.

对于 80～89 岁的老年患者,经口内镜下肌切开术短期临床效果和手术成功率方面与非该年龄段的患者没有显著性差异。然而，围术期不良事件的发生率在 80～89 岁的老年患者中明显升高,特别是重大不良事件和非手术相关的不良事件,因此，对 80～89 岁的老年患者施行经口内镜下肌切开术应谨慎。

引自: *Dig Endosc* 2020, doi: 101111/den13686

例四： Common intraprocedural end points such as voltage abatement, PV disconnection, and exit block persist only in a limited number of patients, even when the outcome is favorable during follow-up. Further investigation will be required to determine whether such data **will have** implications for ablation strategies.

房颤消融术中常用靶点如电压受抑、PV 隔离、PV 传出阻滞等仅出现于少数患者，即使在随访期内结果是有利的。这种资料对消融策略的选择是否有指导价值有待进一步研究。

引自: *Circulation*, 2008, 117(2)：136

（四）语态

"结论"句中较多使用主动语态。为了语篇衔接连贯，在结构性摘要中可直接借助篇章的指向性词汇，采用第三人称形式。而指示性摘要则用第一人称较为普遍，但国外文献中使用第一人称复数也较为常见。

例一： Social support, physical health and self-esteem are protective factors of PTSD, while ICU clinical experience is a risk factor. SES partially mediated the association of SSRS with IES-R.

社会支持、身体健康和自尊水平是 PTSD 保护性因素，而 ICU 工作年限是危险因素。SES 评分在 SSRS 支持评分与 IES-R 间起部分中介作用。

引自:《中华医学杂志》, 2020, 100(1): 32

例二： Thus **we** concluded that increased surface expression of NKCC2 plays an important role in the stimulation of NaCl absorption.

我们的结论是，NKCC2 表面表达水平升高对于刺激 NaCl 吸收起着重要作用。

引自: *Am J Physiol Cell Physiol*, 2006, 7: 280

例三： Although everolimus is currently not indicated for this use, this analysis from EXIST-1 demonstrates its long-term efficacy and safety for the treatment of renal angiomyolipoma in pediatric patients undergoing treatment for TSC-associated SEGA.

虽然目前还没有证明依维莫司（everolimus）的这种用途，但 EXIST-1

试验分析表明，该药在治疗 TSC 相关 SEGA 的儿科患者中治疗肾血管平滑肌脂肪瘤方面具有长期疗效和安全性。

引自：Pediatric Nephrology, 2018, 33: 101

例四：Levosimendan infusion for cardiogenic shock following acute myocardial infarction improved hemodynamic parameters of right ventricular performance. Furthermore, **we** describe the use of right ventricular cardiac power index as a hemodynamic parameter of right ventricular performance.

对于急性心肌梗死后心源性休克患者，左西孟旦输注能改善右心室功能血流动力学参数。此外，我们还采用了右心室功率指数作为右心室工作效能的一个血流动力学参数。

引自：Crit Care Med, 2009, 37(12)：3017

例五：**We** found no evidence of a worthwhile clinical benefit from increasing the three-dose intramuscular Engerix-B vaccine from 40- to 80-μg dose. An unplanned analysis suggested a role of improved protein intake to improve the immune response to hepatitis B vaccine in peritoneal dialysis patients.

未见研究证据证明，三剂肌内注射乙型肝炎疫苗的剂量从 40 μg 增加至 80 μg 能够提高临床治疗效果。随机分析显示，改进蛋白质摄入可以提高腹膜透析患者对乙型肝炎病毒的免疫反应。

引自：Nephrol Dial Transplant, 2010, 25(7)：2303

七、练　　习

7-1　用下列所给的单词和短语，根据意思和意义写出"Conclusion"句，并注意标点符号的使用

1. showed; population characteristics; little association; under the UK; with the quality of primary medical care; incentivised; medical services; contract

2. in long term; and; its; therapeutic superiorty; cost-effectiveness; further; are needed to prove; large multicenter trials and meta-analysis; of; the available data

3. between; the study; in icteric neonates; of UTI; revealed; breast feeding; circumcision and lower prevalence; significant association

4. women do not show; the same benefit; our conclusion; from CABG surgey; is that; that; men do; in a number important QOL measures; and that; cannot be; these differences; attributed to; preoperative differences

5. culture and antimicrobial susceptibility test; moreover; is recommended; after; for resistant cases; the first failure to therapy

6. confirm that; may be related to; the results; this form of hepatitis; high frequency; of; persistent hepatic dysfunction

7. that; a telephone-based; for; findings; with; strongly; disease management program; suggest; can improve; patients; outcomes; a behavioral health problem

8. *H. pylori*; resistance; antimicrobial; could; a; be; *H.Pylori*; major; eradication; of; contributor; to; failure

9. that; in the airways; these; may; findings; enhance; suggest; short term; supplementary oxygen; oxidative stress and inflammation

10. the mortality; being three times; neonates with ARF; higher; demands; of; this entity; a greater awareness; among practitioners; better; and; of this condition; management

7-2　将下列"Conclusion"句中汉语部分译成英文

1. _____（结果表明）that short term supplementary oxygen may enhance oxidative stress and inflammation in the airways.

2. _____（我们的结论是）, this study has extended previous observations of Bid activation during renal ischemia-reperfusion. Importantly, using Bid-deficient mice, _____（结果还表明）a role of Bid in the development of ischemic renal cell injury and renal failure.

3. The present study observations_____（明显表明）ARF is a very common entity among septic neonates.

4. _____（需要进一步研究）to prove the importance of screening in developing countries following vegetarian diet and high incidence of malnutrition.

5. In conclusion, _____（我们的结论证实）Rho-kinase contributes to DSM MLC phosphorylation and there is a higher basal MLC phosphorylation level in diabetic DSM. Our results also suggest that this high basal MLC phosphorylation _____（可能由于）the upregulation of Rho-kinase and CPI-17. Thus Rho-kinase- and CPI-17-mediated Ca^{2+} sensitization might play a role in diabetes-induced alteration of the detrusor contractility and bladder dysfunction.

6. _____（我们的结论是）portopulmonary shunt by splenopneumopexy is an effective procedure for portal hypertension caused by Budd-Chiari syndrome.

7. _____（我们建议）patients undergo a mammographic examination before having a breast biopsy.

8. _____（这一病例说明）although neonatal lupus erythematosus is usually self-limited, SLE may develop in selected patients in future years.

9. Population characteristics _____（表明相关性很小）the quality of primary medical care incentivised under the UK general medical services contract.

10. The advent of MR imaging _____（对早期诊断起重要作用）neonatal disease.

11. _____（数据不能充分证明）routine cytomegalovirus (CMV) screening of donor blood for exchange transfusion in our setting.

12. ＿＿＿＿＿＿＿＿＿＿＿＿＿＿＿（没有发现明显的相互关系）this population between asbestos and smoking at the first visit or longitudinally.

13. ＿＿＿＿＿＿＿＿＿＿＿＿＿（急需进一步研究） to devise strategies to reduce readmission and life threatening events in this group of patients.

14. A reduced MIP is an independent risk factor for MI and CVD death, and a ＿＿＿＿＿＿＿＿（提示）an increased risk for stroke. This＿＿＿＿＿＿＿＿＿＿（与……有关）MIP appeared to be mediated through mechanisms other than inflammation.

7-3 用英文写出下列"Conclusion"句

1. IL-33 可能通过启动 Th2 型免疫反应在 RSV 感染诱导哮喘急性发作小鼠模型中起重要作用。

2. PFN2 蛋白在胃癌组织中高表达可作为胃癌诊断标志和预后的评价指标。

3. 子宫内膜异位症中存在代谢异常，其中 HK2 和 PKM2 表达水平明显升高，可能与其发生相关。

4. 唾液皮质醇浓度与焦虑程度具有一定相关性，唾液皮质醇浓度升高及术前焦虑程度加重增加了妇科腔镜手术后 PONV 的发生风险。

5. 右美托咪定滴鼻用于患儿 CT 或 MRI 检查的镇静成功率更高，且安全性好，但结论仍需高质量的随机对照试验来证实。

6. MMP8 及 MMP9 有望作为判断甲型 H1N1 流感患者疾病严重程度的分子生物学标志物。

7. 抗凝血酶Ⅲ活性可能与患者发生粪便隐血阳性和股静脉血栓有关。抗凝血酶Ⅲ活性是预测 ACLF 患者预后的独立影响因素；当抗凝血酶Ⅲ活性<25%时，患者病死率较高。

8. 3-BP 能增强肝癌细胞 HepG2、SMMC7721 对顺铂诱导的凋亡的敏感性，其机制可能是通过引起细胞内 ATP 缺乏、下调 XIAP 蛋白的表达水平及增加 caspase-3 的活性。

9. Ⅰ型单纯疱疹病毒（HSV-1）能增加炎症因子白细胞介素-6（IL-6）的表达，并对人牙龈成纤维细胞产生影响，可能会导致牙龈炎症的易感性增加。

10. 结果表明 AG 可能通过减轻 ERS 途径从而有助于改善早期 T2DM 小鼠的认知功能。

第八章　医学论文英文摘要写作中的数值表达

医学论文英文摘要的写作中，常涉及许多数值。精确的数值是读者判断文章真实性、可靠性的指标，是获得正确结论的前提。因此，数值的正确表达是医学论文英文摘要写作的一项重要内容。本章就摘要中涉及的英文数值表达举例说明。

一、整合数量的表达

所谓"整合数"是指在数量表达时将同一组属中的各个体（数）以整体形式表达。采用这一表达方式的前提是，整合中的各个体（数）应具有同一类属关系。常用的表示整合数量的短语如下所述。

（1）a series of…：连续数为……

（2）a group of…：一组……

（3）a total of…：总数为……

（4）a number of…：若干……

结构上采用上述"词组+复数可数名词"作句子主语，可以根据侧重点的不同，其谓语形式可以用单数形式，也可以用复数形式。如果将主语内容作为一个整体，谓语动词使用单数；如果将主语内容视作个体累积，则谓语动词用复数形式。

例一： **A series of** randomized controlled trials **has** now shown that enhanced care of major depression in the primary care setting can improve disability outcomes.

一系列的随机控制性试验研究表明，在基层保健环境条件下，加强对严重忧郁患者的护理能有效预防严重后果的发生。

引自：*Brit J Psychiat*, 2005, 14(3): 152

例二： **A total of** 41 patients **were** randomized to the SAL group and 46 patients to the LAL group.

41 例患者随机纳入 SAL 组，46 例患者纳入 LAL 组。

引自：*BJS*, 2019, 106(S4): 5

例三：**A total of** 70 patients with NHLBMI (male:52,femal:18;median age:49 years) **was** studied.

70 例 NHLBMI 中，男性 52 例，女性 18 例，中位年龄 49 岁。

引自：《中华肿瘤杂志》，2000, 22(6): 513

例四：**A number of** recent case reports and series **have** identified a subgroup of atypical fractures of the femoral shaft associated with bisphosphonate use.

近期大量病例报告和系列研究均认为部分患者不典型性股骨干骨折与二膦酸盐的应用有关。

引自：*N Engl J Med*, 2010, 362(19)：1761

二、平均数的表达

为了表示新技术、新方法比传统技术方法具有更好的效果，作者常需通过比较各种技术参数的平均水平是否有较为明显的改善或提高来增强说服力。因而，均数的表达在医学论文英文摘要中应用频繁，是一种有重要意义的数值表达方法。表达平均数常用的英文单词有 average、median 和 mean。值得注意的是，许多作者因对其词义的模糊理解，使用这三个词表达平均数时常会出现词义选择不当。average、median 和 mean 在数理计算上的区别：①average 意为 "**mathematics calculate numerical average**: To calculate a numerical average of something, by finding the total amount and dividing it by the number of members in the group"（*Encarta Dictionary Tools*；指一组数值的平均数，为数值总和除以数目）。例如：4、6、7、11 的总数是 28，数目为 4。28 ÷ 4 = 7，因而 7 是平均数。英文表达是："The average of 4, 6, 7 and 11 is 7."。②mean 意为 "**intermediate value**: a quantity having a value intermediate between the values of other quantities, especially the average obtained by dividing the sum of several quantities by their number."（*The World Book Dictionary*）从该定义中可知，关键问题是 intermediate value 的计算。从严格的统计学考虑，要称一组数的中间数（midpoint），计算方法是将一组数的两个端数相加再除 2。如一组数字 4、6、10、20，平均值为 12，即（4+20）÷ 2=12。但平均数计算为（4+6+10+20）÷4=10。由此看来，average 和 mean 在语境中的词义选择是有区别的。③median 在统计学中有特定的含义，常称中间数、中位数（the middle value in a distribution）。在该词前后有其他数，即一组数字中，一半在前，一半在后。例如，一组数 10、11、12、13、14 中，12 是中位数。平均值是 12，平均数也是 12。

（一）average 及其相关短语表达结构

英文摘要中常用 average 表示均数，常见形式有 "average+名词" 作主语、"average + 名词+ of +数词" 作宾语，还可在 "average" 后加数量词或者是在数量词后直接用 "in average" 来表达均数。

1.　"average +名词"表示：平均……

例一：The **average age** was 47.8 ± 10.7 years; 74.8% were male.

平均年龄为（47.8 ± 10.7）岁，其中 74.8%为男性。

引自：*J Cardiothorac Surg*, 2019, 14: 90

例二：**Average peak BG , CIH duration, and peak insulin requirements** were 199 mg/dL, 6.3 days, and 0.09 units/kg/h, respectively, in patients with CIH.

危重病高血糖（CIH）患者的平均血糖（BG）峰值、CIH 持续时间和胰岛素峰值需要量分别为 199 mg/dl，6.3d 和 0.09 U/(kg·h)。

引自：*J Pediatr*, 2009, 155(5): 734

例三：The **average survival** was 26 months, and 2 patients have remained alive more than 5 years after surgery.

术后平均存活 26 个月，2 例病人存活五年以上。

引自：《中国实用外科杂志》, 2001, 21: 483

2.　"an average +名词+ of +数词"表示：平均……为……

例一：Patients with increased serum CA125 levels had an **average survival rate of 12.5%** at 1 year and 0 at 2 years.

CA125 升高患者的 1 年生存率为 12.5%，2 年生存率为 0。

引自：《中华肿瘤杂志》, 2000, 22(1): 30

例二：There were 1 man and 3 women **with an average age of 34 years**. The average age of the female patients were 27 years.

男、女患者的比例为 1∶3；平均患病年龄 34 岁，其中女性患者平均年龄 27 岁。

引自：《中国医学科学院学报》, 2006, 28(5): 730

例三：…it was significantly elevated by **an average of 2-to 4-fold** as compared with the other groups.

与其他组相比，该组平均升高 2～4 倍。

引自：*J Immunol*, 2005, 174(12): 52

3.　"an average of +数词+名词"表示：平均为……

例一：Patients were studied during the treatment period and were followed up for **an average of 16 months**.

在治疗期间同时对患者进行了研究和随访，随访周期平均为 16 个月。

引自：*Ann Allergy Asthma Immunol*, 2010, 104(3): 253

例二：Readmission cost **an average of $13,392 per patient**, accounting for an estimated annual cost of over $250 million.

再入院费用平均每例患者为 13 392 美元,估计每年费用超过 2.5 亿美元。

引自:Am J Cardiol, 2019, 124(2):205-210

例三: This study investigated whether anxiety characteristics independently predicted the onset of myocardial infarction (MI) over **an average of 12.4 years** and whether this relationship was independent of other psychologic variables and risk factors.

在为期平均超过 12.4 年的观察中,本研究调查了焦虑性格是否独立预测心肌梗死发作及这种联系是否独立于其他心理变量和危险因素。

引自:JACC, 2008, 51(2):113

4. "on (the)average; in average"表示:平均⋯⋯

"in average"现代英语较少使用。"on average"等同于副词 averagely。

例一: Patients with SemD showed the closest association between length of symptoms and stage, taking, **on average**, 10 years to reach the severe stage.

语义性痴呆(SemD)患者的病情与症状持续时间及分期有较大关联性,平均 10 年左右病情会进展到严重程度。

引自:Neurology, 2010, 74(20):1591

例二: Among women drinking **on average** >1 drink of alcohol per day, current HRT users had a 42% increased risk (RR, 1.42; 95%CI, 1.11-1.80) for cataract extraction, compared with women who neither used HRT nor alcohol.

与既未使用激素替代疗法也未饮酒的妇女相比,那些平均每天饮酒大于一杯并且使用激素替代疗法的妇女白内障发病率增加了 42%(RR, 1.42; 95%CI, 1.11~1.80)。

引自:Ophthalmology, 2010, 117(3):424

(二)mean 及其相关表达结构的使用

用 mean 表示均数也较常用,当 mean 作为名词或形容词时,其表达方式较多,通常用"mean +名词(+of+数词)"这一形式来表述,也可以直接在表示范围的数值后用括号内注明的方式呈现平均数。

1. "the/a mean +名词+of+数词"表示:平均⋯⋯为⋯⋯

例一: **The mean survival period of 92** patients was 19.6 months .

92 名患者的平均生存期为 19.6 个月。

引自:《中华肿瘤杂志》, 2000, 22(6):422

例二: During **a mean follow up of 48 ± 25 months**, cardiovascular death occurred in 9% of pts with LVEF <40% and in 2% with LVEF≥40% ($P = 0.014$).

平均（48±25）个月的随访中，LVEF<40%的患者中有9%的患者发生了心血管病死亡，LVEF≥40%的患者中有2%的患者发生了心血管病死亡（$P=0.014$）。

引自：Am J Cardiol, 2019, 124(3):355-361

例三：　There were 2 men and 3 women, with **a mean age of 28 years** (10 to 43 years).

男 2 例，女 3 例，年龄 10～43 岁，平均 28 岁。

引自：《中华外科杂志》, 2001, 39(4): 285

2. 表示平均累积总量的用法：在 **mean** 后加 **total** 表示平均累积总量。

例一：　At 3 months, women in the intervention group had significantly lower **mean total** scores on the HADS than women in the control group.

在 3 个月时，干预组的女性在 HADS 的平均总分明显低于对照组的女性。

引自：Lancet, 2019, 393(10182): 1733

例二：　The **mean total** cost of nebulized therapy was significantly greater for patients receiving RAC than for those receiving LEV.

接受 RAC 喷雾治疗的平均总费用明显高于接受 LEV 的费用。

引自：NMJ, 2007, 74(2): 51

3. 在表示数值范围后用括号内注明的方式来提出平均数。

例：　Eleven consecutive patients (nine females; **mean age 71.7 years**) presented from 1999 to 2009 with acute onset unilateral visual loss.

从 1999 年至 2009 年，连续 11 例患者（9 名女性；平均年龄 71.7 岁）出现急性发作的单侧视力丧失。

引自：Br J Ophthalmol, 2018, 102(12): 333

（三）median 的用法

median 的意思为"relating to, located in, or extending toward the middle"（中间的，趋向中间的）。统计学意义指"the middle value in a distribution, above and below which lies an equal number of values."（中间数值，该值和比它大及比它小的数值是等差的）。

例一：　Sixty-eight children (**median age** 7.3 year, **median weight** 22 kg) underwent 192 procedures.

68 例患儿（中位年龄 7.3 岁，平均体重 22 kg）共接受了 192 次手术。

引自：Paediatr Anaesth, 2010, 20(1): 28

例二：　Between January 1, 2000, and December 31, 2006, 215 patients underwent isolated VSD repair **at a median age of** 10 months (range, 20 days to 18 years) and a median weight of 7 kg (range, 2 to 66 kg).

从 2000 年 1 月 1 日至 2006 年 12 月 31 日，215 例患儿接受了室间隔缺损修补手术，患儿年龄中值为 10 个月（范围：20 天～18 岁），体重中值为 7 kg（范围：2～66 kg）。

引自：Ann Thorac Surg, 2010, 89(2)：544

例三： After **a median follow-up of** 8 months (25th to 75th interquartile range: 3 to 14 months) the mortality rate was 22.1%.

中位随访期为 8 个月（第 25 至 75 的四分位数间距是 3～14 个月），随访发现死亡率为 22.1%。

引自：J Am Coll Cardiol, 2010, 55(11): 1080

例四： **Median survival** of the study group was 517 days (95% CI, 11-626).

研究组的平均生存期为 517 天（95%CI，11～626）。

引自：Am J Gastroenterol, 2010, 105(3): 635

例五： Patient age ranged from 18 to 74 years **with a median duration of** symptoms of 2 days upon presentation and a median Ranson score of 1.

患者的年龄范围为 18～74 岁，就诊前症状持续时间中位数为 2 天，Ranson 评分的中位数为 1。

引自：Ann Surg, 2010, 251(4): 615

三、百分数、比例及率的表达

（一）百分数的表达

百分数的表达可用 percent，也可直接用百分号"%"，现在大多数的英文摘要中都直接用"%"。在用百分数表达时会经常出现以下两种模糊不清并且容易忽视的问题：第一，在百分数值与主题词之间是否要用介词 of。这主要取决于百分数是用来表示主题词所指示内容的一部分还是用来说明主题词的性质，如果是前者则在百分数值与主题词之间应加介词 of，相反如果是后者则不应该用介词 of。例如，"36% 的患者"英文表达为"36% of the patients"，由于 36% 的患者是患者总体中的一部分，所以在 36% 与患者之间用介词 of ；"50% 的葡萄糖"英文则表达为"50% glucose"，因为它只是描述葡萄糖的性质，所以并没有用介词 of。第二，如果同时有几个百分数值连用时，在主题词与百分数值之间一般用逗号隔开（偶尔也可不隔开），在百分数值之后一般用分号表示几个百分数值之间为并列关系，但要注意，最后一个百分数值之后要用句号。

用以引导百分数的结构很多，现将较为常用的引导结构列举如下，同时注意对于"阳性率"或"阴性率"在中外文献中的表达差异。

（1）在医学论文英文摘要写作中，经常会使用某种因素或某个参数指标的阳性率表示各组之间的差异，因而"The positive rates of"和"The percentage of"为最常见的百分数引导结构。

例一： **The positive rates of** B19, ToX, CMV and HSV-2 in 66 case CHD **were**

18.2%, 15.2%, 25.8% and 4.5%, respectively, while that in 38 cases control groups were 0%, 2.6%, 21.2% and 2.6%, respectively.

在 66 例先天性心脏病心肌组织中检测到 B19、ToX、CMV 和 HSV-2 的阳性率分别为 18.2%、15.2%、25.8%和 4.5%。38 例对照中 B19、ToX、CMV 和 HSV-2 的阳性率分别为 0%、2.6%、21.2%、2.6%。

引自:《中华微生物学和免疫学杂志》, 2000, 20(2): 170

例二: With one *vs.* two *vs.* three or more specimens, the **HER2-positive rate** increased from 10.5% to 18.1% to 24.1%, respectively.

与两份、三份或更多标本对比,HER2 阳性率分别从 10.5%上升至 18.1%,最高达 24.1%。

引自: *Am J Clin Pathol*, 2019, 151(5): 461

例三: The **absolute percentage of** LV and LA function improvement was higher for LS than for EF ($P < 0.05$).

LS 的 LV 和 LA 功能改善的绝对百分比高于 EF($P<0.05$)。

引自: *Am J Cardiol*, 2019, 124(2):253-261

例四: All four specimens were unanimously **positive** for K3, -4, and -13 but **negative** for K8 and MUC5AC, suggesting that the keratinocytes were oral mucosa-derived.

所有四个标本中 K3、K4 和 K13 全部呈阳性表达,但 K8 和 MUC5AC 呈阴性,表明角质形成细胞来源于口腔黏膜。

引自: *Invest Ophthalmol Vis Sci*, 2009, 50(10):4660

例五: DET **was positive** for regional wall motion abnormalities in 291 (25%) and negative in 854 (74%) patients.

室壁运动不正常区域的 DET(双嘧达莫超声心动图试验)阳性的患者有 291 例(25%),阴性的患者有 854 例(74%)。

引自: *Eur Heart J*, 2008, 29(1): 79

(2)表示"百分率"的谓语动词除了用 be 表示外,还可以与 reach 等动词搭配。

例一: The rate of excellent and good operative results **reached** 90.63%.

(原位肛门重建术)功能优良率达 90.63%。

引自:《中华整形外科杂志》, 2000, 16(2): 102

例二: **The percentage of** CD34$^+$ cell with the gene transduction at 10 ng/ml Taxol **reached** 38.5%.

在 10 ng/ml 紫杉醇作用下基因转导 CD34$^+$细胞的阳性率可达 38.5%。

引自:《中华血液学杂志》, 2000, 21(3): 234

例三: **The percentage of** patients undergoing surgery with a handover of anesthesiology care progressively increased each year of the study, **reaching** 2.9% in 2015.

接受移交到麻醉科护理的患者比例每年都在逐步增加，2015 年达到 2.9%。

引自：*JAMA*,2018, 319(2): 143

（3）"The incidence of" 和 "The frequency of" 可用来引导某些事件的发生率及频率。例如：

例一： **The incidence of** cerebrovascular disease was not significantly different between groups at 5 years (0.7% in the surgical group *vs.* 1.7% in the nonsurgical group; hazard ratio, 0.69 [95% CI, 0.38-1.25]).

脑血管疾病的发生率在 5 年内组间差异不显著[手术组为 0.7%，非手术组为 1.7%；风险比为 0.69（95%CI，0.38～1.25）]。

引自：*JAMA*, 2018, 320(15): 1570

例二： Of the 240 patients randomly assigned to the 2 treatment groups (120 in each), data for the primary outcome were obtained from 113 pregabalin patients and 115 placebo patients. At both 3 and 6 month postoperatively, **the incidence of** neuropathic pain was less frequent in the pregabalin group (0%) compared with the placebo group (8.7% and 5.2% at 3 and 6 month, respectively; $P = 0.001$ and $P = 0.014$).

将 240 例患者随机分成两个治疗组（每组 120 例），主要结果数据来自于 113 例接受普瑞巴林治疗的患者和 115 例安慰剂患者。术后第 3 个月和第 6 个月，口服普瑞巴林组（0%）的神经性疼痛发生率低于安慰剂对照组（第 3 个月和第 6 个月的发生率分别为 8.7%和 5.2%；$P=0.001$ 和 $P=0.014$）。

引自：*Anesth Analg*, 2010, 110(1)：199

例三： **The frequency of** hypoglycaemic events per month was similar between the groups (0.29 events per month [SD 0.48] in the intervention group *vs.* 0.29 [SD 1.12] in the control group; $P=0.96$).

两组间患者每月发生低血糖的频率基本相似[干预组每月 0.29 次（SD 0.48），对照组每月 0.29 次（SD1.12）；$P=0.96$）]。

引自：*Lancet*, 2019, 393(10176): 1138

例四： Among individuals with CAC = 0, conversion to CAC >0 is nonlinear and occurs **at low frequency** before 4 years. No clinical factor seems to mandate earlier repeat CAC scanning.

在冠状动脉钙化（CAC）评分=0 的患者组中，发生 CAC 评分>0 的改变是非线性的，且在前 4 年内发生率较低。尚无临床因素表明需要对患者早期进行重复 CAC 扫描检查。

引自：*J Am Coll Cardiol*, 2010, 55(11): 1110

例五： **The frequency of** CD34(+) and CD34(+) CD38(−) cells in umbilical cord blood(CB) and the frequency of CD34(+) CD38(−), CD34(+)HLA-DR(+)

cells among CB CD34(+) cells were significantly higher in preterm CB than in term CB(3.14% and 0.76% *vs.* 0.78% and 0.18%; and 9.8% and 20.4% *vs.* 3.9% and 14.6%; *P*<0.001).

脐血 CD34$^+$ 和 CD34$^+$CD38$^-$ 细胞的频率及脐血 CD34$^+$ 细胞中的 CD34$^+$CD38$^-$ 和 CD34$^+$HLA-DR$^+$ 细胞的频率在早产脐血中显著高于足月脐血（分别为 3.14% 和 0.76% *vs.* 0.78% 和 0.18%；9.8% 和 20.4% *vs.* 3.9% 和 14.6%；*P*<0.001）。

引自：《中华医学杂志》，2002, 82：330

（4）在表示表达水平、表达量时，常用"with a yield of""at a level of"等短语来引导。在这些短语后接百分数，也可直接与表达某因素所能达到的具体数值相连用。

例一：In one of 6 bladder cancer specimens and in 4 of 5 colorectal cancer tissues, K20 expression was positive, **at a level of** 41%-77% of the positive control.
6 例膀胱癌组织中，仅有 1 例呈阳性；5 例肠癌组织中，4 例呈阳性，表达量为阳性对照的 41%～77%。

引自：《中华肿瘤杂志》，2000, 22(1): 32

例二：HLAF-1 was effectively expressed in *E.coli* **with a yield of** 88 mg/L.
在 *E.coli* 细胞中高效表达了该因子的重组蛋白，蛋白表达量为 88 mg/L。

引自：《中华肿瘤杂志》，2000, 22(1): 19

（5）与短语动词 account for 搭配使用。

例一：Of these infections, 517,818 (83%) had their onset in the community, and 104,572 (17%) had their onset in the hospital. MRSA and ESBL infections accounted for the majority of the infections (52% and 32%, respectively).
在这些感染中，517 818 人（83%）在社区发病；104 572 人（17%）在医院发病。耐甲氧西林金黄色葡萄球菌（MRSA）和 ESBL 病毒感染占感染的大多数（分别为 52% 和 32%）。

引自：*N Engl J Med*, 2020, 382: 1309

例二：Cryptococcus accounted for 63% (514) of microbiological diagnoses, TB for 28% (227), bacterial meningitis for 8% (68).
微生物诊断的病例中有 63%（514）为隐球菌，28%（227）为 TB，8%（68）为细菌性脑膜炎。

引自：*BMC Infect Dis*, 2010, 10(1): 67

（6）除了上述提到的短语可用来引导百分数外，还可在括号中直接标出所占的百分数，这样既简洁又明了，一目了然，如先表明总数中的具体数值（用…out of…来引导），其百分数值在括号中标出。

例一：Increased serum CA125 levels were observed in **24 out of 66** patients **(36.4%).**
66 例患者中 24 例患者血清 CA125 水平升高，占 36.4%。

引自：《中华肿瘤杂志》，2000, 22(1): 30

例二：Ulcers with active bleeding or visible vessels were found on initial endoscopy in **105 of the 158 patients (66.4%)** with peptic ulcers in the urgent-endoscopy group and in **76 of 159 (47.8%)** in the early-endoscopy group.

接受急诊内镜检查组中的 158 例消化性溃疡患者中有 105 例（66.4%）在初次内镜检查中发现活动性出血或可见血管的溃疡，而早期内镜检查组中的 159 例患者中有 76 例（47.8%）发现溃疡。

引自：*N Engl J Med*, 2020, 382: 1299

（7）可以将百分数直接作为句子的主语使用，但要注意谓语动词应用复数形式。例如：

例一：The mean (SD) age at diagnosis was 32.2 (25.2) years and 62.4% were women.

诊断时平均年龄为 32.2 岁（25.2 岁），女性占 62.4%。

引自：*JAMA*, 2020, 323(13): 1277

例二：Of 124 385 newborns in the screening study, 49.2% were female, 87.6% were of term gestational age, 70.0% were white, and 48.1% were Hispanic.

所筛查的 124 385 名新生儿中，49.2%为女性，87.6%为足月胎龄儿，70.0%为白色人种，48.1%为西班牙裔。

引自：*JAMA*, 2020, 323(12): 1141

（二）比例及率的表达

医学文献中常用 ratio 和 rate 来表示比例和率。需要注意的是，这两个词的概念意义是有区别的。ratio 的意思是 "Relation in degree or number between two similar things"，指的是"对比关系"；而 rate 的意思 "A measure of a part with respect to a whole; a proportion"，特指"部分相对整体形成的比率"。主要有以下几种基本表达方法。

1. "A：B ratio" 表示 "率"

例一：Participants were randomly assigned **in a 1：1 ratio** to self-management, consisting of self-monitoring of blood pressure and self-titration of antihypertensive drugs, combined with telemonitoring of home blood pressure measurements or to usual care.

实验对象按照 1：1 的比例随机分组为自我管理组和常规管理组，自我管理组包括血压的自我监测和抗高血压药的自我滴注，以及家庭血压测量的远程监控。

引自：*Lancet*, 2010, 376(9736): 163

例二：We randomized 35 patients with CHF［age 64±13 years, peak oxygen consumption (pVO$_2$) 14.0±2.7 ml/(kg·min)］to 16 weeks of intravenous iron

(200 mg weekly until ferritin >500 ng/ml, 200 mg monthly thereafter) or no treatment in a **2：1 ratio.**

我们随机给予 35 例慢性心力衰竭患者［平均年龄（64±13）岁，峰值耗氧量（pVO$_2$）（14.0±2.7）ml/（kg·min）］，16 周静脉补铁（每周 200 mg 直至铁蛋白>500 ng/ml，此后改为每月 200 mg）或不予治疗，治疗与非治疗的贫血患者比例为 2：1。

引自：JACC, 2008, 51(2): 103

2. "A/B ratio" 表示 "率"

例一： **TG/HDL-C ratio** is a better predicting index for CHD risk.

TG/HDL-C 比值对于 CHD 诊断是一有临床使用价值的指标。

引自:《中华心血管病杂志》, 2000, 28(1): 33

例二： In this phase 3, randomized, open-label, multicenter study, we assigned 846 patients with chronic-phase Philadelphia chromosome-positive CML **in a 1：1：1 ratio** to receive nilotinib (at a dose of either 300 mg or 400 mg twice daily) or imatinib (at a dose of 400 mg once daily).

在这项 3 期随机开放标签多中心临床研究中，我们共纳入 846 例 Ph 染色体阳性的慢性期慢性粒细胞白血病（CML）患者，按 1：1：1 的比例分配到 3 组，接受不同的治疗（尼罗替尼每次 300 mg 或每次 400 mg，每天 2 次，伊马替尼 400 mg 每天 1 次）。

引自：N Engl J Med, 2010, 362(24): 2251

例三： Patients were randomly assigned **in a 1：1 ratio** to receive targeted intraoperative radiotherapy or whole breast external beam radiotherapy, with blocks stratified by centre and by timing of delivery of targeted intraoperative radiotherapy.

将患者以 1：1 的比例进行随机分组，予以术中靶向放疗或全乳外放射治疗，另外，根据多中心所提供的术中靶向放疗时间进行分层。

引自：Lancet, 2010, 376(9735)：91

3. "ratio of A to B" 表示 "率或比例"

例一： In the 17 cases of SPTCL, **the ratio of male-to-female** was 1：1.1 and the median age was 24 years old.

17 例 SPTCL 男女之比 1：1.1 ，中位发病年龄 24 岁。

引自:《中华病理学杂志》, 2000, 29(2): 103

例二： Hypertension diet, 11.2%; income level of $35 000 or less, 9.3%; higher **dietary ratio of sodium to** potassium, 6.8%; and an education level of high school graduate or less, 4.1%.

高血压饮食占 11.2%；收入水平 35 000 美元或以下占 9.3%；钠钾饮食比

例较高者占 6.8%；高中毕业或以下文化程度占 4.1%。

引自：*JAMA*, 2018, 320(13): 1338

例三： Normal annulus displayed early-systolic anteroposterior ($P<0.001$) and area ($P=0.04$) contraction, increased height ($P<0.001$), and deeper saddle shape **(ratio of height to intercommissural diameter, (15±1)% to (21±1)%; $P<0.001$).**

正常瓣环组显示收缩早期瓣环前后径（$P<0.001$）和瓣环面积（$P=0.04$）较小，高度增加（$P<0.001$），鞍形加深 [高/内连合径之比，（15±1）% *vs.* （21±1）%；$P<0.001$]。

引自：*Circulation*, 2010, 121(12): 1423

4. "ratio of A/B" 表示 "率或比值"

例一： The ratio of the geometric mean of values obtained at weeks 4 and 8 to the baseline value was 0.53 in the sacubitril–valsartan group as compared with 0.75 in the enalapril group.

在第 4 周和第 8 周沙库巴曲/缬沙坦组测得的几何平均值与基线值的比值为 0.53，而在依那普利组为 0.75。

引自：*N Engl J Med*, 2019, 380: 539

例二： Chronotropic incompetence was defined as the ratio of increase in HR during exercise to age-predicted maximal increase in HR <0.6.

（心脏）变时机能不全界定为运动期间心率增加与年龄预测的最大心率增加之比（HR< 0.6）。

引自：*Br J Anaesth*, 2019, 123(1):17-26

5. 在表达率的名词前用些修饰成分来表示 "××率"

例一： The 1-,3-,5-year **survival rate** was 96.6%,92.8% and 71.4%, respectively.

1、3、5 年生存率明显提高，分别为 96.6%、92.8% 和 71.4%。

引自：《中华肿瘤杂志》, 2000, 22(1): 77

例二： **Two-year event rate** was 15% for H/M ≥1.60 and 37% for H/M <1.60.

H/M≥1.60 的患者两年的心脏病发病率为 15%，H/M<1.60 的患者则为 37%。

引自：*J Am Coll Cardiol,* 2010, 55(20)：2212

例三： The **annual mortality rate** was 5.2% in the I-Preserve trial.

I-Preserve 试验期间，年死亡率为 5.2%。

引自：*Circulation*, 2010, 121(12)：1393

6. 用 "proportion" 表示比例

例一： The median **proportion** of LOEA recommendations was 7.9% (25th-75th percentiles, 0.9%-15.2%).

LOEA 建议的中位数比例为 7.9%（第 25～75 百分位数，0.9%～15.2%）。

引自：*JAMA*, 2019, 321(11): 1069

例二：Atherothrombotic patients throughout the world had similar risk factor profiles: a high **proportion** with hypertension (81.8%), hypercholesterolemia (72.4%), and diabetes (44.3%).

全世界动脉粥样硬化血栓形成患者具有相似的危险因素，即高血压（81.8%）、高胆固醇血症（72.4%）及糖尿病（44.3%）的比例高。

引自：*JAMA*, 2006, 295: 180

例三：A significantly greater **proportion** of patients in group 3 graded their overall satisfaction as satisfactory compared with group 1 (43% *vs.* 23%, *P*=0.010), and the proportion was similar to that in group 2 (43% *vs.* 35%, *P*=0.133).

第 3 组与第 1 组相比绝大部分患者将总满意度评为满意（43% *vs.* 23%，*P*=0.010），与第 2 组接近（43% *vs.* 35%, *P*=0.133）。

引自：*Am J Gastroenterol*, 2010, 105(6)：1319

7. 与"率"有关的几个名词的用法问题

（1）**morbidity**：患病率，意为："the rate of incidence of a disease"（发病率，发生疾病的概率）或"the condition of being diseased"（患病状况）。因此，morbidity rate 意为某一特定期间每 1000、10 000 或 100 000 人口中患有某指定疾病的病例数，其统计方法应是"The morbidity rate（or attack rate）is the number of cases of a specific disease divided by the total population at risk for that disease."（某种疾病的病例数除以有患该病风险的总人数得出的结果）。

例一：As compared with singleton gestations, twin pregnancies are associated with a significantly higher risk of preterm birth and maternal complications as well as fetal and neonatal **morbidity** and mortality.

早产、母体并发症、胎儿和新生儿发病率及其死亡率的风险，双胎妊娠明显高于单胎妊娠。

引自：*Am J Obstet Gynecol* 2019, 221(3):253.e1-253.e8.

例二：In addition to the considerable **morbidity** and mortality associated with COPD, this disease incurs significant healthcare and societal costs.

除了与慢性阻塞性肺疾病（COPD）相关的相当高的发病率和死亡率外，这种疾病还会带来巨大的医疗和社会成本。

引自：*Int J Chron Obstruct Pulmon Dis*, 2006, 1(3): 219

例三：Our aim was to investigate the epidemiological effect of this city-wide sanitation programme on diarrhoea **morbidity** in children less than 3 years of age.

我们的目的是调查覆盖全市的卫生项目对小于 3 岁儿童的腹泻发病率的

流行病学的影响。

引自: *Lancet*, 2007, 370(9599): 1622

（2）**mortality**：死亡率，意为 "All deaths reported in a given population"（某种疾病的死亡人数）。mortality rate 与 death rate 同义。其统计学计算方法为 "The number of deaths is a particular population divided by the size of that population at the same time"（特定人群的死亡数除以同期该人群人数得出的结果）。表示死亡率时，需要注意区别 "case fatality" 或 "case fatality rate"（病死率），其意义为 "The proportion of people or animals who die from a disease to the total number of patients or animals suffering the disease within a certain period of time, which is used to describe the severity of a particular disease. "。

例一： The relapse rate and early **mortality** was 13.8% and 10.3% respectively in type L group being significantly lower than those in the type S group.

L 型的复发率及早期病死率分别为 13.8%、10.3%，显著低于 S 型。

引自:《中华内科杂志》, 2000, 39(1): 31

例二： Both low EF and diastolic dysfunction were independently related to higher levels of BNP. At 6 months, **mortality** was 16% for both preserved and reduced EF (age- and sex-adjusted hazard ratio, 0.85; 95% CI, 0.61-1.19; $P = 0.33$ for preserved *vs.* reduced EF).

EF 降低及舒张功能不全均与 BNP 水平升高独立相关。EF 正常者及降低者 6 个月死亡率均为 16%（对年龄和性别进行校正后风险比为 0.85；95%CI, 0.61～1.19；*P*=0.33）。

引自: *JAMA*, 2006, 296: 2209

例三： Perioperative **mortality** decreased steadily over time and accounted for 68.4% of all deaths.

围术期死亡率随着时间稳定下降，占全部死亡的 68.4%。

引自: *Circulation*, 2008, 117(1): 85

例四： **Case fatality rate** was similar in both sexes; increasing with age; 0.03% were <15 years of age, 0.1%, 15-24 year-old, and 0.5%, ≥25 years.

男性与女性的病死率相似；随着年龄增长；0.03%为年龄<15 岁，0.1%为年龄 15～24 岁，0.5%为年龄≥25 岁。

引自: *Scandinavian Journal of Infectious Diseases*, 2020, 29(1): 87

（3）**incidence（rate）**：发病率；（疾病）发生率。意指："the rate of occurrence of new cases of a disease or condition, or the ratio of the number of new cases of a condition to the total number of persons in the population at risk for the condition during a specific period"（指的是根据一定时期内某一人群中新发生新的病例数来衡量患病情况的指标）。

例一： Age-specific **incidence rates** were higher in participants with youth-onset diabetes mellitus at all ages.

在所有年龄组中，青年糖尿病患者糖尿病性终末期肾病（ESRD）的特定年龄发病率较高。

引自：JAMA 2006, 296(4): 421

例二： Computed tomography excluded pulmonary embolism in 1505 patients, of whom 1436 patients were not treated with anticoagulants; in these patients the 3-month **incidence** of VTE was 1.3%.

1505 例患者通过 CT 检查排除了肺栓塞，其中 1436 例未予抗凝治疗，这些患者 3 个月内静脉血栓栓塞的发生率为 1.3%。

引自：JAMA, 2006, 295(2): 172

例三： The **incidence of** perioperative visual loss after nonocular surgeries ranges from 0.002% of all surgeries to as high as 0.2% of cardiac and spine surgeries.

非眼科术后围手术期视力丧失的发生率在所有手术中为 0.002%，在心脏和脊柱手术中高达 0.2%。

引自：American Journal of Ophthalmology, 2008, 145(4)：604

（4）**prevalence**：患病率；流行率。意思指的是 "the measure of the existing number of cases, or the proportion of existing cases of a condition in the given population at risk at a specific point in time"（某一特定时间里在给定数目的人群中所有患病的人数或有某种疾病病例的数目）。

例一： The estimated number of AIP patients in 2016 was 13,436, with an overall **prevalence rate** of 10.1 per 100,000 persons.

据估计，2016 年急性胰腺炎患者人数为 13 436 人，总患病率为 10.1/100000 人。

引自：J Gastroenterol, 2020, 55: 462

例二： Our analyses found that the **prevalence** of HTN (17.66%) was greater than that of DYS (12.33%).

结果显示，HTN 的患病率（17.66%）高于 DYS（12.33%）。

引自：Clin Ther, 2008, 30(6): 1145

例三： The **prevalence** of nonalcoholic fatty liver disease was 38% among variant-allele carriers and 0% among wild-type homozygotes ($P<0.001$).

变异等位基因携带者中非酒精性脂肪肝的患病率是 38%，野生型纯合子（未携带该基因变异体）的患病率为 0%（$P<0.001$）。

引自：N Engl J Med, 2010, 362(12)：1082

（5）**frequency**：频数；频率分布。其意为 "the ratio of the number of times an event occurs in a series of trials of a chance experiment to the number of trials of the experiment performed"（一系列实验中偶然现象次数与所做的一系列实验的次数的比率）。

例一：However, lower specificity and the need for preceding small-bowel radiography (due to the high **frequency** of asymptomatic PSBO) may limit the utility of CE as a first-line test for Crohn's disease.

然而胶囊内镜（CE）的特异度较低，且通常需要先通过小肠放射学检查才能应用（因为无症状性的部分小肠梗阻的发生率高），这些缺点都限制了 CE 作为诊断克罗恩病的一线检查方法的应用。

引自：*Gastrointest Endosc*, 2008, 68(2): 255

例二：When compared with 733 control samples from the same population, the **overall frequency** of these rare variants in SCN5A was significantly higher in the SCD cases (6/60, 10.0%) than in controls (12/733, 1.6%; $P=0.001$).

与 733 个来自相同人群的对照样本相比，SCN5A 罕见突变的整体频率在 SCD 患者显著增高（6/60，10.0% *vs*. 12/733，1.6%；$P=0.001$）。

引自：*Circulation*, 2008, 117(1): 16

例三：The primary objective was to compare average change in HbA $_{1c}$ from baseline to 6 months. Safety was assessed by the **frequency** of hypoglycaemic events.

主要目的是比较从基线到 6 个月 HbA$_{1c}$ 的平均变化。以低血糖发生频率评估安全性。

引自：*Lancet*, 2019, 393(10176): 1138

四、数量增减的表达

（一）直接表达法

在医学论文英文摘要中，常需说明某一变量的增减。用于表示数字增减的常用动词有 increase、rise、decrease、fall、decline、drop、reduce 等。用这样的动词作句子的谓语，表示数量的增减，被视为直接表达法。需要注意的是，以上动词后所用的介词不同，其所表达的意思亦有所不同的。其主要有两种情况：①表示增减的动词后直接加数字或者是与介词 by 连用，用来表示"增加了多少"或"减少了多少"；②用介词"to"与表"增减"的动词相搭配，用来表示"增减到"某个数值。

例一：The 5-year survival rate of gastric cancer and liver cancer **increased 8.8% and 29.3%** from 1988 to 1990, respectively.

胃癌、肝癌 1990 年的 5 年生存率，比 1988 年分别增加了 8.8% 和 29.3%。

【析】"… increased 8.8%，增加 8.8%"与 "… increased by 8.8%，增加 8.8%"意思相同。

引自：《中华肿瘤杂志》, 2000, 22(3): 311

例二：The proportion of NARST **increased from** 19% in 1999 **to** 54% in 2006.

萘啶酸抗伤寒沙门氏菌（抗药性）比例从 1999 年的 19% 增至 2006 年的 54%。

引自：JAMA, 2009, 302(8): 859

例三： Their invasive capability was **decreased by** 46.7%.

　　人肝癌细胞侵袭能力降低了 46.7%。

　　【析】"…decreased by" 表示"降低了……"。

引自：《中华肿瘤杂志》, 2000, 22(3): 287

例四： The total fraction time of bile reflux **decreased from** 15.7%±7.8%, 17.0%±16.3%, and 16.9%±15.6% **to** 4.9%±4.5% ($P<0.01$), 0.8%±0.9% ($P<0.01$), 1.2%±2.3% ($P<0.01$) respectively.

　　24 小时胃内胆汁反流总时间百分比由治疗前的 15.7%±7.8%、17.0%±16.3% 和 16.9%±15.6% 降至 4.9%±4.5%（$P<0.01$）、0.8%±0.9%（$P<0.01$）和 1.2%±2.3%（$P<0.01$）。

　　【析】"decreased from…to" 表示"由……降至……"。

引自：《中华消化杂志》, 2000, 20(2): 105

例五： Among all youths, the adjusted mean total cholesterol level **declined from** 164 mg/dl(95% CI, 161 to 167 mg/dl) in 1999-2000 to 155 mg/dl.

　　在所有青年人群中，调整后的总胆固醇水平从 1999～2000 年的 164 mg/dl（95%CI，161～167 mg/dl）降至 155 mg/dl。

引自：JAMA, 2019, 321(19): 1895

（二）间接表达法

在表达数量/数字的增减、大小时，还可直接用形容词的比较级形式来表示。

例一： There was **higher** concentration of EGF with an average of 0.50 μg/L in HFF group compared with human serum (0.26μg/L, $P<0.05$).

　　卵泡液中 EGF 的含量为 0.50 μg/L，血清中为 0.26 μg/L，两组比较，有显著性差异（$P<0.05$）。

引自：《中华妇产科杂志》, 2001, 36(2): 215

例二： Confirming and extending previous reports, carriers of the 719Arg allele of KIF6 have **34% higher** risk of myocardial infarction and 24% higher risk of CHD compared with non-carriers among 25, 283 women from the WHS.

　　在 WHS 的 25 283 名女性中，与非携带者相比，KIF6 的 719Arg 等位基因携带者心肌梗死的风险高达 34%，冠心病的风险高达 24%，这证实并丰富了以前的报道。

　　（注：WHS: Women's Health Study，女性健康研究）

引自：JACC, 2008, 51(4): 444

例三： The area under the receiver operating characteristic curve for E/EDT (0.947±0.035) was statistically **significantly greater than** that for E/A (0.753±0.068) (P = 0.004).

在 E/EDT（0.947±0.035）ROC 曲线下的面积显著大于 E/A（0.753±0.068）（P=0.004）。

引自：*J Am Soc Echocardiogr*, 2009, 22(10): 1159

五、极限数的表达

对于极限数的表达，我们可以选用表示最大数、最小数的名词（如 "a maximum of、a minimum of"）或者是用表示极限的形容词（maximal）来表示，还可用一些词组（如 "as…as+数词" "be up to +数词" "at least +数词" 等）来表示。

（一）maximal size 表示：最大尺寸

例一： Gross examinations of the specimens at 6 months after implantation revealed that there was neocartilage formation; the **maximal size** was 8 mm × 8 mm.

6 个月后聚乳酸支架维持良好，所有植入块的边缘均有不同程度的新生软骨形成，软骨细胞增生活跃，最大为 8 mm×8 mm。

引自：《中华整形外科杂志》, 2000, 16(6): 333

例二： Infections were evenly divided between invasive bacterial and fungal infections unresponsive to **maximal** antibiotic and/or antifungal therapy.

将感染（患者）均等分为两组——侵袭性细菌感染组和真菌感染采用最大剂量抗生素和（或）抗真菌药物治疗无效组。

引自：*Haematologica*, 2009, 94(12)：1661

例三： With careful monitoring of haemodynamics, the dose was increased stepwise by 0.5 mg/kg every 4-6 h **up to a maximum of** 2 mg/kg.

仔细监测血流动力学的同时，按照 0.5 mg/kg（每4～6小时）逐步增加剂量，最大剂量为 2 mg/kg。

引自：*Eur J Cardiothorac Surg*, 2010, 38: 71

例四： Patients received **a minimum of** 3 and **a maximum of** 6 cycles with 1 cycle beyond stable radiographic and fluorodeoxyglucose positron emission tomography (FDG-PET) scans.

患者接受为期 3～6 个疗程的治疗，其中 1 个疗程实施常规放疗和 FDG-PET 扫描。

引自：*Blood*, 2010, 115(15)：3017

（二）"as … as+数词" 的应用

例一：The prevalence of CVD-related mortality in total CRF death was **as high as 44.2%**.

CVD 相关死亡人数占 CRF 总死亡人数的 44.2%。

引自:《中华肾脏病杂志》, 2001, 17(2): 91

例二：The incidence of perioperative visual loss after nonocular surgeries ranges from 0.002% of all surgeries to **as high as 0.2%** of cardiac and spine surgeries.

非眼科手术后围手术期视力丧失的发生率在所有手术中为 0.002%，在心脏和脊柱手术中高达 0.2%。

引自: *Am J Ophthalmol*, 2008, 145(4): 604

例三：In humans, such cells have been found to persist in maternal blood **as long as 27 years** postpartum.

在人类，这种细胞在产后母体血液中可存在长达 27 年之久。

引自: *STEM CELLS*, 2003, 21: 131

（三）"up to +数词" 表示：达到……

例一：Major or clinically relevant nonmajor bleeding was observed in **up to 4.7%** of those receiving osocimab, 5.9% receiving enoxaparin, and 2% receiving apixaban.

在接受奥西单抗治疗的患者中，高达 4.7%的患者出现了严重或临床相关的非大出血，依诺肝素组为 5.9%，阿哌沙班组为 2%。

引自: *JAMA*, 2020, 323(2): 130

例二：There was a decrease in BMI in both treatment groups **up to week 12**, thereafter stabilizing with orlistat but increasing beyond baseline with placebo.

观察至 12 周时，两组 BMI 均有下降，此后，奥利司他组体重维持稳定，而安慰剂组则超过基线。

引自: *JAMA*, 2005, 293: 2873

例三：Participants were recruited 5-10 years after their first delivery and followed annually for **up to 9 years**.

所招募的参与者为第一次分娩后 5～10 年，每年随访，长达 9 年之久。

引自: *Am J Obstet Gynecol*, 2019, 221(4):333.e1-333.e8

（四）"at least +数词" 表示：下限值。at least 是副词词组，常与数词连用，起修饰作用

例一：A total of 2005 men met inclusion criteria and completed the baseline and **at**

least 1 postbaseline survey (median age, 64 [59-70] years).

共 2005 位男子达到了纳入标准,完成了基线调查和至少 1 次基线后调查 [中位年龄 64 岁(59~70 岁)]。

引自: *JAMA*, 2020, 323(2): 149

例二: The mean follow-up was (18.1±13.3) months, during which 209 (67.6%) patients had **at least** 1 detected high atrial rate episode consistent with AF.

平均随访时间为(18.1±13.3)个月,其间有 209 例(67.6%)出现至少 1 例检测到高房率发作伴心房颤动。

引自: *Am Heart J*, 2008, 155(1): 94

例三: Among trials of **at least** one year's duration (mean 2.7 years), the rate ratio for vascular events was 1.45(1.12 to 1.89; *P*=0.005).

在至少持续 1 年的试验中(平均 2.7 年),血管病变的比率是 1.45(1.12~1.89; *P*=0.005)。

引自: *BMJ*, 2006, 332: 1032

六、倍数的表达

英语中增加几倍的说法,与汉语稍有不同,主要是要考虑是否包括原来的底数在内。倍数通常应用 times、fold 等词汇来表达,一般用法是在具体的数值后加上 times、fold,用来表示多少倍。但"一倍"不说 one time,而应说 once;"两倍"不说 two times,应说 twice;三倍以上才说 three(four, five…)times。如果是"2~3 倍",可以翻译成"two or three times"或者是"2 or 3 times"。医学论文英文摘要中,如果遇到"一倍半"、"两倍半"时,可译成"1.5 times"、"2.5 times"。

(一)直接表达法

例如:"A 的长度是 B 的三倍",可以直接译成"the length of A is 3 times the length of B",当然可以用 that 代替后一个 the length 使句子简洁,即"the length of A is 3 times that of B"。汉语中,对于这两个英语句还可译成"A 比 B 长两倍"。

例一: Compared with NG group, PKC activity increased significantly in HG group (**3.3 times**).

HG 组细胞膜 PKC 活性较 NG 组升高 3.3 倍。

引自:《中华肾脏病杂志》, 2001, 1794: 247

例二: Compared with nondiabetic participants, the death rate was **3.0 times as high** in individuals with youth-onset diabetes mellitus (95% CI, 1.1-8.0) and **1.4 times as high** in individuals with older-onset diabetes mellitus.

与非糖尿病受试者相比,青年型糖尿病患者的死亡率为前者的 3 倍

（95%CI，1.1~8.0），老年型糖尿病患者的死亡率是其 1.4 倍。

引自: JAMA, 2006, 296: 421

例三： However, rheumatoid arthritis is **5 times** more likely to develop after delivery than at any other time.

但是，产后出现类风湿关节炎的可能性较其他时期高出 5 倍。

引自: JAMA, 2005, 294: 2751

（二）使用比较级

例如："A 的长度是 B 的三倍"或者"A 比 B 长两倍"可以译成"A is three times longer than B"。

例一： The chemotherapeutic sensitivity of Lovo and LS174T cancer cell lines with wild-type p53 was **5-10 times higher than** that of 4 other cell lines with mutated p53.

Lovo 和 LS174T 癌细胞株对化疗药物的敏感性，p53 野生型高出 p53 突变型的 5~10 倍。

引自:《中华肿瘤杂志》, 2000, 22(5): 389

例二： We investigated the effect of diet plus pravastatin treatment on cardiovascular events in 5356 women during the 5-year follow-up. The incidence of cardiovascular events in those women was **2 to 3 times lower than that** in men.

在 5 年随访期内,进行饮食控制加普伐他汀治疗的 5356 例女性患者心血管事件发生率女性比相应的男性患者低 2~3 倍。

引自: Circulation, 2008, 117(2): 205

（三）使用"as...as"句型

例如："A 的长度是 B 的三倍"或者"A 比 B 长两倍",可以译成"A is 3 times as long as B"。

例一： The cumulative risk rate of gastric cancer in males was **3 times as high as** that of females.

男性胃癌发病率为女性的 3 倍。

引自:《中华肿瘤杂志》, 2000, 22(3): 311

例二： The concentration of iodine in the thyroid gland can increase to **as much as 25 times** that of the blood.

甲状腺中的碘浓度可增至血液中的 25 倍之多。

引自: Bariatric Times 2015, 12(4): 14

（四）表示增减的动词用于倍数表达

前文提过， increase、rise、decrease、fall、decline、drop、reduce 等可用来表示数字的增减。用这样的动词作句子的谓语，后面接 "…times" 或 "…fold"。如上文 "A 的长度是 B 的三倍" 或者 "A 比 B 长两倍"，可以译成 "A increases 3 times"。但当 times、fold 与 increase、decrease 等动词搭配时，注意与之连用的介词 to 和 by。用介词 to 时，表示包括有底数在内，相当于汉语的 "到" 字，意即 "增加到多少倍"。而介词 by 则表示实际增加的净数，不包括底数在内，表示增加多少，不管是百分数还是倍数最好用 by，就不容易发生误解。但用百分数时，一百之内无所谓底数，如 "增加 15%"，可以说成 "increase by 15%"，也可以说成 "increase 15 per cent" 都不会发生误解。在年龄比较中也有这种情况，如 "他比我大五岁"，可以说成 "He is older than I by five years"，也可以不用 "by" 而说成 "He is five years older than I"。此外，上述动词间或使用其名词形式，表达同样的概念。

例一： Six weeks after apoA-I GT, HDL cholesterol levels were increased by 1.6-fold (*P*<0.001) compared with diabetic controls injected with the Ad.

Apo A-I 基因转移（GT）后 6 周，与注射腺病毒载体 (Ad) 的糖尿病对照组相比，HDL-C 水平增加了 1.6 倍(*P*<0.001)。

引自：*Circulation*,2008, 117:1563

例二： The average integral optical density of mRNA for TGF-β and TIMP-1 **increased by 8 and 7 folds** (*P*<0.001).

（增生性瘢痕组织中 TGF-β 和 TIMP-1）平均积分光密度分别增加了 8 倍和 7 倍（*P*<0.001）。

引自：《中华整形外科杂志》，2000, 16(1): 34

例三： In the longitudinal subgroup, fibrate and statin use increased to 10.4% and 36.5%, respectively, over 5 years.

在纵向研究小组，（患者）使用非诺贝特和他汀 5 年后，（周围神经病变）可分别增至 10.4% 和 36.5%。

引自：*Diabetologia*, 2008, 51(4): 562

七、其他数值表达

（一）剂量表达

常用 dose 或 dosage 来表示药品及射线等的剂量。这两个词在其所表示的意义上有差异，不可互换。dose 指 "A specified quantity of a therapeutic agent, such as a drug or medicine, prescribed to be taken at one time or at stated intervals."（剂量），一种特定的治疗

方法的用量，如药剂或药物等一次或一定间隔的剂量。Dosage 则指 "Administration of a therapeutic agent in prescribed amounts; the determination and regulation of the size, frequency, and number of doses"（服用的药量；处方以一定剂量配给的药），即指 "剂量学"。常用搭配有 "in a dose, each dose"（每次剂量）；"daily dosage"，"the dosage in a day"（每天剂量）；"the initial dose"，"the initial dosage"（首次剂量）；the total dose/dosage of（总剂量）。

例一：Oral vitamin D supplementation between 700 to 800 IU/d appears to reduce the risk of hip and any nonvertebral fractures in ambulatory or institutionalized elderly persons. An oral vitamin D **dose of** 400 IU/d is not sufficient for fracture prevention.

口服补充维生素 D（700～800 IU/d）可以降低尚能活动的老人或慈善机构收容的老年人发生髋部骨折和脊椎以外骨折的危险，每天口服 400 IU 维生素 D 并不足以预防骨折。

引自：JAMA, 2005, 293: 2257

例二：We randomly assigned 247 adults with nonalcoholic steatohepatitis and without diabetes to receive pioglitazone **at a dose of** 30 mg daily (80 subjects), vitamin E **at a dose of** 800 IU daily (84 subjects), or placebo (83 subjects), for 96 weeks.

随机对 247 例非酒精性脂肪肝且无糖尿病的成年患者予以吡格列酮治疗，日剂量为每天 30 mg（80 例），维生素 E 每天 800 IU（84 例），或安慰剂（83 例），为期 96 周。

引自：N Engl J Med, 2010, 362(18)：1675

例三：Early intensive and sustained vasodilation was a comprehensive pragmatic approach of maximal and sustained vasodilation combining individualized doses of sublingual and transdermal nitrates, **low-dose** oral hydralazine for 48 hours.

早期强化和持续血管扩张采用综合实用、最大和持续血管扩张方法，结合个性化剂量差异，舌下和透皮硝酸盐给药，低剂量口服肼屈嗪 48 小时。

引自：JAMA, 2019, 322(23): 2292

例四：Tocilizumab treatment led to **dosage-related** decreases in the absolute neutrophil count, with a median decrease of 38% in the 4 mg/kg **dosage** group and 56% in the 8 mg/kg dosage group.

Tocilizumab 治疗导致剂量相关性的绝对中性粒细胞计数下降，4 mg/kg 剂量组下降 38%（中位数），8 mg/kg 剂量组下降 56%（中位数）。

引自：Arthritis Rheum, 2010, 62(2): 542

例五：The **daily dosage** of levodopa could be reduced by 68%.

左旋多巴每天剂量可减少 68%。

引自：Exp Med, 2003, 3: 37

例六：　In patients with NASH and control subjects, we randomly dispensed one 1 g L-carnitine tablet after breakfast plus diet and one 1 g tablet after dinner plus diet for 24 weeks or diet alone at the same dosage and regimen.

我们让 NASH 患者和对照受试者随机早餐后服用 1 片 1 g 的 L-肉碱加上饮食，以及晚餐后服用 1 片 1 g 的 L-肉碱加上饮食，为期 24 周，或者仅接受相同剂量和方案的饮食。

引自：*Am J Gastroenterol*, 2010, 105(6)：1338

（二）持续时间的表达

摘要写作中常需要交代研究所持续的时间过程，从短的时间数小时到天、月、年及多年等。研究过程中持续时间表达主要借助介词加具体时间，常用介词有 during、between、from…to、over 等，如介词 during 后接持续时间长短的范围（如 12～24 h；during a 5 year period），或 over+持续时间（如 over a period of 5 years）；between+持续时间（如 between May，2002 and September，2006）；in+持续时间（如 in 2003—2006；in the years 2003—2006）；from +持续时间（如 from 2003—2007）等。

例一：　After IR, myocardial levels of expression of ICAM-1 mRNA were increased significantly and reached a peak at 6 h; but the ICAM-1 protein peaked during 12-24 h. Number of PMNs and infarction size also increased and peaked after reperfusion 12-24 h.

心肌再灌注时，ICAM-1 表达明显上调，其 mRNA 表达至 6 小时达高峰，而蛋白质表达水平、PMNs 浸润数和梗死范围改变于 12～24 小时达高峰。

引自：《中华心血管病杂志》，2000, 28(1): 65

例二：　Cross-sectional study of 2310 healthy Icelandic adults who were divided equally into 3 age groups (30-45 years, 50-65 years, or 70-85 years) and recruited from February 2001 to January 2003.

于 2001 年 2 月至 2003 年 1 月从冰岛入选 2310 名健康成人，平分至 3 个年龄组（30～45 岁，50～65 岁，70～85 岁），进行横断面研究。

引自：*JAMA,* 2005, 294: 2336

例三：　The clinicopathological features and prognosis of 2417 patients with sporadic primary colorectal cancer who underwent an operation at the Asan Medical Center between January 1998 and December 2002 were examined.

选取 1998 年 1 月至 2002 年 12 月期间在 Asan 医疗中心接受手术治疗的 2417 例散发原发性大肠癌患者，就其临床病理特征及预后情况进行研究。

引自：*Dis Colon Rectum*, 2010, 53(4)：377

例四：　Data were obtained from records from general practices who had registered patients with the UK's Health Improvement Network database between 1987 and 2004.

所有资料来自在 1987～2004 年间英国健康促进网络数据库中注册的全科医师的病例记录。

引自: Lancet, 2006, 367(9516): 1075

例五：During a median follow-up of 21 months, 46 events occurred (31 cardiac deaths, 15 non-fatal MI).

为期 21 个月的中期随访, 发生死亡患者 46 例(31 例患者为心源性死亡, 15 例患者为非致死性心肌梗死)。

引自: Eur Heart J, 2008, 29(3): 377

例六：Over an 18-month treatment period in patients with type 2 DM, pioglitazone slowed progression of CIMT compared with glimepiride.

与格列美脲比较, 在为期 18 个月的治疗期间, 匹格列酮减缓了 2 型糖尿病患者 CIMT 的进展。

引自: JAMA, 2006, 296: 2572

例七：Rifaximin significantly reduced the risk of an episode of hepatic encephalopathy, as compared with placebo, over a 6-month period (hazard ratio with rifaximin, 0.42; 95% confidence interval [CI], 0.28 to 0.64; $P<0.001$).

在 6 个月期间, 与服用安慰剂组比较, 服用利福昔明明显降低了肝性脑病的发作风险 (应用利福昔明危险比为 0.42; 95%CI: 0.28～0.64; $P<0.001$)。

引自: N Engl J Med, 2010, 362(12) : 1071

（三）数值范围的表达

数值范围的表达可用 range、vary, 或由 range、vary 所组成的短语后接数词来表示 (range 可做动词或名词使用, 但结构不同)。常见表达有 "ranged from A～B" "range: A～B" "ranged from A to B" "range between…and…" "with a range of…to…" "vary from…to…" "from…to…"。这些结构可用于年龄范围、各种变量变化等表达。

例一：Follow-up data were available from 151 patients for 29.7 months (range, 6-78 months), and clinical outcome was assessed.

收集 151 例随访患者资料, 随访时间平均 29.7 个月 (6～78 个月不等), 并评价临床疗效。

引自: Clin Gastroenterol Hepatol, 2010, 8(2) : 151

例二：The ages of the participants ranged from a median of 31 to 72 years. The proportion of males ranged from 3% to 97%.

参与者的年龄 31～72 岁, 男性的比例从 3% 至 97% 不等。

引自: Am J Cardiol, 2019, 124(2):262-269

例三：The range of the discrepancy varied from a worsening in thresholds up to 20 dB and improvement in thresholds up to 45 dB.

阈值的差异范围从 20 dB(恶化）到 45 dB(改善）不等。

引自：Otolaryngol Head Neck Surg, 2010, 142(1)：36

例四： Follow-up ranged between 1 (82 eyes) and 7 years (13 eyes) (mean, 35.3±20.7 [standard deviation] months per eye).

随访期为 1 年（82 眼）至 7 年（13 眼）不等（35.3±20.7，SD:月/眼）。

引自：Ophthalmology, 2008, 115(4)：608

例五： In sensitivity analyses, however, the deviation score varied from −72% (using raw baseline disability status scale scores, rather than applying a "no improvement" algorithm) to 156% (imputing missing data for year two from progression rates for year one).

然而在敏感度分析中，偏差分数则为从−72%至156%不等（使用原始基线数据对残疾状况进行评分取代"无改善"计算法；利用第 1 年数据和进展速率进行计算以补充第 2 年丢失的数据）。

引自：BMJ, 2009, 339：b4677

（四）约略数的表达

约略数的表达通常以含有"约略"含义的词或词组与一个确定的数值搭配。表示"约略"含义的词或词组大多为副词，如 approximately、about、some、or so、almost、nearly、over、above、more than、greater than、less than 等。

例一： Among adolescents and young adults with ADHD who were receiving prescription stimulants, new-onset psychosis occurred in **approximately** 1 in 660 patients.

在接受处方兴奋剂治疗的患有注意力缺陷多动症的青少年和年轻成年人中，约 660 例患者中有 1 例出现新发精神病。

引自：N Engl J Med, 2019, 380: 1128

例二： The stability of the kit could be maintained at 4℃ for **more than** 3 months.

制成的药盒在 4℃条件下可保存 3 个月（之久）。

引自：《中华核医学杂志》, 2001, 22: 314

例三： The degree of LV and LA remodeling by LS is **almost** twice that of EF. Remodeling was similar for both genders.

通过 LS 重塑 LV 和 LA 的程度几乎是 EF 的两倍，但两性的重塑相似。

引自：Am J Cardiol, 2019, 124(2):253-261

例四： Unlike Brazil, China, and Mexico, communicable diseases still account for nearly half of deaths in India in children aged 5–14 years (73 920 [46.1%] of 160 330 **estimated** deaths in 2016).

与巴西、中国和墨西哥不同，传染病仍然占印度 5～14 岁儿童死亡人数的近一半（73 920，46.1%，2016 年估计死亡人数为 160 330 人）。

（五）大数目中的小数目

表达"某…中的一部分""在…例中有…例"，大数目中的小数目，可用 of、out of 或 among 来表示。

1. 介词 of 常用句式为"数字＋of＋数字"

例一： Nine **of** 16 cases had clinical infection.

16 例中有 9 例为临床感染。

引自：《中华器官移植杂志》, 2001, 22(3): 224

例二： Of 149 healthy, long-term trained cross-country skiers from three different age groups who were invited, 122 and 117 participated in the studies in 1976 and 1981, respectively.

149 位来自不同国家、长期训练的健康越野滑雪者应邀请参与了本研究，这些参与者处于 3 个不同的年龄段。另外，1976 年和 1981 年分别有 122 人和 117 人参与了研究。

引自：*Eur J Cardiovasc Prev Rehabil*, 2010, 17(1): 100

2. 词组 out of 常用句式为"数字＋out of＋数字"

例一： ARF had recovered in 22 **out of** 49 neonates in whom data was available; three patients had left against medical advice.

对于现有资料统计后发现，49 例急性肾衰竭新生儿中有 22 例康复，3 例擅自出院。

引自：*Ind J Pediatr*, 2006, 73: 19

例二： 50 out of 52 patients were followed-up for 100.1 ± 70.9 months.

52 例患者中有 50 例接受了（100.1±70.9）个月的随访。

引自：*J Cardiothorac Surg*, 2019, 14: 82

3. 介词"among"，常用句式为"among＋数字，数字"

例一： Among 759 patients with BCNE, a causative microorganism was identified in 62.7%, and a noninfective etiology in 2.5%.

759 例血培养为阴性的心内膜炎（BCNE）患者中，62.7%的患者的病因为细菌所致，非感染性病因占 2.5%。

引自：*Clin Infect Dis*, 2010, 51(2) : 131

例二： The prevalence of HPV was higher in HIV-positive women than in HIV-negative women in all age groups. **Among** HIV-infected women, 69%

were positive for ≥1 HPV type, 46% for a carcinogenic HPV type, and 10% for HPV-16.

在所有年龄组，HIV 阳性妇女的 HPV 感染率都高于 HIV 阴性的妇女。在感染 HIV 的妇女中，69% 的患者呈阳性的 HPV 类型 ≥1 种，46% 的患者致癌 HPV 类型呈阳性，10% 的患者 HPV-16 呈阳性。

引自：*J Infect Dis*, 2009, 199(12)：1851

4. 介词 in 常用句式为 "数字+in+数字"

例一： During the open-label phase, clinical and hematologic responses were observed in 17 of 19 patients (89%) and were sustained for 48 weeks in 14 of 19 patients (74%).

在开放标签阶段，19 例患者中有 17 例（89%）观察到临床和血液学反应，19 例患者中有 14 例（74%）持续 48 周。

引自：*N Engl J Med*, 2019, 380：1336

例二： Percutaneous coronary intervention was adjudicated as successful in 58 of 60 attempts.

PCI 手术 60 例，有 58 例成功。

引自：*Am Heart J*, 2008, 155(1): 121

（六）余数的表达

"另有多少例"，"其余多少例" 可以用下述方式表达。

1. "another+数词+名词"

例一： Two patients (50%) had urinary or enteric compressive complaints, while **another 2 patients** had no clinical symptoms.

2 例患者（50%）有泌尿系统或肠道压迫症状，另 2 例患者无临床症状。

引自：《中国医学科学院学报》, 2006, 28(5): 730

例二： In **another 20 patients** (20%), CsA was considered beneficial; however, it was required for a longer period of time, 5-10 years for some of the cases.

另外 20 例（20%）患者环孢菌素 A（CsA）治疗有效，但治疗周期较长，一些病例需要治疗 5～10 年。

引自：*Allergy*, 2018, 65(11): 1478

2. "the other +数词+名词"

例一： **The other 5 cases** of cerebral necrosis and 2 cases with postoperative cerebral malacia demonstrated FDG uptake defects

另 5 例术后放射治疗后脑损伤患者和 2 例术后软化灶 ^{18}F-FDG PET 影像

均显示局部放射区为放射性局部缺损或明显低下。

引自:《中华核医学杂志》, 2001, 22(1): 14

例二: Inflammatory genes were more markedly upregulated in coronary arteries than **the other 2 arteries.**

冠状动脉炎性基因上调比其他两条动脉(颈动脉及胸主动脉)更为显著。

引自: *Arterioscler Thromb Vasc Biol*, 2008, 28(2): 359

3. "数词+others"

例: After follow-up for an average of 2 years , only 1 of the 8 patients did not recover as a result of psychosis and **7 others** had no symptoms but normal endocrine results.

术后 8 例均获得随访,平均 2 年,除 1 例患者伴有神经官能症,症状未减,余 7 例血压及内分泌检查皆恢复正常。

引自:《中华外科杂志》, 2001, 39(9): 787

4. "the remaining +数词+名词"

例一: Four patients have been registered for transplantation, and **the remaining three patients** show signs of severe cholestasis.

4 位患者正在等待肝移植,剩下的 3 位患者也有严重的胆汁淤积的症状。

引自: *Endoscopy*, 2008, 40(3) : 214

例二: 27 out of 52 associate with simple cardiac abnormalities, 20 out of 52 associate with complex cardiac malformations, **the remaining 5 patients** without cardiac abnormalities.

52 例患者中, 27 例与单纯心脏异常有关, 20 例与复杂心脏畸形有关,其余 5 例无心脏异常。

引自: *J Cardiothorac Surg*, 2019, 14: 82

例三: Fifty-nine patients had surgically documented CP and comprised group 1; **the remaining 41 patients** with RMD comprised group 2.

59 例外科发现的 CP 患者构成组 1,剩下的 41 例 RMD 患者构成组 2。

引自: *JACC*, 2008, 51(3): 315

5. 其他表达方式

除上述表达外, 还可以借助其他英语词来表示。这些词国内作者写作时较少使用。但国外文献较多见。

例一: Blood was the most useful specimen, providing a diagnosis for 47.7% of patients by serological analysis (mainly Q fever and Bartonella infections).

Broad-range polymerase chain reaction (PCR) of blood and Bartonella-specific Western blot methods diagnosed **7 additional cases**.

血液是最佳标本，47.7%的患者可通过血清学分析获得确诊（主要为 Q 热和巴尔通氏体感染）。其他 7 例患者通过血液广谱聚合酶链式反应（PCR）和巴尔通氏体特异性蛋白质印迹法确诊。

【析】借助 additional 表示，需要注意的是，数词要放在 additional 之前。

引自：Clin Infect Dis, 2010, 51(2)：131

例二：Stent insertion was successful in 9 of 10 patients. Failure to control bleeding was observed in 3 patients (2 with gastric varices), with control of bleeding in the **remainder**.

10 例患者中 9 例支架置入成功。3 例出血无法控制（2 例伴有胃静脉曲张），其余患者成功止血。

【析】使用 remainder 表示，Remainder 意为 "Something left over after other parts have been taken away."，通常与定冠词 the 连用。

引自：Gastrointest Endosc, 2010, 71(1)：71

例三：Investigators diagnosed complete remission in 24% and marked improvement in **further 57%** of patients with isotretinoin treatment, in contrast to remission in 14% and marked improvement in 55% of patients treated with doxycycline.

采用异维 A 酸治疗的患者中，研究者确认有24%的患者完全缓解，另有57%的患者明显改善；而采用多西环素治疗的患者中，14%的患者完全缓解，55%的患者明显改善。

【析】使用 further 表示，Further 意为："additional"。

引自：J Dtsch Dermatol Ges, 2010, 8(7): 505

（七）年龄的表达

年龄的表示多种多样，本节主要讲述医学文摘中经常使用的表示方法。常用的表达方式如下所述。

1. 准确年龄表达

1）"of+数词+years old（或 of age）"，如 "a patient of 27 years old"。

2）"aged+数词+years"，如 "a patient aged 27 years"。

3）"at（the）age of+数词"，如 "a patient at the age of 27（years）"。

2. 不确定性年龄表达

1）"（限制语）+ 数词+years of age"，如 "over the age of 40 years；over 40 years of age；under the age of 40 years；above the age of 40 years；below the age of 40 years；after the age of 40 years; more than 40 years old; less than 40 years old; younger/older than 40 years"。

2）"aged+数词+years+（限制语）"，如"aged 40 years and over"。

3）"at+数词+years of age"，如"at 40 years of age or less"。

例一： To identify risk factors in early life (up to **3 years of age**) for obesity in children in the United Kingdom.

确定英国儿童在幼儿期（3 岁以下）发生肥胖的危险因素。

引自：*BMJ*, 2006, 321: 1744

例二： Incidence rate of diabetic ESRD and mortality **between 25 and 55 years of age**, according to age at onset of type 2 diabetes mellitus.

根据 2 型糖尿病的发病年龄，计算 25～55 岁糖尿病 ESRD 的发病率和死亡率。

引自：*JAMA*, 2006, 296: 421

例三： Longitudinal population-based study conducted between 1965 and 2002 in Pima Indians from the state of Arizona. Participants were divided into 2 groups: (1) youth-onset type 2 diabetes mellitus (onset **<20 years of age**) and (2) older-onset type 2 diabetes mellitus (onset **20-55 years of age**).

于 1965～2002 年在 Arizona 比马印第安人中进行人群纵向研究。参试者分为两组：青年型 2 型糖尿病（发病年龄<20 岁）和青中年型 2 型糖尿病（发病年龄 20～55 岁）。

引自：*JAMA*, 2006, 296: 421

例四： Prospective cohort study of 15 632 initially healthy US women **aged 45 years or older** (interquartile range, 48-59 years) who were enrolled between November 1992 and July 1995.

对 15 632 例入选时处于健康状态的美国妇女进行前瞻性队列研究。1992 年 11 月至 1995 年 7 月入组时年龄≥45 岁（四分位范围 48～59 岁）。

引自：*JAMA*, 2005, 294: 326

例五： At entry, the cross-sectional sample had a mean±SD **age of 63.8±11.3 years**, 48.7% were men.

入组时，横向样本年龄均数±SD 是（63.8±11.3）岁，48.7%是男性。

引自：*Diabetologia*, 2008, 51(4): 562

例六： A prospective, population-based study of infants **aged 0 to 90 days** who resided in areas in 8 US states with active laboratory surveillance for invasive *S. pneumoniae* infections from July 1, 1997, to June 30, 2004.

从 1997 年 7 月 1 日至 2004 年 6 月 30 日，对居住在美国 8 个州的出生后 0 至 90 天婴儿进行了前瞻性、基于人群的研究，利用各州实验室，对侵袭性肺炎链球菌感染进行主动监测。

引自：*JAMA*, 2006, 295(14): 1668

例七：We conducted a population-based United States cohort study of patients **over 65 years of age** to examine use and determinants of prediagnosis surveillance in patients with HCC who were previously diagnosed with cirrhosis.

基于人群的美国队列研究，研究对象为 65 岁以上的患者，旨在分析先前被诊断为肝硬化的 HCC 患者的诊断前监测到的用药情况及遗传因素。

引自: Hepatology, 2010, 52(1)：132

例八：The study group included 16 patients who had been diagnosed as having idiopathic PAH when they were **younger than 15 years old**; all were **younger than 20 years of age**.

研究组包括 16 例 15 岁之前已诊断为特发性肺动脉高压（PAH）患者，所有研究对象年龄均小于 20 岁。

引自: Circ J, 2010, 74(2): 371

（八）间隔频率的表达

医学论文摘要中，通常需要对间隔时间予以描述，尤其在实验研究中更为常见。间隔时间的表达主要有下述两种方式。

1）"at intervals of+数词"或"at+数词+intervals"：每隔多久。

2）"every+数词+时间数（天、星期、月等）"：每隔……天等。注意 every 表示间隔频率的概念，如 every fourth day "每隔三天"（即"每第四天上"；every fifth day "每隔四天"（即"每第五天上"），依此类推。

例一：Thyroid function and antithyroid antibody levels were examined regularly **at 6-12-month intervals** and when there were clinical signs of thyroid dysfunction.

甲状腺功能出现异常临床症状时，间隔 6～12 个月定期检查甲状腺功能和甲状腺抗体水平。

引自: Circ J, 2010, 74(2): 371

例二：After standardized intraocular Collamer lens (ICL) implantation, patients underwent complete ophthalmologic examinations before surgery and **at 1 week, 1 month, 3 months, 6 months, and at yearly intervals** thereafter.

按标准植入 ICL 后，患者分别在手术之前，术后 1 周、术后 1、3、6 个月及随后的每一年接受系统的眼科检查。

引自: Ophthalmology, 2010, 117(8)：1506

例三：Non-invasive ambulatory BP measurements **at 15 min intervals** were performed.

无创动态血压监测每隔 15 分钟测血压 1 次。

引自: Eur Heart J, 2008, 29(3): 401

例四： Semen analysis was performed **every 3 months** during pre-treatment and the first year of combined therapy.

前期治疗期间及综合治疗期的第 1 年，每 3 个月（对患者）进行一次精液分析。

引自：*J Endocrinol Invest*, 2010, 33(9): 618

例五： Maintenance dosing was 40 mg **every other week** in 88% of patients.

88%的患者治疗维持剂量为 40 mg，每隔 1 周 1 次。

引自：*Am J Gastroenterol*, 2009, 104(12) : 3042

（九）多组数值联合的表达

英文摘要写作中，尤其对研究结果的描述，通常涉及多组数值。从简洁策略手段，这些数值可以按一定的范畴和逻辑关系先给出主要数值，次要（带有补充说明性质的）数值可用括号或分号罗列其后。

例一： 31 patients were included. Sentinel node was identified in 21 patients (detection rate 67.7%). The detection rate was significantly higher in women undergoing immediate vs. delayed staging (88.9% *vs.* 41.7% *P*=0.003). Four patients had positive nodes. In all the patients with lymphatic dissemination, a positive sentinel node was identified (sensitivity:100%, false-negative-rate:0%, negative-predictive-value:100%). One (3.2%) intra- and 2 (6.5%) post-operative grade I complications occurred.

纳入 31 例患者。21 例患者检出前哨淋巴结（检出率 67.7%）。在接受即时分期和延迟分期的妇女中，检出率明显更高（88.9% *vs.* 41.7% *P*=0.003）。四例患者有阳性淋巴结。在所有淋巴扩散的患者中，检出阳性前哨淋巴结（敏感度：100%，假阴性率：0%，阴性预测值：100%）。术后出现一级并发症 1 例（3.2%），二级并发症 2 例（6.5%）。

引自：*Am J Obstet Gynecol*, 2019, 221(4): 324.e1-324.e10

例二： There were 146 cases of IPD, 89 before and 57 after PCV7 introduction. Isolated bacteremia occurred in 94 cases(64%), pneumonia in 27 (18%), meningitis in 22 (15%), and septic arthritis and /or osteomyelitis in 3 (2%). Mean rates of IPD for infants aged 0 to 90 days decreased 40% from 11.8 (95% confidence interval [CI], 9.6-14.5) to 7.2 (95% CI, 5.6-9.4; *P*=0.004) per 100 000 live births following PCV7 introduction. Among black infants, mean rates of IPD decreased significantly from 17.1 (95% CI, 11.9-24.6) to 5.3 (95% CI, 2.8-10.1; *P*=0.001) per 100 000 live births, with a nonsignificant decrease from 9.6 (95% CI, 7.3-12.7) to 6.8(95% CI, 4.9-9.4) per 100 000 live births for white infants rates of PCV7—serotype isolates decreased significantly from 7.3 (95% CI, 5.3-10.1) to 2.4 (95% CI, 1.6-3.8; *P*<0.001) per 100 000 live births, while rates of non-PCV7 serotypes remained stable (*P*=0.55).

侵袭性肺炎球菌疾病（IPD）患儿共发现 146 例，七价肺炎球菌结合疫苗（PCV7）接种计划实施之前有 89 例，实施之后有 57 例。单纯菌血症患儿 94 例（64%），肺炎患儿 27 例（18%），脑膜炎患儿 22 例（15%），化脓性关节炎患儿和（或）骨髓炎患儿 3 例（2%）。PCV7 接种计划实施之后，出生后 0～90 天婴儿的 IPD 平均发病率下降了 40%，从 11.8/10 万例活产儿（95%CI：9.6～14.5）下降至 7.2/10 万例活产儿（95%CI 5.6～9.4；*P*=0.004）。黑人婴幼儿的 IPD 平均发病率的下降非常显著，从 17.1/10 万例活产儿（95%CI：11.9～24.6）下降至 5.3/10 万例活产儿（95%CI：2.8～10.1；*P*=0.001）；而白人婴幼儿的发病率则下降不明显，仅从 9.6/10 万例活产儿（95%CI：7.3～12.7）下降至 6.8/10 万例活产儿（95%CI：4.9～9.4）。PCV7 血清型分离株出现率显著降低，从 7.3/10 万例的活产儿（95%CI：5.3～10.1）下降到 2.4/10 万例的活产儿（95%CI：1.6～3.8；*P*<0.001），而非 PCV7 血清型分离株的出现率则基本稳定（*P*=0.55）。

引自：*JAMA*, 2006, 295(14): 1668

八、练　习

8-1　将下列句子译成英语

1. 我们对总数 180 例患者随访了 1～5 年，随访平均时间为 3.2 年。

2. 在 8 例小细胞癌患者中，有 5 例口服药物有效。

3. 我们用氨苄青霉素治疗这位患者，剂量为每天 4 g。

4. 我们对 78 例施行曲张静脉减压术的肝硬化患者进行了研究。

5. 在 1981～2000 年冠心病死亡率下降 54%。

6. 年龄≥45 岁的新发直肠出血患者中 1/10 有结肠肿瘤。

7. 在 38 例已做内脏血管造影的 Zolllinger-Ellison 综合征患者中，仅 2 例确诊为原发性胰腺肿瘤；另有 4 例虽然通过适当的检查，但不能最后确诊。

8. 在 122 例患者中，有 25 例发生原发性高血压，他们的平均体重并不明显超过其余的人。

9. 住院平均年龄为 60 岁，男女比例为 3∶1。

10. 从皮肤和呼吸道丧失的水分为约 700 ml。

11. 经过 30～220 分钟的反复灌注，正常心肌活力降低了 63%，而短暂性心肌缺血的心肌活力降低了 15.3%。

12. 外科术后心房颤动［Post-operative atrial fibrillation（POAF）］是心脏外科术后的常见并发症，发生率在 30%～50%。

8-2　将下列句子中的部分中文译成英文

1. _____（平均年龄）at loss of ambulation was 8.1y but at the time of the study.

2. _____（总数为）232 seizure episodes occurred in ninety babies _____（平均）2.58 seizure episodes per baby（range 1 to 7 episodes）in first 28 days of life.

3. Fifty two babies （57.8%）developed first seizure within first 48 hours of life, _____（其中）which 20 babies had seizure in _____（不足）12 hours of life.

4. _____（一组）almost 30 students has been meeting monthly to discuss articles from Psychosomatic Medicine and is still going strong.

5. Rakoff-Nahoum and colleagues studied the interaction of TLRs and commsensal organisms in _____（一系列）experiments with mice.

6. _____（5%～10%的出生时体重不足 1500 g 的婴儿）will develop NEC and the incidence increases with decreasing gestational age.

7. Complement protein concentrations increase after birth and _____（接近）mean adult values _____（16～18 个月大小）。

8. The incidence of neonatal seizures as reported by various studies _____（在 0.1%～0.5%）in term neonates and 10%-22.7% in preterm neonates.

9. Of 93 children, 62（66.6%）were MDRTF. 24 cases were _____（5 岁以下），26 between 5-10 years and 12 were above 10 years. _____（男女比例为 1.85：1）.

10. Triclofos was used _____（每公斤体重 50 mg）for inducing sleep where needed.

11. A retrospective review of charts for all patients referred to the pulmonary clinic for evaluation of recurrent chest infection _____（1993 年 1 月至 2005 年 8 月）at King Faisal specialist hospital.

12. A "new" prescription was defined by an_____（间隔至少 120 天）since last use of an antidepressant (based on prescription date and intended duration of use).

13. There were 11 （55%）men, and the_____（平均年龄 72 岁）(range, 53 to 84 years).

14. _____（高达 64%的人）who have experienced a stroke have some degree of cognitive impairment.

15. _____（24 个培养为阳性的患者中）enrolled in our study, _____[14 人为男性（58.33%），10 人为女性（41.67%）]. _____（患者年龄范围）was _____（分别为 3.5～14 岁,中位年龄为 9.5～10 岁）.

16. _____（1999 年 4 月至 2005 年 10 月间），consecutive patients with high-grade carotid stenosis（_____（70%有症状的患者和 90%无症状的患者）assessed with ultrasound）were treated with CAS after a prospective protocol at our institution.

17. Clinically apparent cardiomyopathy was first evident_____（10 岁后）

and _____（发病率随年龄上升）, being present in all patients_____
（18 岁以上）.

18. The incidence of neonatal seizures as reported by various studies_____
（0.1%～0.5%）in term neonates and 10%～22.7% in preterm neonates.

19. In the current case series family history was _____（仅 1/3 为阳性）number of cases.

20. _____（发病率最高）（30.6%）seen in the _____
（2～5 岁年龄组）。_____［第二次发病高峰
（25.8%）见于 7～10 岁年龄组］. It was seen only in a one infant. 22（35.5%）cases were females and 40（64.5%）cases were males. Therefore, _____（男女比例为 1.85∶1）.

21. In the susceptible group, _____（2/11 的患者主诉有阳性病史）of peptic ulcer in their families.

22. Moreover, AICAR has been used for the treatment of Lesch-Nyhan syndrome_____
_____（剂量按每公斤体重 100 mg）in humans without any side effects.

23. Children with neurofibromatosis type 1 and symptomatic inoperable plexiform neurofibromas received oral selumetinib_____（每天 2 次，剂量 25 mg）per square meter of body-surface area.

24. Vitamin B6_____（每天 50～100 mg 的剂量）was used to mitigate hematologic toxicity.

25. Haematology, biochemistry, and CD4-cell counts were done_____（每 12 周）.

第九章　医学论文英文摘要语法修辞

语法是语言的组织规律，它是关于词的形态变化和用词造句的规则。广义上，英语语法不仅涉及词法、句法，而且涉及文体。所谓文体指的是风格，即说话、做事、表达及表演的一种方法（The way in which something is said, done, expressed, or performed）。目前已出版的介绍英语语法的著作种类繁多，只要读者需要，可以博取众家之长，参考起来非常方便。本章仅从医学论文英文摘要写作的实际需要出发，从科技文体的角度阐述主谓一致、非谓语动词、平行结构、复合句、否定句、比较结构等在写作中的应用及标点符号的正确使用。

一、主　谓　一　致

一致是一个语法范畴，指句子成分之间在人称、数、格、性等方面保持一致。人称、格和性的一致性比较简单，本章不再赘述。句子的主语和谓语在数上保持一持，也称为主谓一致，一般遵循三个基本原则：①语法一致（grammatical concord），即形式上一致；②意义一致（notional concord），即表达意义或意念一致；③邻近原则（concord of proximity），即指谓语的动词形式与邻近的名词一致。

（一）单数名词

单数名词作句子主语时，句子的谓语动词采用单数。但是，需要注意的是，医学英语由于其词源的多样性，不同名词尾缀代表了不同的名词形式。例如：acidosis（酸中毒）、arthritis（关节炎），其词尾的-osis、-itis 分别表示某种病态和炎（症），形式上是单数名称；而 ganglia（神经节）、protozoa（原虫）、bronchi（支气管）这 3 个词不同的词尾却体现的是复数名词形式，其对应的单数形式分别是 ganglion、protozoon、bronchus。除此之外，还有相当多的尾缀形式变化需要引起重视，因为它们会影响到句子的主语和谓语形式的一致性。对于此类名词词尾变后的形式意义，学习并掌握它们不是十分困难，此处不多做赘述，本节重点介绍某些特殊结构在主谓一致中的应用。

1. "one or two+复数名词"作主语

本结构作主语，谓语动词用复数形式。

例一： **One or two** color monoclonal antibodies directly labeled with immunofluorescence **were** used to analyze the surface and cytoplasma antigens by flow cytometry, and an antibody integral system was developed for the immunologic classification.
用一种或两种直接免疫荧光标记的彩色单克隆抗体，通过流式细胞仪分析表面抗原和细胞质抗原，建立抗体积分系统进行免疫分类。

引自:《中华血液学杂志》, 2001, 22(12): 633

例二： The postoperative 3-, 5-, and 7-year overall survival rates of HCC patients with CD151(high)/MMP9(high)/MVD(high) were significantly lower than those of the CD151(low)/MMP9(low)/MVD(low) group or groups in which only **one or two** of CD151, MMP9, and MVD **were** highly expressed.
CD151（高）/MMP9（高）/MVD（高）组肝细胞癌患者术后 3、5 和 7 年总体生存率显著低于 CD151（低）/MMP9（低）/MVD（低）组患者或 CD151、MMP9 和 MVD 中存在一项或两项高度表达的患者。

引自: *Hepatology*, 2010, 52(1): 183

例三： One third of those transfusions in which **one or two** antigen-mismatched platelets **were** used were failures.
使用一种或两种抗原不匹配的血小板输血时，1/3 是失败的。

引自: *Blood Banking and Transfusion Medicine* (Second Edition), 2007

2. "单数名词+with 等（along with/together with/except/as well as/as much as/rather than/more than/no less than）+名词"结构作主语

本结构作主语，谓语动词的数与第一个名词保持一致。

例一： These changes, **together with** a significant decrease in the frequency of circulating plasma cells, **suggest** a specific effect of tocilizumab on autoantibody-producing cells.
这些变化，连同浆细胞循环频率的显著下降，表明 tocilizumab 对自身抗体产生细胞的特异性作用。
【析】These changes 为主语，together with 引导的内容属于补充说明，所以谓语用复数形式 suggest。

引自: *Arthritis Rheum.*, 2010, 62(2): 542

例二： This paucity of knowledge about the importance and presence of COPD, **as well as** its treatment, **is** seen among patients.
患者普遍对慢性阻塞性肺疾病（COPD）的重要性缺乏认识，甚至不知晓是否已患 COPD 及该如何治疗。

【析】paucity 在句子中作主语，as well as 后的内容为补充信息，所以谓语动词用单数 is。

例三：The remarkable variation in definitions and recommendations, **along with** scarce details of the methods used to reach this advice, **makes** the available sources of drug information ill suited for clinical use.

由于定义和建议条款存在极大差异，以及无详细方法指导该如何获得这些建议，这使得现有药物信息源非常不适于指导临床应用。

【析】句子的主语是 variation，谓语用单数 makes。

例四：Improved technology and surgical procedures **along with** changes in clinical practice **were** likely factors linked with enhanced and sustained seizure-free outcomes in the post-1997 series.

技术完善、手术方法改进及临床实践的改观是提高和维持 1997 之后组癫痫控制的主要因素。

【析】主语用的是并列名词 "…technology and…procedures"，故谓语用复数形式 were。

例五：Fenofibrate, particularly administered **together with** metformin, **is** superior to metformin and lifestyle intervention in exhibiting beneficial effects on systemic inflammation, hemostasis, and monocyte secretory function in type 2 diabetic patients with mixed dyslipidemia.

非诺贝特对于 2 型糖尿病患者伴混合性血脂异常，在控制全身性炎症、止血及单核细胞分泌功能方面的效果优于单纯使用二甲双胍和生活方式干预。若与二甲双胍联用，效果更为显著。

【析】主语是 "Fenofibrate"，药品名，为单数形式，故谓语用单数 "is"。

例六：Surgical treatment **rather than** radiation **was** also associated with better survival, although we could not control for confounders that may bias treatment selection.

虽然不能控制能够使治疗选择产生偏倚的混杂因素，但手术治疗而不是放射治疗也可提高生存率。

【析】主语为 "….treatment"，与 "rather than" 连用，谓语用单数 "was"。

例七：Chronic spontaneous urticaria (CSU) lasting **more than** 6 weeks **is** one of the most disabling types of urticaria and often results in severely impaired quality of life.

慢性自发性荨麻疹（CSU）持续 6 周以上，为该病最常见的致残类型之一，且易严重影响生活质量。

【析】主语 chronic spontaneous urticaria 是疾病名称，为单数形式，故谓语同样用单数 is。

引自：*Ann Allergy Asthma Immunol*, 2010, 104(3)：253

（二）复数形式名词作主语

规则变化的名词，其复数名词大多以-s 或-es 形式结尾，在句中作主语要求谓语动词与复数对应，但不表示以-s 结尾的名词作主语，谓语一定要用复数。

1. 表示时间、距离、重量的复数名词作主语

此类复数形式名词作主语，谓语用单数形式。

例一：The **length** of mechanical ventilation was 7.5±12.8 days. The median duration of follow-up was 37 months.

机械通气时间为（7.5±12.8）天。平均随访时间为 37 个月。

引自：*Transplantation*, 2008, 86(4)：515

例二：Postoperative **half year is** high incidence stage of incision hernia and all inducing factors should be avoided.

术后半年内是腹壁切口疝发生的高峰期，应特别注意保护，尽量避免一切诱发因素。

引自：《中国实用外科杂志》, 2001, 21(2): 91

2. 外来的复数名词作主语

此类复数形式名词作主语，谓语动词用复数，典型的例子如 the data 作主语。

例一：The **data** of 56 cases of portal hypertension treated with portoazygous devascularization and shunt from April 1987 to April 1999 **were** summarized.

总结 1987 年 4 月至 1999 年 4 月采用断流加分流术治疗 56 例门静脉高压症的经验。

引自：《中国实用外科杂志》, 2001, 21(2): 147

例二：Patient-level **data were** pooled from 5 prospective, double-blind, randomized trials of PES versus bare-metal stents (BMS) (n = 3513).

患者水平资料来自 5 个 PES 对比金属裸支架（BMS）（n=3513）的前瞻性双盲随机试验。

引自：*JACC*, 2008, 51(7): 708

特别提示：以"-s"结尾的某些表示疾病的名词作句子的主语时，因此类名词属于单数性质，故谓语动词只能采用单数形式。例如：

例一： **Statistical analysis was performed** using χ^2 test to determine the association between normal or dysplastic tissues and tumors.

采用χ^2检验分析正常组与组织发育不良和肿瘤组的差异。

引自：*World J Gastroenterol*, 2002, 8: 200

例二： **Splenic vein (SV) hyperdynamics is** the main source of increased portal blood flow.

脾静脉高动力循环是门静脉血流量增加的主要来源。

引自：《中国实用外科杂志》, 2001, 21(2): 149

（三）并列主语

几个名词作句子的并列主语，谓语动词一般用复数形式，但下列情况例外。

1. "名词+and+名词"结构作主语

本结构作主语，若表示同类事物或单一概念，谓语动词用单数形式。

例一： **Breast-conserving surgery and radical radiation therapy is** effective for patients with early stage of carcinoma of breasts.

早期乳腺癌患者接受保乳综合治疗可以取得满意的临床效果，可成为早期乳腺癌的首选治疗方法。

引自：《中国实用外科杂志》, 2001, 21(9): 547

例二： **Early diagnosis and treatment is** the key point to decrease the death rate.

早期确诊、及时治疗是降低病死率的关键。

引自：《中国实用外科杂志》, 2001, 21(3): 218

2. "名词（代词）+ or+名词（代词）"结构作主语

本结构作主语，如果 or 只连接两个并列单数名词，谓语动词的数一般与 or 后的名词（代词）保持一致；若 or 的前面出现了由 and 连接的两个并列主语，此时倾向使用复数形式谓语。

例一： A cerebral performance category of **1 or 2 at hospital discharge was** recorded in 7.5% of patients in the manual CPR group and in 3.1% of the LDB-CPR group (*P*=0.006).

出院时脑功能分级 1～2 级者比例在人工 CPR 组为 7.5%，LDB-CPR 组为 3.1%（*P*=0.006）。

【析】主语中心名词是 category，故谓语用单数 was。

引自：*JAMA*, 2006, 295(22): 2620

例二： **A total of 546 patients with implantable cardioverter-defibrillators(ICDs) and prior documented malignant ventricular tachycardia(VT) or**

ventricular fibrillation(VF) were enrolled between October 2001 and August 2004.

在 2001 年 10 月至 2004 年 8 月间, 共纳入 546 例病历记载曾有恶性室性心动过速（VT）或心室颤动（VF）的植入埋藏式心脏复律除颤器（ICD）患者。

【析】主语中心名词是 patients, 故谓语用复数 were。

引自：JAMA, 2006, 295(22): 2613

例三： **In patients with known or suspected CAD, DET result by wall motion criteria and CFR are** additive and complementary for the identification of patients at risk of experiencing hard events.

对于已知或可疑的 CAD 患者, DET 测定室壁运动和 CFR 为识别不良事件提供了有力的补充依据。

【析】主语中心名词是 patients, 故谓语用复数 are。

引自：Eur Heart J, 2008, 29(1) : 79

3. 由连词短语 "either…or…/neither…nor…/not only…but（also）…" 连接的并列主语

本结构作主语, 通常根据就近一致原则, 即按与动词最近的那个名词来确定谓语动词的数, 请注意观察体会。

例一： **Sixty-eight patients (29.7%) either were** on AT **or** had AT initiated during follow-up.

随访期间 68 例（29.7%）患者接受或开始 AT 治疗。

引自：Circulation, 2010, 121(1) : 20

例二： **Neither patients nor investigators or their teams were** masked to treatment assignment.

无论是患者或研究者还是研究小组, 均不知治疗方案。

引自：Lancet, 2010, 376(9735) : 91

例三： We propose that an immediate consequence of the unfolded protein response (UPR) **not only limits** the accumulation of misfolded proteins **but also protects** tissues from harmful exogenous stresses.

我们认为 UPR 的直接结果不仅限制了未折叠蛋白的蓄积, 也保护组织免受外源有害应激的损害。

引自：EMBO J, 2009, 28(9): 1296

（四）表示部分的 "名词+of+名词" 结构作主语

谓语动词的数需要从下述几个方面考虑。

1. "a series+of+名词" 结构作主语

本结构作主语，谓语动词用复数形式，如果当成一个整体看，则谓语动词可用单数形式。

例一： In recent years, **a series of publications have demonstrated** a potentially important role for magnetic resonance imaging in the pre-mortem diagnosis of sporadic Creutzfeldt-Jakob disease.

近年来，一系列报道证实了 MRI 在预诊断散发性 Creutzfeldt-Jakob 病的重要性。

引自：Brain, 2009, 132(Pt 10)：2659

例二： **A series of 50 patients with bacterial wound infection were treated** with antibiotic Cefotaxime, of which 46 were reported satisfactory.

对 50 例细菌性伤口感染患者采用抗生素头孢噻肟治疗，其中 46 例疗效满意。

引自：Statistics for the Life Sciences(5th Edition),Chapter9.2

例三： **A series of 104 consecutive patients with a fracture of the coccyx was studied.** The mechanism, level, characteristics of the fracture line and complications were recorded.

对 104 名尾骨骨折的患者进行了研究。记录骨折机制、水平部位、特征和并发症。

引自：Eur Spine J, 2019, doi:10.1007/s00586-019-06188-7

2. "number、average" 作句子主语

"a number+of+复数名词" "an average（total）+ of +复数名词"结构作句子的主语，谓语动词用复数；"the number+of+复数名词" "the average（total）+ of +复数名词"结构作主语，谓语动词用单数。

例一： However, **the number of fat cells stays** constant in adulthood in lean and obese individuals, even after marked weight loss, indicating that **the number of adipocytes is** set during childhood and adolescence.

然而，不管是消瘦者，还是肥胖者，甚至体重显著减轻后，成年人脂肪细胞数量仍保持不变，这提示脂肪细胞数量在儿童和青少年就已固化。

引自：Nature, 2008, 453(7196)：783

例二： Despite adequate epicardial artery reperfusion, **a number of patients with STEMI have** a poor prognosis because of microvascular damage.

尽管有足够的心外膜动脉再灌注，但很多 ST 段抬高心肌梗死（STEMI）患者因为微循环受损而预后较差。

引自：J Am Coll Cardiol, 2008, 51(5): 560

例三： **There are a number of types** of PAH, one of which is pulmonary veno-occlusive disease (PVOD).

肺动脉高压（PAH）有许多种类型，其中之一是肺静脉闭塞性疾病（PVOD）。

引自：*Chest*, 2009, 135(6)：1462

例四： **A total of 2318 cord blood units (CBU) were** collected, among which, 1240 CBUs met all tests and standards. The average volume of collected qualified cord blood was (98.31±26.95) ml, the average amount of nucleated cells after separation was $(1.22\pm0.47)\times10^9$, and the average recovery percentage of nucleated cells (88.90±9.65)%.

共采集 2318 份脐血，合格 1240 份，合格率为 53.5%，合格脐血采集的平均容积为（98.31±26.95）ml，分离后脐血有核细胞为（1.22±0.47）$\times10^9$，回收率为（88.90±9.65）%。

引自：《中华血液学杂志》，2001, 22(4): 411

例五： **Average of Cobb's angle before operation**, 1 year after operation, 2 year after operation **was** 66.2 degree, 36 degree and 36 respectively.

手术前，手术后 1 年，手术后 2 年的 Cobb 角平均分别为66.2°，36°和36°。

引自：《中华小儿外科杂志》，2001, 22(3): 197

例六： **An average of seven losartan molecules were** successfully coupled to M6PHSA.

平均有 7 个氯沙坦分子成功地与 M6PHSA 耦合。

引自：*Hepatology*, 2010, 51(3)：942

3. "percent（百分数）+ of + 名词"结构作主语

本结构作主语，如果名词为单数，则谓语动词用单数形式；如果名词为复数，则谓语动词用复数形式。

例一： **The percent of the positive cells** expressed IL-4, IL-5, IL-10 and IFN-γ mRNA **were** 64%, 36%, 45%, 0%。

表达 IL-4，IL-5，IL-10 及 IFN-γ mRNA 的细胞阳性率分别为 64%、36%、45%、0%。

引自：《中华儿科杂志》，2001, 39(2): 98

例二： Less than **7 percent of patients** with a new diagnosis of CRC **were** detected via a screening test.

通过筛检而首次诊断的患者少于7%。

引自：*Dis Colon Rectum*, 2008, 51(5)：573

例三： The **percentage** of hepatocytes containing TCC neoantigen in NH **was** much greater than that in non-NH liver disease, and there was no overlap between the groups.

新生儿血色病（NH）病例中含终末补体级联（TCC）抗原的肝细胞比例比非 NH 肝病大得多，且两组间无重叠。

引自：*Hepatology*, 2010, 51(6)：2061

本结构偶然也有跟单数谓语的情况。例如：

Fifteen percent of all deaths was associated with an HAI.

15%的死亡与医院获得性感染相关

引自：*Gastroenterology*, 2008, 135(3)：816

4.“分数+of+名词”作主语

名词词组是分数，后跟 of-属格，采用意义一致的原则来确定谓语动词的单、复数形式，即如果名词为单数，则谓语动词用单数形式；如果名词为复数，则谓语动词用复数形式，但是，如果直接用百分数做主语时，则用复数形式谓语。

例一： Multivariable analysis of survival data indicates a better outcome for younger children and for those with better systolic function at presentation, but overall, **one third of children die or require** transplantation within 1 year of presentation.

存活数据的多变量分析结果提示，低龄、收缩功能较好的儿童具有更好的预后。但总体而言，1/3 的儿童在出现症状后一年内死亡或需要进行移植。

引自：*Circulation*, 2008, 117(1): 79

例二： **More than one third of patients** in this large, population-based trial **were cured**.

大样本人群试验显示，治愈的患者超过了 1/3。

引自：*J Clin Oncol.*, 2010, 28(14)：2339

例三： **One-third of soft tissue sarcoma (STS) metastasize** and current risk-stratification **is** suboptimal, therefore, novel diagnostic and prognostic markers would be clinically valuable.

1/3 的软组织肉瘤（STS）可发生转移，而目前的危险分层方案不佳。因此，能够体现诊断和预后的新指标势必具有非常重要的临床意义。

引自：*BMC Genomics*, 2007, 8: 73

5.“数量词/百分数+of+名词”结构作主语

本结构谓语动词用复数。

例一： In total, **22,383** of the 33,858 enrolled women **were** 30 years or older with intraepithelial lesions or malignancies (NILM) cytology.

纳入的 33 858 名女性中，总共有 22 383 名为 30 岁或以上，细胞学检查为上皮病变或恶性肿瘤（NILM）患者。

引自：*Am J Clin Pathol*, 2019, 151(4): 433

例二： **76% of** the surgical and 75% of the nonsurgical patients **were** female.

76%的手术患者和 75%的非手术患者是女性。

引自：JAMA, 2018, 320(15): 1570

例三： **8 of the patients were** found to have gastroesophageal reflux (GER).

8 例患者出现胃食管反流。

引自：《中华小儿外科杂志》, 2001, 22: 288

6. "most+ of+名词"结构作主语

本结构作主语，谓语动词用复数。

例一： **Most of these cases were** pancytopenia with normal or decreased bone marrow cellularities and increased normoblasts.

这些病例大多为全血细胞减少症，骨髓细胞正常或减少，晚幼红细胞增多。

引自：《中华血液学杂志》, 2001, 22(1): 79

例二： **Most of these DNIEMD lesions are** found on the lower extremities of women and men, and they have an increased association with MM, DN and NMSC.

大多数 DNIEMD 患者的病变部位位于下肢，且与 MM、DN 及 NMSC 关系密切。

引自：J Cutan Pathol, 2009, 35(12): 1148

7. half + of the

"half + of the" 如果后接单数名词，谓语动词用单数，若后跟复数名词，则用复数谓语动词，这一用法包括另一结构："The rest of the…"。

例一： In the community, more than **half of patients with HF have preserved** EF, and isolated diastolic dysfunction is present in more than 40% of cases.

社区中半数以上的心力衰竭患者 EF 值正常，40%以上的患者存在单纯舒张功能不全。

引自：JAMA,2006, 296: 2209

例二： At three weeks, **half of the patients were** randomly assigned to continue in their originally assigned group for an additional three weeks.

在第 3 周，一半的患者随机分配到初始试验组中，再继续治疗 3 周。

引自：BMJ, 2008, 336(7651): 999

例三： **The rest of the patients are** anomalous origin of left pulmonary artery (AOLPA).

其余患者为左肺动脉异常起源（AOLPA）。

引自：J Cardiothorac Surg, 2019, 14: 82

（五）代词作主语

代词作主语，其谓语动词数的要求与名词作主语时数的要求基本相同，但有些代词作主语时情况特殊。

1. all 作主语

all 作主语时谓语动词用复数。All 也可用作形容词，做前置定语，使用时不要将其混淆。

例一： **All patients** who survived to hospital discharge were followed up for a minimum of 2 years.

所有存活到出院的患者均接受了至少 2 年的随访。

引自：*JAMA Intern Med*, 2018, 178(12): 1681

例二： Rats infused long term with Ang II exhibited higher levels of activated Rac1, phospho-STAT3, collagen synthesis, and atrial fibrosis in the atria, **all of which were** attenuated by oral losartan and simvastatin.

长期灌注 Ang Ⅱ 的大鼠心房中，激活的 Rac1、磷酸化 STAT3、胶原合成和心房纤维化等均处于较高水平，这些变化可以被口服氯沙坦和辛伐他汀所减轻。

引自：*Circulation*, 2008, 117: 344

2. "each of +复数名词"结构作主语

本结构作主语，谓语动词一般用单数。

例一： For each biomarker, **each of the three upper quartiles was** compared to the lowest quartile.

对于每一个生物标志物，将 3 个四分位数中的每一个与最低四分位数进行比较。

引自：*PLoS Med*, 2008, 5(10): e203

例二： **Each of these groups was** then subdivided into two groups (*n*=12) that allowed for simulated mortality.

然后将这些组中的每一组再分成两组（*n*=12），用其模拟死亡率。

引自：*Br J Anaesth*, 2019, 123(1): 81-87

3. "None of …" 和 "of"

"None of …" 和 "of" 后接单数宾语，谓语动词用单数；of 后接复数宾语时，谓语动词采用单数还是复数，主要依据说话人大脑中联想到的是复数还是单数概念，即出于个体考虑还是整体考虑。

例一： Fourteen patients (18%) required further ICD-related surgery; **none of these**

operations were attributed to abandoned leads.

14 例（18%）接受了与埋藏式心脏复率除颤器（ICD）有关的手术，但（再次）手术，均不是导联失效所致。

引自: Heart Rhythm, 2009, 6(1)：65

例二：Pulmonary embolism was ruled out **if none of the three criteria were** met and the D-dimer level was less than 1000 ng per milliliter.

如果三个标准都不符合，并且 D-二聚体水平低于每毫升 1000 ng，则排除肺栓塞。

引自: N Engl J Med, 2019,380: 1139

二、非谓语动词

非谓语动词是动词的非谓语形式，传统语法分类包括动词不定式、动名词和分词。现代语法分类为动词不定式、-ed 分词和 -ing 分词。无论是何种分类，均有一个共同特征，即动词丧失了其固有功能，动词在句中不能用作谓语，因而并无语法上的主语，不受主语人称和数的限制，但其有逻辑主语。非谓语动词既有动词性质，又有非动词性质。非谓语动词的动词性质表现：①有时态和语态的变化；②及物动词须有宾语。非动词性质表现在所承担的句子成分上：①相当于名词；②相当于形容词；③相当于副词。

（一）动词不定式

动词不定式可用作主语、表语、宾语、定语、同位语、状语和补语。

1. 动词不定式作主语

动词不定式可在句中充当主语，但当代英语常用 it 作为语法上的主语，这种用法称作"先行"it。将真实主语不定式放在谓语之后。

例一：**It is common practice to restore and maintain** sinus rhythm in patients with atrial fibrillation and heart failure.

心房颤动和心力衰竭患者的常规治疗方法是恢复和保持窦性节律。

引自: N Engl J Med, 2008, 358(25)：2667

例二：**It will be necessary to determine** the cause and extent of such abnormalities and wether they also occur in human induced pluripotent stem cells (hiPSC) generated using different reprogramming methods.

有必要确定这些异常情况的诱因和程度，以及运用不同的重编程序法来诱导人多能干细胞（hiPSC）是否也会出现这些情况。

引自: Stem Cells,2010, 28(4): 704

例三：**It was successful to establish** a rat multiple organ dysfunction syndrome (MODS) model that was useful for basic study on serious trauma and therapeutic drug screening test.

本研究的复制方法是成功的，复制的大鼠多器官功能障碍综合征模型适于创伤及药物筛选所用。

引自：《中华实验外科杂志》, 2001, 18(9): 506

2. 动词不定式作表语

例一：　The purpose of this study was to compare the early and late results of percutaneous and surgical revascularization of left main coronary artery stenosis.

本研究旨在比较冠状动脉左主干狭窄经皮介入和外科血运重建术的早期和晚期结果。

引自：*J Am Coll Cardiol*, 2008, 51(5): 538

例二：Our aim was to investigate whether acute infections transiently increase the risk of venous thromboembolism.

本研究的目的是确定急性感染是否会短暂增加静脉血栓栓塞的风险。

引自：*Lancet*, 2006, 367(9516): 1075

3. 动词不定式结构作名词或代词修饰语

动词不定式作名词或代词修饰语时，通常只能置于其所修饰的名词或代词之后，动词不定式与所修饰的名词或代词可能是主谓关系。

例一：Clopidogrel is widely used in diabetic patients after vascular events; however, the ability of this **thienopyridine to yield** additional antiplatelet protection on top of aspirin has never been explored in a controlled study with comprehensive assessment of platelet activity.

氯吡格雷目前已被广泛应用于治疗糖尿病患者伴心血管事件，但它在抗血小板作用上是否比阿司匹林更有效，尚未经综合测定血小板活性对照试验所证实。

引自：*Am Heart J*, 2008, 155(1): 93

例二：**Failure of aspirin to suppress** platelet aggregation in women is one hypothesized mechanism.

其中一个可能的机制是由于阿司匹林无法抑制女性血小板聚集。

引自：*JAMA*, 2006, 295(12): 1420

4. 动词不定式作目的状语

动词不定式作目的状语，其逻辑主语通常是全句的主语，有时候为了强调这种目的状语，动词不定式前常加"in order"或"so as"，或将动词不定式、"in order +动词不定式"置于句首。

例一：In order to identify genetic factors related to thyroid cancer susceptibility, we adopted a candidate gene approach.

为了查明与甲状腺癌易感性相关遗传因素，我们采取了候选基因方法。

引自：*PLoS Genet*, 2009, 5(9)：e1000637

例二： We queried the National Inpatient Sample Database years 2002-2015 **to identify** hospitalizations with Prinzmetal angina.

我们查询了 2002～2015 年国家住院样本数据库，以确定 Prinzmetal 心绞痛患者的住院情况。

引自：*Am J Med*, 2019, 132(9): 1053-1061

5. 动词不定式作主语或宾语补足语

主语与用作主语补足语的动词不定式短语构成复合主语，二者在逻辑上是主谓关系。动词不定式在句中充当宾语补足语，宾语与充当宾语补足语的动词不定式构成复合宾语，二者在逻辑上是主谓关系。

例一： 4230 people were asked **to fulfill the questionnaire.**

入户问卷调查 4230 人。

引自：《中华内科杂志》, 2001, 40(9): 597

例二： Participants were required **to meet** published appropriate use criteria.

参与者必须符合已公布的适当使用标准。

引自：*JAMA*, 2019, 321(13): 1286

6. "疑问代词/疑问副词+动词不定式"结构

疑问代词"who、what、which"，或疑问副词" when、where、how"后加动词不定式可构成一种特殊的动词不定式短语，它可在句中作主语、宾语、表语等。

例一： To investigate the ways **how to decrease** the morbidity and mortality of pancreaticoduodenectomy.

探讨降低胰十二指肠切除术并发症发生率及手术死亡率的措施。

引自：《中国实用外科杂志》, 2001, 21(3): 295

例二： It is important that physicians recognise the clinical signs of IMDs and know **when to propose** advanced laboratory testing or referral to a higher centre for better patient management.

对于医生，熟知遗传性代谢性疾病（IMDs）的临床症状和表现，并能确定何时应建议患者到设备先进的实验室做进一步检测或将患者转诊至上级中心以获得更好的治疗，这些都是很重要的。

引自：*Eye*, 2010, 24(4): 507

7. 动词不定式的被动式

当动词不定式逻辑上的主语是这个动词不定式所表示的动作的承受者时，动词不定式要用被动式。

例一： This set-up enabled full agonist concentration-response curves to be constructed on a single population of cells.

这种设置可以在单个细胞群体上构建完全激动剂浓度－反应曲线。

引自：*Br J Pharmacol*, 2019, 176(16): 2894-2904

例二： Those with cognitive impairment or frailty in AF had higher predicted risk for stroke and higher observed mortality, yet were less likely to be treated with OAC.

心房颤动（AF）伴认知障碍或体质虚弱者中，发生卒中的风险及死亡率更高，但接受 OAC 治疗的可能性较小。

引自：*Am Heart J*, 2019, 211: 77-89

例三： Pancreatic cancer is a deadly disease characterized by late diagnosis and resistance to therapy. Much progress has been made in defining gene defects in pancreatic cancer, but a full accounting of its molecular pathogenesis remains to be provided.

胰腺癌是一种致命性疾病，具有难以早期诊断和对治疗不敏感的特点。尽管在确定胰腺癌基因缺陷方面的研究已经取得了很大进展，但是胰腺癌的分子发病机制仍需进一步探索。

引自：*Cancer Cell,* 2009, 15(3)：207

（二）动名词

动名词是由动词原形加词尾-ing 构成，其构成方法与现在分词一样。因而其既具有动词性质，又具有名词性质。动名词在句中可作主语、表语、宾语或介词的宾语。在现代英语语法分类中，语法学家们将动名词和现在分词归为 V-ing 分词。此外，动名词既可独立用作主语，也可与名词连用，此时，其后的名词从逻辑关系上属于该动名词的逻辑宾语。

1. 动名词作主语

例一： Comprehensive **monitoring** and correct management, perioperation usage of artificial liver support system, etc. are all major factors that related to success.

围手术期的严密监测与正确处理，人工肝的辅助治疗等是肝移植成功的重要条件。

引自：《中国实用外科杂志》, 2001, 21(1)：48

例二：**Strengthening** the management of perioperation can improve the security of the operation and decrease the postoperative complications.

加强围手术期处理，可提高手术的安全性，减少并发症的发生。

引自：《中国实用外科杂志》，2001, 21(9): 664

2. 动名词作表语

例一：Other risk factors for pesticide poisoning with mixed preparation were **smoking or taking** food during spraying, **leaking** or breakdown of sprayers, without washing their whole body as soon as possible after spraying, poor personal protection, **spraying** for a long time, **spraying** by women and spraying pesticide on cotton.

农药中毒的其他危险因素还有：工间吸烟或进食、喷雾器发生故障或滴漏、施药后不能尽快清洗全身、个人防护不严密、长时间施药、女性施药和棉花上的农药。

引自:《中华预防医学杂志》，2001, 35(1): 13

例二：Selective digestive tract decontamination (SDD) and selective oropharyngeal decontamination (SOD) are infection-prevention measures used in the treatment of some patients in intensive care, but reported effects on patient outcome **are conflicting**.

选择性消化道净化（SDD）和选择性口咽净化（SOD）是感染预防措施，用于重症监护中的一些患者的治疗，但对患者预后的报告结果不一致。

引自: *N Engl J Med*, 2009, 360(1): 20

3. 动名词作宾语

例一：These findings suggest that CRP in plaques or found **circulating** in CVD patients can influence DC function during atherogenesis.

研究表明，在动脉粥样硬化形成过程中，CRP 在斑块中或在心血管疾病患者的血液循环中可以影响 DC 的功能。

引自: *Arterioscler Thromb Vasc Biol* , 2008, 28(3) : 412

例二：The meta-analysis software, REVMAN3.1, was applied for **investigating heterogeneity** among individual studies and summarizing effects across studies.

应用 REVMAN3.1 软件对各研究结果进行一致性检验和数据合并。

引自:《中华预防医学杂志》，2001, 35(6): 408

4. 动名词复合结构

名词所有格或物主代词后+动名词，即构成动名词的复合结构。在动名词的复合结构中，名词所有格或物主代词是动名词的逻辑主语。这种复合结构在句中多用作主语或宾语。当然，现代英语中，动名词复合结构用作宾语时，其名词亦可用通格，代词也可用宾格。例如：

例一： Living liver transplantation shortens the waiting time of liver transplantation and alleviates **patient's suffering.**

活体肝移植的开展缩短了受体等待肝移植的时间。

引自：《中华外科杂志》, 2001, 39(11): 861

例二： …a patient's prior experience with antithrombotic therapy affects **their understanding** of the process.

患者先前的抗血栓治疗经历会影响到他们后期对治疗过程的理解。

引自：*J Am Coll Cardiol*, 2019, 132(4): 525

（三）动名词与动词不定式的比较

虽然动名词和动词不定式都可用作主语、宾语、表语和同位语，但两者在起同一语法作用时，所表达的含义仍然存在一定的区别。动名词通常表示泛指、概括意义；抽象或经常性的动作；已经成为过去的动作。而动词不定式则表示具体的或特定的一次性动作，同时还有提示时间意义的功能，即表示现在或未来的动作。此外，在某些动词之后只接动名词（如 keep、avoid、deny、prevent 等），而另一些动词后只能接动词不定式（如 fail、expect、refuse 等），还有些动词既可接动词不定式也可跟动名词（如 try、need 等）。至于这类特殊用法要求，建议作者在写作中若不能把握时，最佳方法是查阅词典或语法专著。

例一： **Comparing** baseline, pre-flare, and at-flare values indicated that neither C3 nor C4 levels decreased pre-flare, but both decreased on average significantly at flare.

基线水平、发作前和发作时的测定值比较发现，C3 和 C4 水平在发作前都没有降低，而在发作时都有显著下降。

【析】动名词 comparing 在句中作主语，表示泛指，同时暗示这是一个过去的动作。

引自：*Lupus*, 2010, 19(11): 1272

例二： The rituximab-based regimen was more efficacious than the cyclophosphamide-based regimen for **inducing** remission of relapsing disease.

对诱导复发疾病的缓解，基于利妥昔单抗方案比基于环磷酰胺方案更有效。

引自：*N Engl J Med*, 2010, 363(3): 221

例三： A total of 2003 patients expected **to require** mechanical ventilation for 24 hours or longer were randomized.

（我们）总共随机选择了 2003 例需要机械通气 24 小时或 24 小时以上的患者。

【析】动词不定式 "to require" 表示具体的动作，同时提示目前状况。

引自：*JAMA*, 2008, 300(7)：805

例四：The purpose of this article **is to describe** the features, treatment, and risk factors for relapse of children with mature teratoma (MT) and immature teratoma (IT) to assist future treatment plans.

本文的目的旨在描述儿童成熟畸胎瘤（MT）和未成熟畸胎瘤（IT）的特征、治疗和复发危险因素，以期指导后续治疗方案的制订。

【析】动词不定式 "to describe" 表示本次研究，而非持续性行为。

引自：*J Clin Oncol*, 2008, 26(21)：3590

（四）分词

分词是动词的一种非限定形式。它分为两种，一种是现在分词，另一种是过去分词。现代语法通常将现在分词和动名词统归为 "-ing" 分词。现在分词由动词原形加词尾 "-ing" 构成，过去分词由动词原形加词尾 "-ed" 形式构成。这两种分词在句子中的功能基本相同，主要起形容词或副词作用，可以用作定语（包括前置形容词和后置形容词）、表语、状语或宾语补足语。例如：

例一：Non-invasive evaluation of left ventricular **filling pressure** has been scarcely studied in critically ill patients.

关于非侵入性评估危重患者左心室充盈压的研究罕有报道。

【析】前位修饰名词 pressure。

引自：*Crit Care*. 2008, 12(1): R18

例二：A total of 1102 adult patients with congenital heart disease (age 36.0±14.2 years) **attending our institution** between 1999 and 2006 had creatinine concentration measured.

1999 年至 2006 年间，对入住我院的 1102 例先天性心脏病患者［（36.0±14.2）岁］进行了血肌酐浓度测定。

【析】后位修饰 patients。

引自：*Circulation*, 2008, 117(18)：2320

例三：Platelet reactivity was assessed by light transmittance aggregometry **using adenosine 5'-diphosphate, arachidonic acid, and collagen.**

采用 5'-腺苷二磷酸、花生四烯酸和胶原透光率集合度测定血小板反应性。

【析】现在分词短语"using…"在句中作状语。

引自：*J Am Coll Cardiol*, 2008, 52(9)：734

例四：In this 3-year prospective study, 321 subjects **aged above 25 years** with impaired glucose tolerance (IGT) were included.

对 321 例（年龄>25 岁）糖耐量低减（IGT）人群进行 3 年前瞻性研究。

【析】过去分词短语"aged…"在句中作后置定语。

引自:《中华内分泌代谢杂志》, 2001, 17(2): 131

1. 现在分词和过去分词作形容词用时在功能上的区别

现在分词和过去分词，无论是用作前位修饰还是后位修饰，其主要差异为现在分词表示主动行为动作或正在发生的行为动作，而过去分词表示被动动作或已经完成的动作。例如：

例一： Ventilation rates were high, with 60.9% of **segments containing** a rate of more than 20/min.

通气频率较高，60.9%的时段频率超过 20 次/分。

【析】分词 containing 和其逻辑主语 segments 形成主谓关系。

引自: *JAMA*, 2005, 293: 305

例二： In 252 460 **patients treated** with lipid-lowering agents, 24 cases of hospitalized rhabdomyolysis occurred during treatment.

252 460 例采用降脂药物治疗的患者中，24 例住院治疗期间发生横纹肌溶解症。

【析】"patients treated with…" = "patients who were treated with…"。过去分词 treated 和其逻辑主语构成被动关系。

引自: *JAMA*, 2004, 292(21): 2585

例三： The presence of left ventricular thrombus was not associated with an **increased risk** of systemic thromboembolism

左心室血栓的存在与系统性血栓栓塞风险的增加无关。

【析】"increased risk" 表示业已完成的动作状态。

引自: *Am J Med*, 2019, doi:10.1016/j.amjmed.2019.02.033

例四： Two hundred forty-two consecutive **patients undergoing** elective PCI with undetectable preprocedural cTnI were recruited.

纳入本研究的是 242 例行选择性 PCI、术前未检测到 cTnI 的患者。

【析】"…patients undergoing…" = "patients who were undergoing…" 表示本研究在当时存在的状况。另外，要注意的是，进行体亦可表示一段时间内存在的状态或连续行为。

引自: *Circulation*, 2009, 119(6) : 820

例五： Idiopathic pulmonary fibrosis (IPF) /usual interstitial pneumonia is a **ravaging condition** of progressive lung scarring and destruction.

特发性肺纤维化（IPF）/普通型间质性肺炎能导致肺部瘢痕形成及结构破坏等进行性的肺损伤。

【析】分词 ravaging 作前置定语修饰 condition，同时具有主动意思。

引自: *Proc Natl Acad Sci U S A*, 2010, 107(32): 14309

例六： Twenty-three children (age, 3.2-14.3 years) with **IgE-mediated** peanut allergy confirmed by positive double-blind, **placebo-controlled** food challenge (DBPCFC) received OIT following a rush protocol with roasted peanut for 7 days.

一共 23 位（年龄 3.2～14.3 岁）通过双盲、安慰剂对照的阳性测试（DBPCFC），确认患有由 IgE 介导的花生过敏症，并计划食用烤制花生7 天后接受口服免疫治疗（OIT）。

【析】"IgE-mediated peanut allergy" 与 "placebo-controlled food challenge" 两个短语中分别构成合成词作定语，起形容词作用并表示被动意义。

引自：*J Allergy Clin Immunol*, 2010, 126(1)：83

2. 作表语用的分词

现在分词和过去分词均可用作表语。作表语用时，现在分词多表示主语所具有的特征，过去分词多表示主语所处的状态。

例一： Previously, we found that mast cell tryptases and carboxypeptidase A3 (CPA3) **are differentially expressed** in the airway epithelium in asthmatic subjects.

先前我们发现哮喘患者气道上皮内存在肥大细胞类胰蛋白酶和羧肽酶 A3（CPA3）的差异表达。

【析】过去分词 expressed 表示"肥大细胞类胰蛋白酶和羧肽酶 A3（CPA3）"的状态。

引自：*J Allergy Clin Immunol*, 2010, 125(5)：1046

例二： Total serum IgE levels are frequently **elevated** in patients with chronic urticaria and these are **associated** with disease severity and duration.

慢性荨麻疹患者总血清 IgE 水平经常升高，并与疾病严重程度及持续时间呈相关性。

【析】过去分词 elevated 和分词短语 "associated with" 同样表示其主语所处的状态。

引自：*Int Arch Allergy Immunol*, 2010, 153(3)：288

例三： Although neutropenia may limit the maximum dosage of tocilizumab in patients with SLE, the observed clinical and serologic responses are **promising** and warrant further studies to establish the optimal dosing regimen and efficacy.

虽然中性粒细胞减少可能会制约 tocilizumab 治疗系统性红斑狼疮患者的最大剂量，但是从临床和血清学反应来看是有希望的，值得进一步研究，以确定最佳剂量方案和疗效。

【析】现在分词 promising 作表语，表示主语的特征。另外，需要注意的是，摘要写作不同于论文主体部分写作，所以，现在分词用作表语的状况较少，一般用于背景及结论。

引自：*Arthritis Rheum*, 2010, 62(2): 542

3. 分词用作状语

分词不仅可用作定语，同时也可用作状语，修饰或说明句中谓语动词的动作或整个句子所表达的意思。作状语用的分词通常为分词短语，表示原因、时间、伴随性状况、条件或结果等。此时，分词短语在句中相当于一个状语从句的功能。注意：①分词短语可以扩展为状语从句，但鉴于英文摘要写作的简洁性要求，故分词短语在摘要写作中使用较为普遍；②分词短语的位置可以在句首、句中或句末，放在句首位置较多，表示结果时常置于句末；③分词短语所表示的动作可能发生于谓语动词的动作之前或之后，亦可能与谓语动词同时发生；④使用分词短语作状语时应注意分词短语的逻辑主语，即逻辑主语应与主句主语保持一致，否则会导致悬空分词（dangling participle）错误。

例一：These data indicate that ADSC strongly inhibit PDAC proliferation, both *in vitro* and *in vivo* and induce tumor cell death **by altering cell cycle progression**.

这些数据表明，ADSC 在体外和体内能高度抑制 PDAC 增殖、通过改变细胞周期的进程诱导肿瘤细胞死亡。

【析】分词短语 by altering cell cycle progression 表示伴随状况。

引自：*PLoS One*, 2009, 4(7): e6278

例二：In the other blood pressure difference trials (excluding CHD events in trials of beta blockers in people with CHD), there was a 22% reduction in CHD events (17% to 27%) and a 41% (33% to 48%) reduction in stroke for a blood pressure reduction of 10 mmHg systolic or 5 mmHg diastolic, similar to the reductions of 25% (CHD) and 36% (stroke) expected for the same difference in blood pressure from the cohort study meta-analysis, **indicating that** the benefit is explained by blood pressure reduction itself.

在其他血压差异性试验中（冠心病患者服用 β 受体阻滞剂试验中冠心病发作不在此列），随着收缩压降低 10 mmHg 或舒张压降低 5 mmHg，冠心病发作减少 22%（17%～27%），脑卒中发生率减少 41%（33%～48%），与队列研究经荟萃分析所预期的降压效果基本接近（冠心病发作下降 25%；脑卒中发生率下降 36%）。这一结果显示得益于降压。

注："indicating that…"为分词短语作状语，提示结果。

引自：*BMJ*, 2009, 338: b1665

例三：**Compared with controls**, case patients were less likely to have undergone any attempted colonoscopy (adjusted conditional odds ratio [OR], 0.69 [95% CI, 0.63 to 0.74; $P < 0.001$]) or complete colonoscopy (adjusted conditional OR, 0.63 [95%CI, 0.57 to 0.69; $P < 0.001$]).

与对照组相比，病例组结肠癌患者接受结肠镜检[调整条件比值（OR），0.69(95%CI, 0.63～0.74, $P < 0.001$)]或完全结肠镜检[OR, 0.63(95%CI, 0.57～0.69, $P < 0.001$)]的可能性较小。

【析】分词短语在句首，起条件状语作用。Compared with controls = If case

patients were compared with the controls…

引自：*Ann Intern Med*, 2009, 150(1)：1

例四： **Despite being involved in** cell death of several cell types, virtually nothing is known about the function of LL-37 in keratinocyte apoptosis.

尽管 LL-37 参与若干种类型细胞的凋亡，但我们对其在角质形成细胞凋亡中所起的作用几乎知之甚少。

【析】分词短语 "Despite being involved in …" 在句中起让步状语功能，修饰全句。

引自：*J Invest Dermatol*, 2009, 129(4)：937

例五： Having established facial and hind-paw allodynia as a useful animal surrogate of headache-associated allodynia, we next showed that blocking pain-facilitating processes in the rostral ventromedial medulla (RVM) interfered with its expression.

首先建立大鼠面部和后爪异常性疼痛的模型。该动物模型可模拟与头痛相关的疼痛。我们随后发现，干扰基因表达可阻断延髓头端腹内侧区（RVM）的疼痛易化进程。

【析】分词短语 "Having established …" 提示时间先后关系，即 establish 先于 show。此外，主句中的主语 we 亦为分词短语 "Having established…" 的逻辑主语。若该句写成："Having established facial and hind-paw allodynia as a useful animal surrogate of headache-associated allodynia, blocking pain-facilitating processes were shown in the rostral ventromedial medulla (RVM) interfered with its expression."。就会造成悬空分词错误，即分词短语的逻辑主语和主句中主语不一致现象，从而导致逻辑关系混乱。

引自：*Ann Neurol*, 2009, 65(2)：184

4. 分词用于复合结构

分词用于复合结构，亦为宾语补足语。通常只用于两类带宾语的动词之后。第一类为感官动词；第二类为"使役"动词。同样，现在分词在这类结构中表示动作正在进行，意义主动。过去分词表示动作完成，意义被动。

例一： Population-based, prospective 7-year cohort study in 4 US communities using the Atherosclerosis Risk in Communities Study database. Participants ($n=$ 11,612, aged 49 to 73 years) **had retinal photographs taken** between 1993 and 1995.

应用动脉粥样硬化危险社区研究资料库，在美国 4 个社区进行了长达 7 年的人群前瞻性队列研究。参试者（$n=$11 612，年龄 49～73 岁）于 1993～1995 年间拍摄了视网膜照片。

【析】分词 taken 逻辑上的主语 retinal photographs 与其为被动关系。

引自：*JAMA*, 2005, 293(1)：63

例二：Nevertheless, we observed a significant association between PD and nondystonic pain, beginning after the onset of parkinsonian symptoms (odds ratio, 2.1; 95% confidence interval, 1.4-2.9).

然而，我们观察到在帕金森病症状发生之后，帕金森病（PD）与非张力疼痛之间存在显著相关（比值比，2.1；95%CI，1.4～2.9）。

【析】分词短语 beginning 与主句动词 observed 同步。

引自：*Arch Neurol*, 2008, 65(9)：1191

5. 分词短语用作独立结构

分词短语作状语时，其本身没有主语，句子的主语便是分词结构的逻辑主语。例如：Having safely piloted the new technique of single-dose targeted intraoperative radiotherapy with Intrabeam(=After we have safely piloted…)，we launched the TARGIT-A trial on March 24, 2000.[使用新技术光子放射治疗仪（Intrabeam）安全地进行了单次剂量靶向术中放疗小规模试验后，我们于 2000 年 3 月 24 日启动了 TARGIT-A 试验]。但有时分词也可以有自己的独立主语。这种主语加分词短语的结构称为独立结构（absolute construction）。另外，现代语法中，由介词短语 "with+宾语+现在分词/过去分词" 也被看作独立结构。

例一：The overall postoperative morbidity rate was 51.9%, pulmonary complications (37%) being the most frequent.

术后所有并发症的死亡率为 51.9%，肺部并发症（37%）是最常见的并发症。

【析】主句的主语为 "morbidity rate"，独立结构的主语为 "pulmonary complications"。其完整结构为 "pulmonary complications (37%) were the most frequent."。

引自：*Eur J Cardiothorac Surg*, 2008, 33(6): 1096

例二：However, despite thorough preoperative assessment being applied in the selection of the candidates for surgery (=However, despite thorough preoperative assessment had been applied in the selection of the candidates for surgery), a practical and reliable individual risk-analysis stratification is still lacking.

尽管在选择手术候选人时进行了充分的术前评估，但我们仍缺乏一个确实可行的个体化风险评估系统。

引自：*Eur J Cardiothorac Surg*, 2008, 33(6): 1096

例三：Thirty-nine percent of the LGG patients were severely fatigued, with older patients being most affected.

低级别胶质瘤（LGG）患者中有 39% 的患者为严重性疲劳，且更易发生于老年患者。

【析】with +宾语（older patients）+过去分词（affected），这一结构表示已完成的被动意义。

引自：*J Neurooncol*, 2009, 92(1): 73

例四： We believe this pattern reflects the multidifferentiation pathway of MAC, with eccrine/sebaceous differentiation occurring at deeper levels of the dermis.

我们认为，由于小汗腺/皮脂腺分化发生在真皮深层，这种情况反映了微囊肿附属器癌（MAC）的多向分化。

【析】with +宾语（differentiation）+现在分词（occurring），这一结构表示正在发生的或进行的主动意义。

引自：*Am J Dermatopathol*, 2010, 32(3): 257

例五： In 62% (n=72) of patients the aetiology was identified ("secondary DBN"), the most frequent causes being cerebellar degeneration (n=23) and cerebellar ischaemia (n=10).

62%（n=72）的患者病因得以确定（"继发性 DBN"），最常见的原因是小脑变性（n=23）和小脑缺血（n=10）。

【析】分词独立结构 "the most frequent causes being cerebellar degeneration 和 cerebellar ischaemia" 在句中作同位语，对前面的情况加以补充说明。

引自：*J Neurol Neurosurg Psychiatry*, 2008, 79(6): 672

三、平 行 结 构

平行（parallelism）是写作中常用的一种修辞手段。首先，我们看看关于平行的英文定义，其定义为 "in rhetoric, component of literary style in both prose and poetry, in which coordinate ideas are arranged in phrases, sentences, and paragraphs that balance one element with another of equal importance and similar wording. The repetition of sounds, meanings, and structures serves to order, emphasize, and point out relations. In its simplest form parallelism consists of single words that have a slight variation in meaning:'ordain and establish'or'overtake and surpass'. Sometimes three or more units are parallel." 笼统地讲，平行结构是指修辞上的一种写作技巧，即用类似的语法结构形式来表达相同或相似的概念。具体地说，平行结构要求：当一个句子的某些部分并列使用或由关联词连接时，句子的这些部分必须保持相同的语法结构。常用的平行结构大体上有三种类型：①单词平行并列；②短语平行并列；③从句平行并列。这种语言结构的并列是变换句型的重要手段之一。它不仅能在同句中扩充句意，而且能合并句子，从而使语言表达简练、紧凑、文笔流畅。

1. 单词平行并列

例一： To examine the developmental trajectory of obesity in adolescence in relation to **sex, ethnicity, and socioeconomic status.**

观察与性别、种族和社会经济状况相关的青春期肥胖症的发展曲线。

引自：*Cardiology*, 2007, 3: 1671

例二： **Body mass index (BMI), waist hip ratio (WHR), glucose, blood pressure, lipid profile and estradiol levels** were measured.

测量体重指数（BMI）、腰臀比（WHR）、血糖、血压、血脂和雌二醇水平。

引自：*Maturitas*, 2010, 66(3)：285

2. 短语平行并列

例一： The ability of angiotensin-converting enzyme inhibitor therapy **to preserve ventricular function** and **improve somatic growth and outcomes** in these infants is unknown.

对于婴儿，血管紧张素转换酶抑制剂疗法是否具有保护心室功能、改善身体发育和结果的能力尚不清楚。

引自：*Circulation*, 2010, 122(4)：333

例二： The leukemia incidences (1950～1995) **in 27011 medical diagnostic X-ray workers and in 25782 non-radiation workers in hospital employed** between 1950 and 1980 in China were compared by O/E.

用 O/E 程序分析了我国 1950～1980 年在职的 27011 名医用诊断 X 线工作者和 25782 名医院其他科室医务工作者 1950～1995 年白血病的发病资料。

引自：《中华血液学杂志》, 2001, 22(4)：344

例三： Randomized, double-blind, placebo-controlled trial conducted at 95 urology clinics in the United States **involving men 40 years or older who had a total International Prostate Symptom Score of 12 or higher and, an International Prostate Symptom Score quality-of-life (QOL) item score of 3 or higher, a self-rated bladder condition of at least moderate bother, and a bladder diary documenting micturition frequency (>or=8 micturitions per 24 hours) and urgency (>or=3 episodes per 24 hours), with or without urgency urinary incontinence.**

在美国 95 家泌尿诊所中开展随机、双盲、安慰剂对照试验。纳入的男性患者均≥40 岁，国际前列腺症状评分（International Prostate Symptom Score）总分≥12 分，国际前列腺症状评分中生活质量（quality-of-life, QOL）评分≥3 分，膀胱状况自测结果为至少带来中度困扰，排尿日记中记录有尿频（24 小时排尿次数≥8 次）和尿急（24 小时出现≥3 次）情况，伴或不伴有急迫性尿失禁。

引自：*JAMA*, 2006, 296：2319

3. 从句平行并列

例一： Mounting evidence suggests **that statins possess antiarrhythmic properties and (that) inhibit atrial fibrillation (AF).**

越来越多的证据显示他汀类药物具有抗心律失常特性，并可以抑制心房颤动。

例二： In conclusion, these data indicate **that LV pressure in patients with CCTGA affects the degree of TR** and **that septal shift caused by changes in LV** and RV pressure is an important mechanism.

总之，这些数据表明，先天性心脏病患者的左心室压力影响室间隔缺损的程度，由左心室和右心室压力变化引起的室间隔移位是一个重要的机制。

例三： To determine **which children are susceptible to critical illness hyperglycemia (CIH)** and **whether CIH severity and duration correlate with diagnosis or illness severity.**

确定哪些儿童易发生危重病高血糖（CIH），以及 CIH 的严重程度和持续时间是否与诊断或疾病严重程度相关。

4. 平行结构中代词、介词或冠词省略时应注意的问题

利用平行结构行文时，为了文体的简练起见，相同的代词、介词或冠词等通常可以省略。

例一： Infants with single-ventricle physiology have poor growth and are at risk for abnormalities in ventricular systolic and diastolic function.

单心室婴儿会发生发育不全，且存在心室收缩和舒张功能异常的风险。

【析】diastolic function 前省略了介词 in。

例二： Each patient without papilledema was matched to the patient with papilledema who was closest to his/her age and sex. （sex 之前省略了限定代词 his/her）

将每例无视盘水肿患者和一名年龄与性别与其最接近的视盘水肿患者进行配对。

例三： we examined a total of 1,575 Japanese subjects in a genome-wide association study (stage 1) and a subsequent study (stage 2).

我们对 1575 名日本人进行了第一阶段的全基因组关联研究和随后的第二阶段研究。

【析】介词短语后的两个并列短语前分别都带有不定冠词 a，尤其是第二个短语前的 a 不能省略。一旦省略，就会造成意思上的混乱，即传递的信息为同一个研究。例如："A doctor and assistant were performing the surgery." 表示的意思为"医生同时又是助手"。这显然是不可能的事，

因此应改为 "A doctor and an assistant were performing the surgery." 。

引自: Proc Natl Acad Sci U S A, 2009, 106(31): 12838

例四: The adverse outcomes of assisted fertilisation that we noted compared with those in the general population could therefore be attributable to the factors leading to infertility, rather than to factors related to the reproductive technology. 因此,与普通人群相比,我们观察到仅有辅助受精的妇女出现妊娠不良结果可能是导致不孕症的因素,而与生殖技术因素无关。

【析】试想一下,若将本例后半部分写成"attributable to the factors leading to infertility, rather than factors related to the reproductive technology",不仅导致语法错误,同时造成表意混乱不清。

引自: Lancet, 2008, 372(9640): 737

四、复 合 句

复合句由一个主句和一个或一个以上的从句构成。从句分主语从句、表语从句、宾语从句、同位语从句、定语从句和状语从句六类。由于主语从句、表语从句和宾语从句在句中的功用相当于名词,故这三种从句又统称为名词性从句。医学论文英文摘要中使用较多的从句为宾语从句和定语从句。

(一)宾语从句

用作宾语的从句称作宾语从句。引导宾语从句的关联词有从属连词、疑问代词、疑问副词、缩合连接代词、缩合连接副词。

1. 从属连词引导的宾语从句

引导宾语从句的从属连词有 whether、that、when 等。

例一: Our data demonstrated **that higher levels of cystatin C are associated with an increased risk of HF and that such association may be limited to hypertensive individuals**.
研究表明,仅在高血压患者中,高 cystatin C 水平增高心力衰竭风险。高血压与 cystatin C 对心力衰竭风险的影响有待进一步研究。

引自: Am Heart J, 2008, 155(1): 82

例二: Colorectal cancer is a leading cause of cancer death in North America; studies have shown **that screening improves survival**.
在北美,结直肠癌是癌症死亡的一个主要病因;已有研究显示筛检可以提高生存率。

引自: Dis Colon Rectum, 2008, 51(5): 573

2. 疑问副词引导的宾语从句

引导宾语从句的疑问副词有 when、where、why、how 等。

例一： To explore **why pancreaticoduodenectomy was not performed at the initial operation in 7 patients with periampullary carcinoma who underwent at reoperative PD.**
探讨 7 例再次剖腹手术行壶腹部癌根治性切除的病人在第一次手术时未行根治性切除的原因。

引自:《中国实用外科杂志》, 2001, 21(6): 483

例二： Non-small-cell lung cancer with sensitive mutations of the epidermal growth factor receptor (EGFR) is highly responsive to EGFR tyrosine kinase inhibitors such as gefitinib, but little is known about **how its efficacy and safety profile compares with that of standard chemotherapy.**
非小细胞肺癌伴易感性表皮生长因子（EGFR）突变患者对 EGFR 酪氨酸激酶抑制剂，如吉非替尼等高度敏感。但与标准化疗相比，其疗效和安全性资料还知之甚少。

引自: *N Engl J Med*, 2010, 362(25): 2380

（二）定语从句

用作定语的从句称作定语从句。定语从句通常置于它所修饰的名词或代词之后，被修饰的这种名词或代词称作先行词。引导定语从句的关联词为关系代词和关系副词。引导定语从句的关系代词 who、whom、whose、which、that 等在从句中可用作主语、宾语、定语等。引导定语从句的关系副词 when、where、why 等在从句中只充当状语。

1. 关系代词引导的定语从句

引导定语从句的关系代词有 who、whom、whose、that、which 等。Who、whom、whose 指人，who 是主格，在从句中用作主语或宾语；whom 是宾格，在从句中用作宾语；whose 是属格，在从句中用作定语（有时亦可指物）。that 在从句中既可用作主语，亦可用作宾语（非正式文体中可以省去），既可指人亦可指物，但在当代英语中多指物。which 在从句中既可作主语亦可作宾语，一般指物。此外，as、than、but 亦可用作关系代词。

例一： We conducted a randomized, double-blind, placebo-controlled, 104-week trial to evaluate verubecestat at doses of 12 mg and 40 mg per day, as compared with placebo, in patients **who had memory impairment and elevated brain amyloid levels** but **whose condition did not meet the case definition of dementia.**

我们进行了一项随机、双盲、安慰剂对照试验，为期 104 周，以评估患有记忆障碍和脑淀粉样蛋白水平升高但病情不符合痴呆病例定义的患者，采用每天剂量为 12 mg 和 40 mg 的 verubecestat 与安慰剂对比治疗效果。

引自：*N Engl J Med*, 2019, 380: 1408

例二： Ninety patients (41%) were adjudicated with acute myocardial infarction as rescue eligible of **whom 68 were referred for rescue PCI.**

90 例（41%）符合补救 PCI 治疗条件，68 例接受 PCI 治疗。

引自：*Am Heart J*, 2008, 155(1)：121

例三： Prospective, multicenter, randomized trial of 384 patients with in-stent restenosis **who were enrolled between February 2003 and July 2004 at 26 academic and community medical centers.**

对 384 例支架内再狭窄患者进行前瞻性、多中心、随机试验。患者选自于 2003 年 2 月至 2004 年 7 月 26 家医疗机构及社区医疗中心。

引自：*JAMA*, 2006, 295: 1264

例四： T cell vaccination (TCV) may decrease host autoimmunity, **which seems related to the changes of T lymphocyte subsets and thymus and prophylactic effect on diabetes.**

T 细胞接种（TCV）可以降低宿主对自身免疫的反应性，这种作用可能与宿主脾脏、胸腺淋巴细胞亚群的变化和对糖尿病的预防效应有关。

引自：《中华内分泌代谢杂志》, 2001, 17(1): 11

2. 关系副词引导的定语从句

关系副词 when、where、why 等亦可用来引导定语从句，when 在从句中用作时间状语，其先行词是表示时间的名词；where 在从句中用作地点状语，其先行词是表示地点的名词；why 在从句中用作原因状语，其先行词只有 reason。

例一： The reason **why some deposit fat in the liver whereas others do not** is poorly understood.

为什么一些脂肪沉积于肝脏而其他的不沉积原因还不清楚。

引自：*Arterioscler Thromb Vasc Biol*, 2008, 28(1): 27

例二： Parallel nested case-control studies among women ［Nurses' Health Study (NHS)］ and men ［Health Professionals Follow-up Study (HPFS)］ **where 246 women and 259 men** who developed incident CHD were matched to controls (1：2) on age and smoking.

巢式平行病例对照研究。其中女性［护士健康研究体系（NHS）］和男性［卫生专业人员随访研究（HPFS）］中分别有 246 名女性和 259 名男性存在冠心病发作，并在年龄和吸烟方面与对照组（1：2）相匹配。

引自：*Eur Heart J*, 2008, 29(1): 104

3. 限制性和非限制性定语从句

定语从句可分为限制性定语从句和非限制性定语从句。限制性定语从句与先行词关系密切，如果从句缺少会影响全句的意义，且从句前一般不用逗号。非限制性定语从句与先行词有一种松散的修饰关系，从句前用逗号隔开。因此从句中的关系代词不能省略。that 一般不引导非限制性定语从句。

例一：SMC sheet transplantation allows for controlled and localized delivery of cells **that possess angiogenic potential directly to ischemic tissues.**

SMC 片移植可以控制并移植具有新生血管潜能的细胞到局部缺血组织。

引自：*Arteriosclerosis Thrombosis and Vascular Biology*, 2008, 28(4): 637

例二： Interferon-γ inhibits the growth and function of thyrocytes induced by thyroid-stimulating antibody (TsAb), **which suggests that interferon-γ might regulate thyroid function in Graves' disease.**

γ干扰素可抑制 Graves 病的自身抗体甲状腺刺激抗体对甲状腺细胞生长和功能的刺激作用，推测γ干扰素在 Graves 病的发病中起一定调节作用。

引自：《中华内分泌代谢杂志》, 2001, 17(2): 111

例三：Pulmonary embolism was classified as unlikely in 2206 patients (66.7%). The combination of pulmonary embolism unlikely and a normal D-dimer test result occurred in 1057 patients (32.0%), **of whom 1028 were not treated with anticoagulants.**

2206 例患者（66.7%）分类为肺栓塞可能性小组。在 1057 例肺栓塞可能性小且 D-二聚体结果正常的患者（32.0%）中，有 1028 例未予抗凝治疗。

引自：*JAMA*, 2006, 295: 172

例四： Carotid artery intima-media thickness (CIMT) is a marker of coronary atherosclerosis and independently predicts cardiovascular events, **which are increased in type 2 diabetes mellitus (DM).**

颈动脉内膜中层厚度（CIMT）是冠状动脉粥样硬化的一种标志物，可以独立地预测心血管疾病的发生。

引自：*JAMA*, 2006, 296: 2572

例五： The study population consists of 6425 subjects, **of whom 2931 were born before 37 weeks of gestation and 2176 had a birth weight <2500 g.**

一共纳入 6425 名受试者，其中 2931 名于妊娠 37 周前出生，2176 名出生体重低于 2500 g。

引自：*Circulation*, 2008, 117(2) : 205

例六：Carcinoembryonic antigen-related cell adhesion molecule 1 (biliary glycoprotein; CEACAM1) is expressed in normal bladder urothelium and in angiogenically activated endothelial cells, **where it exhibits proangiogenic properties.**

癌胚抗原相关的细胞黏附分子 1（胆汁糖蛋白; CEACAM1）在正常膀胱尿

路上皮和血管原性激活内皮细胞中表达，并表现出促进血管形成的特性。

引自：*Eur Urol*, 2010, 57(4): 648

五、省略与替代

省略（ellipsis）即避免重复，是一种语法修辞手段。狭义上，是指省略句子中的某个要素是必要的，但不会影响意义传递，却能保持语言简洁。广义上，省略包括略去冗词，尤其是冠词等某些虚词。替代（substitution）也和省略一样，是避免重复、连接语篇的手段之一。所谓替代就是用替代词（pro-form）去代替特定语境中已经出现过的词语。

（一）省略

1. 冠词的省略

在题名写作中，首要任务是简洁，因此，写作题名时，尽可能略去冗词，特别是标题首冠词。一般说来，可数名词复数和不可数名词可以不加冠词表示泛指。例如：

例一： An experimental study on correlation between postmortem intervals and 5'-NT or ACP in the rats' liver.

大鼠离体肝脏 5'-NT、ACP 活性与 PMI 的相关性研究。

【析】该题名中，题首不定冠词 an 和 in the rats' liver 中的定冠词均可略去。不定冠词可以用来表示类属关系，题名中 study 之前有了 experimental 限定，冠词 an 就显得多余；其次，表示动物的名词一般均为可数名词，用复数形式或在单数形式前加定冠词都表示泛指。该题名宜修改为"Experimental study on correlation between postmortem intervals and 5'-NT or ACP in rats' liver."同样的道理，下例题名也可按此方法修改。

例二： The clinical and mammographic characteristics of phyllodes tumor.

乳腺分叶状肿瘤的临床及钼靶 X 线分析

【析】修改为"Clinical and mammographic characteristics of phyllodes tumor."。

2. 主语的省略

在并列结构中，如果通过语境可以找到后一个分句的主语，此时，后一个分句的主语可以省略。例如：

例一： We propose that SHP functions as a novel tumor suppressor in the development of HCC. These findings provide new insight into the molecular mechanisms leading to this common cancer and they may have both diagnostic and therapeutic applications.

研究者提出 SHP 可能是肝细胞癌发展过程中一个新的肿瘤抑制基因，它可能为肝细胞分子机制提供新的研究方向，并且有望运用于诊断和治疗。

【析】该句中的第二个分句使用了代词 they，从两个分句之间的关系看，代词 they 指代的是 these findings，因而可以略去，将其改为"These findings provide new insight into the molecular mechanisms leading to this common cancer and may have both diagnostic and therapeutic applications. "。

例二：These polymorphisms were genotyped in 262 celiac patients and there were 214 controls.

这些多态性在 262 名腹腔疾病患者中进行了基因分型，其中 214 名作为对照组。

【析】两个并列句中实际上主语相同，均是 polymorphisms，故此句应写为 " These polymorphisms were genotyped in 262 celiac patients and 214 controls."。

3. 谓语动词的省略

句子中如果存在并列宾语，而并列宾语无论从动词搭配（动词与名词等搭配使用）还是动词形式（包括时态、语态一致）均处于同一逻辑关联时，其后的动词可以省略，甚至主谓可同时省略。例如：

例一：This article reviews the basic science evidence, animal experiments, and reviewed human clinical data supporting the existence of an "insulin-resistant cardiomyopathy" and proposes specific potential therapeutic approaches.

该文章回顾了支持"胰岛素抵抗心肌病"存在的基础科学证据，动物实验和人类临床数据，并提出潜在的治疗方法。

【析】句中的谓语动词为 reviews，从整个语篇分析无论是搭配关系还是动词形式均处于同一语篇层面，因此，后面的谓语动词不仅在原句中动词形式改变不当，而且还可以省略，改为"This article reviews the basic science evidence, animal experiments, and human clinical data supporting the existence of an 'insulin-resistant cardiomyopathy' and proposes specific potential therapeutic approaches. "

例二：The protocol included fetal echocardiograms performed weekly from 16 to 26 weeks' gestation and (the protocol included fetal echocardiograms performed) biweekly from 26 to 34 weeks.

该方案包括 16～26 周每周进行一次、26～34 周每两周进行一次胎儿超声心动图检测。

【析】句中括号内的成分为可以省略的部分。但需要注意的是，若存在不同的动词搭配或时态、语态时，谓语动词则不能省略。如下例。

例三：We **estimated the effectiveness** of vitamin D supplementation in preventing hip and nonvertebral fractures in older persons and **conducted the investigation** as such.

评估补充维生素 D 在预防老年髋骨骨折和非脊椎骨折方面的效果，并做了类似研究。

【析】所使用的搭配动词不同，另一个谓语动词不可省略。

例四：The use of statins **had been suggested** to protect against AF in some clinical observational and experimental studies but **has remained** inadequately explored.

一些临床观察和实验研究提示他汀具有抗 AF 作用，但未得到充分验证。

【析】时态和语态不同，第二个分句的谓语动词应保留。

例五：A strategy of early revascularization resulted in a 13.2% absolute and a 67% relative improvement in 6-year survival **compared with** initial medical stabilization.

与早期药物保守治疗相比，早期血运重建使6年生存率绝对增高13.2%，相对增高67%。

【析】句中 compared with 之前略去了包括引导状语从句的连接副词 when。略去的部分为 "when improvement in 6-year survival was compared with…"。英语中，由 when、while、if、as、though、although、whether 等引导的状语从句，如果从句中的谓语动词包含 be 动词，从句的主语和主句的主语为同一逻辑关联，或从句中的主语为代词 "it+be" 这一结构，或从句中的主语为代词 they 等指代的是主句中的主语即 "they+be" 结构时，be 动词包括 it/they 均可省略。例如：

例六：Patient age, gender, Barrett's segment length, and follow-up were similar, though they were not identical, in both cohorts.

尽管不是完全相同，两队列的患者年龄、性别、Barrett 节段长度和随访期均相似。

【析】该句可以改写为 "Patient age, gender, Barrett's segment length, and follow-up were similar, though not identical, in both cohorts."。

例七：We included 396,077 patients aged 66 years or older who had a history of cardiovascular disease or diabetes while **(they were)** undergoing medical treatment and who were alive on April 1, 2006.

研究共包括396 077 例年龄≥66 岁，正在接受内科治疗，截至2006 年4月1 日仍然存活的有心脏病史或糖尿病史的患者。

【析】注意句中括号内为略去的成分。

（二）替代

所谓替代，也称为置换，即用另一种表达去置换前一种表达内容。英语中常见的替代手段有如下几种。

1. 名词性替代

用替代词取代名词词组或名词中心词，这一语法现象称作名词性替代。名词性替代词主要有 one/ones（one 替代单数名词，ones 替代复数可数名词）；the same（可以用作整个名词词组的替代词，可指共指对象或非共指对象）；the kind/the sort（通常替代不可数名词）；不定代词 each、none、all、some、any、either、neither、both；代词 that/those；名词词组 the former、the latter 等。此外，还可以利用词的上、下级关系替代同一类属事物。例如：在特地语境中我们可以用 animal 替代 rat、mouse，用 agent 替代具体的药物，disease 替代具体的病症等。

例一：Animal models have repeatedly demonstrated the existence of an insulin-resistant cardiomyopathy, **one** that is characterized by inefficient energy metabolism and is reversible by improving energy use.

动物模型已反复证明胰岛素抵抗性心肌病的存在，其特征为能量代谢效率低下，但可通过改善能量运用而逆转。

【析】句中的 one 替代了前文中的 "insulin-resistant cardiomyopathy"，使得句子更为简洁，避免了不必要的重复。

例二：Nonpolypoid colorectal neoplasms containing carcinoma were smaller in diameter as compared with the polypoid **ones.**

含恶性肿瘤的非息肉状结直肠肿块的直径小于含癌的息肉状肿块。

【析】由于前文中被替代的词 neoplasms 为复数形式，故此，使用相应的词形 ones 保持语法一致。

例三：We directly sequenced the entire coding region and splice junctions of 5 cardiac ion channel genes, SCN5A, KCNQ1, KCNH2, KCNE1, and KCNE2, in 113 SCD cases from 2 large prospective cohorts of women (Nurses' Health Study) and men (Health Professional Follow-Up Study). Controls from **the same** population were then screened for the presence of mutations or rare variants identified in cases, and sequence variants without prior functional data were expressed in *Xenopus* oocytes to assess their biophysical consequences.

从女性（护士健康研究）和男性（健康职业随访研究）的两个大型前瞻性队列研究中，我们直接对 113 例 SCD 患者的 5 个心肌离子通道基因的整个编码区和剪切点进行测序，包括 SCN5A、KCNQ1、KCNH2、KCNE1 和 KCNE2，对照选自相同人群，对这些对照人群进行罕见突变筛查，将没有既往功能资料的突变序列表达于爪蟾卵母细胞，以评价其生物学结果。

【析】众所周知，英语中名词可以用作定语，故此，句中利用 "the same" 替代了前文中的 "women（Nurses' Health Study）and men（Health Professional Follow-Up Study）"。

例四：The absolute unadjusted difference in 7-year survival between regions providing the highest rates of both invasive and medical management strategies and those providing the lowest rates of **both** was 6.2%.

介入和药物治疗策略采用率最高的地区与介入和药物治疗采用率最低的地区，两者未经校正的 7 年绝对生存率差异为 6.2%。

【析】用代词 both 替代 survival。

例五： In this review, we propose 2 primary subtypes of AHF: (1) acute decompensated cardiac failure, characterized by deterioration of cardiac performance over days to weeks leading to decompensation; and (2) acute vascular failure, characterized by acute hypertension and increased vascular stiffness. Registry data suggest that **the latter** is the more common form of AHF in the general population, although **the former** is often overrepresented in studies focused in academic tertiary care centers.

在此我们提出急性心力衰竭的两个基本亚型：①急性失代偿性心力衰竭，以心功能数天或数周内恶化导致失代偿为特征；②急性血管性衰竭，以急性高血压和血管弹性下降为特征。研究显示，尽管人们更为重视第一种亚型，但在一般人群中第二种亚型更为常见。

【析】句中利用 the latter、the former 替代前文提及的两种假设，从而避免重复过于烦琐的内容。

例六： Although these differences did not reach statistical significance, the overall risk reductions were similar to **those** in men.

尽管上述差异没有统计学意义，但是这些心血管危险性的降低与男性患者相似。

【析】本句为比较关系，借助代词 those 替代前文复数词组 "risk reductions"。

例七： Heart failure with preserved EF is associated with a high mortality rate, comparable to **that** of patients with reduced EF.

与 EF 降低的心力衰竭患者相似，EF 正常的心力衰竭患者死亡率也较高。

【析】与例六一样，利用代词 that 替代前文的单数词组 "high mortality rate"。

2. 动词性替代

用动词替代词去替代动词词组（即谓语）或动词词组中心词（即谓语动词）这一语法现象称作动词性替代。动词性替代通常由 do 的相应变化形式担任。do 的功能：一是替代动词词组即整个谓语；二是替代动词词组中心词即谓语动词。例如：

例一： In the NHS we did not find an inverse association between alcohol and CHD in B2 non-carriers (*P* trend: 0.5), but **did** among B2 carriers.

在 NHS 研究中，我们未发现在酗酒和没有 B2 携带的冠心病患者之间存在负相关（*P*：0.5），但在 B2 的携带者中却存在。

【析】did 替代的是 "find an inverse association between alcohol and CHD"。

例二： Of 110 patients, 25% evolved in LV remodeling and 75% **did not**.

110 名患者中，25% 的患者发生了 LV 重塑，75% 的患者未发生重塑。

【析】"did not" 替代的对象为 "evolved in LV remodeling"。

例三： Children conceived by medically assisted reproduction had worse outcomes than **did those** conceived naturally.

通过医学辅助生殖受孕的儿童比自然受孕的儿童结局更差。

【析】本句中用 did 为替代 outcomes，此外，用 those 替代 children。

例四： The IMR correlated significantly with the peak creatinine kinase (CK) while the other measures of microvascular dysfunction **did not**.

微循环阻力（IMR）指数与肌酸激酶（CK）峰值显著相关，而微血管功能障碍的其他指标则不相关。

【析】同上例一样，根据结构和语境分析可知，其完整内容应是 "...dysfunction **did not correlated significantly with the peak creatinine kinase**."。

3. 分句性替代

用替代词去替代名词性分句，这一手段称作分句性替代。英语中常用 so 替代肯定陈述分句，用 not 或词性、语义相似的词替代否定陈述分句，但这类替代在摘要写作中由于语篇上的差异，尤其在结构性摘要中使用得较少。

例一： Diabetes increased myocardial AGE deposition in patients with reduced LVEF (from 8.8 ± 2.5 to 24.1 ± 3.8 score/mm^2; $P=0.005$) and **less so** in patients with normal LVEF (from 8.2 ± 2.5 to 15.7 ± 2.7 score/mm^2, $P=$NS).

LVEF 下降的患者，糖尿病增加 AGE 在心肌中沉积〔（8.8±2.5）～(24.1±3.8) score/mm^2；$P=0.005$〕、而在 LVEF 正常患者则 AGE 沉积减少（8.2±2.5）～(15.7±2.7) score/mm^2，$P=$NS）。

【析】句中的 less 和 so 替代的是 "diabetes increased myocardial AGE deposition."。即后一分句的完整意思为 "diabetes increased myocardial AGE deposition in patients with normal LVEF."。又如下例：

例二： Such an increase in HO activity reflected induction of HO-1. HO-1 mRNA was markedly induced in the maleate-treated kidney at 8 h and progressively **less so** at 18 and at 24 h.

HO 活性增加反映 HO-1 的诱导。在用顺丁烯二酸治疗的肾脏内，HO-1mRNA 在治疗 8 小时时明显被诱导，而这一诱导在治疗 18、24 小时时逐渐递减。

六、简明与冗余

简明与冗余本为矛盾的对立关系。简明（brevity, conciseness）的原则即是仅用少量词语准确地表达更多内容（expressing much in few words; clear and succinct），而冗余（redundancy）却是赘言、冗长不必要的重复（unnecessary repetition）。鉴于医学论文英文摘要的写作特点，如何处理好这一矛盾关系，对于以汉语为母语的作者来说，确实难以驾驭。掌握并使用一门语言，本身就不是一蹴而就的，它需要通过长期不断阅读、揣摩、反复写作实践，了解并掌握医学英语的文体特点。英文摘要写作中，我们应注意如下几个方面。

（一）删繁就简

英语语言的特点之一是灵活多样性，不仅体现在一词多义、一词多性（speech），而且对于同一概念意义具有多种表达。但写作摘要时应采用简洁、简化的表达形式。

例一：Children were followed for 12 months **in order to** determine overall counts of diarrheal episodes and respiratory tract infections.

为了确定腹泻和呼吸道感染发生的频率，（我们）对被研究儿童进行了为期 12 个月的随访。

【析】句中用 "…in order to determine overall counts of diarrheal episodes and respiratory tract infections." 表示目的，从简洁角度看，可以将其简化为 "…to determine overall counts of diarrheal episodes and respiratory tract infections."。

例二：Little is known **with regard to** the factors that influence these rates.

对影响其发生率的因素还知之甚少。

【析】"with regard to" 的意思是 about、concerning。因此，该句中完全可以用 about 或 concerning 替代 "with regard to"，从而简化文字。

医学论文英文摘要写作中，涉及此类表达很多。为了方便读者掌握，特将其归类如下：

1. 表示目的类

冗词赘语	简洁措辞
in order to	to
with a view to	to
for the purpose	for
on behalf of	for

2. 表示方法、行为类

冗词赘语	简洁措辞
It has been reported by us that	we now report that
be referred to as	be called

续表

冗词赘语	简洁措辞
take into consideration	consider
through the use of/by means of	through/by/with
in a position to	can
are found to be	are
as far as the observations are concerned	we observed
by means of	by/with
fall off	decline
give rise to	cause
It necessitates the inclusion of	It needs/requires

3. 表示原因、结果类

冗词赘语	简洁措辞
due to the fact that	because/due to
on account of the fact that	because
despite/in spite of the fact that	although/though
for the reason that	because/since
with regard to	about/concerning
with the result that	so that
accounted for the fact that	because
are in agreement to/with	agree to/with
as a consequence of	because of
be capable of being attributed	due to
on the basis of	from/by/because

4. 表示时间、过程类

冗词赘语	简洁措辞
at this point of time	now
at the present time	now
during the same time that	during/while
during the course of	during
prior to	before
at all times	always
in the near future	soon
subsequent to	after

5. 表示结论类

冗词赘语	简洁措辞
bring all this to a conclusion	conclude
in consequence of this fact	therefore/consequently
It appears that	apparently
The conclusion we can draw from	we conclude

6. 表示数量类

冗词赘语	简洁措辞
a majority of	most
a number of	many/several
a small number of	a few
an innumerable number of	innumerable/countless/many
in close proximity to	near

7. 描述及其他类

冗词赘语	简洁措辞
it is clear that	clearly
if it is necessary	if necessary
it is obvious that	obviously
are known to be	are
if it is assumed that	if
in all cases	invariably
it is likely that	likely
it is possible that	possibly
it is worth pointing out that	note that
Red in color	red

（二）擅用名词词组

　　构成名词词组的中心词可以是单字名词，也可以是复合名词（compound noun）。复合名词词组是指词组的中心为名词，通常是由两个或更多的词结合在一起组成一个整体概念的名词。针对名词中心词的修饰语与中心词的相对位置关系来说，分为前置修饰语（pre-modifier）和后置修饰语（post-modifier）。某些名词词组中，其所修饰的前置或后置名词可以易位，尤其是后置的带有 of 或 with 的修饰语，改变修饰位置但不会改变其意义，从而简化对同一概念的表达。例如："infection of upper respiratory tract"可以写作"upper respiratory tract infection"。在现代英语中，复合名词该如何书写，迄今无一定的准则可循，常见构成主要包括：①连成一个词，如 heartbeat、stomachache。②词与词之间使用连字符"-"连接，如 birth-control、dose-dependency。③名词与名词之间分开写，前一名词起前位修饰功能，如 heart failure、vascular endothelial growth factor。

　　例一： Analysis of data from a randomised trial. Impaired kidney function was defined as **low rate of glomerular filtration.**
　　对一项随机试验的资料进行分析。低肾小球滤过率界定为肾功能受损。
　　【析】"rate of glomerular filtration"可以为前位修饰，即"low glomerular filtration rate"。

　　例二：In patients of critically ill, use of the PAC neither increased overall mortality or days in hospital nor conferred benefit.

对于重症患者而言，PAC 的使用既不增加总体死亡率或住院天数，也没有给患者带来益处。

【析】从简洁角度看，"in patients of critically ill"宜修改为"in critically ill patients, …"。

例三： **In 37 recipients undergone anemic heart transplant**(31 male/59.1±10.3 years/hemoglobin<12.0 g/dl), complete anemia work-up was performed including erythropoietin determination.

对 37 例贫血的心脏移植受者[31 例男性，（59.1±10.3）岁，血红蛋白<12.0 g/dl]进行包括促红细胞生成素测定在内的贫血全系列诊断检查。

【析】根据其语法及逻辑关系，句中"In 37 recipients undergone anemic heart transplant"可以借助复合名词的构成方式将中心词词组改为"In 37 anemic heart transplant recipients…"。

那么，在何种情况下可以改变名词修饰语的位置，利用复合名词替代复杂的表达方式呢？鉴于医学概念属性，英语中的复合名词大体可以分类如下：

1）以"患者"作中心名词，加前位修饰语构成。例如："in-hospital patient"（住院病人）；"high-risk patient"（高危患者）；"rheumatoid arthritis patients"（类风湿关节炎患者）；"DMARD-treated patients"[疾病修饰抗风湿药物（DMARD）治疗的患者]等。

2）以"疾病"作中心名词，加前位修饰词组成。例如："coronary heart disease"（冠心病）；"acute coronary syndrome"（急性冠脉综合征）；"conduction system disease"（传导系统病）；"high-grade dysplasia cancer"（高分化异型增生癌）；"hematopoietic acute radiation syndromes"（造血急性辐射综合征）；"stress-induced myocardial perfusion defects"（负荷诱导的心肌灌注缺损）等。

3）以各种"测定量"为中心名词，加前位修饰词组成。这类中心名词包括"含量、浓度、水平"等。例如："protein concentration"（蛋白质含量）；"serum IgE levels"（血清 IgE 含量）；"cholesterol saturation index"（胆固醇饱和指数）；"cellular A3G levels"（细胞 A3G 水平）；"cartilage glycosaminoglycan content"（软骨糖胺聚糖含量）；"recurrence rate"（复发率）等。

4）以各种"机能、组织结构"为中心词，加前位修饰词构成。例如："plasma protein extravasation"（血浆蛋白外渗）；"plasma angiotensinase activity"（血浆的血管紧张素酶活性）；"megaspore mother cell"（大孢子母细胞）；"serum carcinoembryonic antigen"（血清癌胚抗原）；"High-fidelity intracardiac pressure"（高保真心内压力）；"left ventricular ejection fraction"（左心室射血分数）等。

5）以各种"检测""治疗"措施为名词中心词。例如："exploratory biopsy"（探查性活组织检查）；"X-ray television macrofluorscope"（电视 X 线放大透视）；"Aspirin-clopidogrel antiplatelet dual therapy"（阿司匹林 – 氯吡格雷抗血小板双重治疗）；"orthotopic liver transplantation"（原位肝移植）；"hormone replacement therapy"（激素取代疗法）；"percutaneous coronary intervention"（经皮冠状动脉介入治疗）等。

6）其他类型。例如："civilian trauma population"（普通创伤人群）；"post-myocardial infarction remodeling"（心肌梗死后重塑）；"Paclitaxel-eluting coronary stents"（紫杉醇涂层冠脉支架）；"a potent, low-molecular-weight, nonpeptide, direct renin inhibitor"（一种有效的低分子量非肽直接肾素抑制剂）；"valve-related re-operations"（瓣膜相关的再手术）等。

（三）借助英语词法、句法功能

为了达到简洁，避免冗余，写作时要尽可能利用英语的某些特殊句法功能，如灵活运用非谓语动词简化句子结构，避免使用冗词等。这类写作技巧和要求在整个章节基本都有描述，故不赘述。

（四）含蓄否定

"否定"是相对"肯定"而言，凡是肯定的事物都有与其相反的否定的事物。"否定"是英语语言应用很广的一个逻辑范畴。从表达的内容来说，"否定"可分为一般否定（包括完全否定、基本否定、部分否定、单项否定及多项否定）和特殊否定（包括强意否定和委婉否定）；从表达方式上，英语的否定主要有：①使用否定词，如 no、not 等；②带有否定词缀的词，如 abnormal（不正常的）；③用含有"否定"语义的词，如 fail（不，没能）；④用含有"否定"语义的句式。出于英文摘要写作简洁的考虑，对于"否定"意义的表达，应尽可能利用英语的含蓄否定，即形式上貌似肯定，而意义上却为否定。此类否定如果应用得当，会极大地提高我们的措辞能力。这类否定的词如下所述。

1. 名词或名词词组

常用的表达含蓄否定的名词或名词词组有 absence（不在，缺乏）、freedom（没有）、failure（未能）、lack（缺少）、in the absence of（在缺少……的情况下）。

例一： The **absence of symptoms** correlated well with documented freedom of AF.
无症状与记录到的无 AF 复发存在较强的相关性。

例二： In early survivors, actuarial **freedom from death or transplantation** was 93.7%, 89.9%, 87.3%, and 82.6% at 5, 10, 15, and 20 years, respectively.
早期幸存者中，5、10、15、20 年内准确统计到的无死亡或心脏移植者分别为 93.7%、89.9%、87.3%和 82.6%。

例三： There is a **lack of** potent, selective antagonists at most subtypes of P2Y receptor.
大多数亚型 P2Y 受体无有效、选择性拮抗剂。

2. 动词或动词词组

带有含蓄否定的动词或动词词组有 fail（不，没能）、decline（拒绝）、miss（未……）、

deny（否认）、refuse（拒绝）、exclude（排除）、mismatch（不匹配）、withhold（拒给）、（prevent、keep、hinder、protect、save）from（防止，避免）等。

> **例一：** Finally, analyzing 11 single-nucleotide polymorphisms from the GeneChip Mapping 500K Array, genotyped in 1644 controls and 753 cases, **failed to provide evidence for association.**
> 最后，对 1644 个对照和 753 例患者进行基因芯片 500K 分析，未能提供相关性的证据。

> **例二：** **Missed opportunities for immunization** were documented for approximately 50% of patients with AHB who reported cohabitation with HBV carriers and for 70% of those who reported injection drug use.
> 有资料显示：在错过免疫机会的 HBV 患者中，大约 50% 的患者称与 HBV 携带者共同居住，有 70% 的患者称注射毒品。

> **例三：** **Anticoagulants were withheld from** patients classified as excluded, and all patients were followed up for 3 months.
> 排除肺栓塞的患者不予抗凝治疗。所有患者均随访 3 个月。

3. 形容词或形容词词组

带有含蓄否定的形容词和形容词词组有 free of（没有）、far from（远非）、clear from（不含）、rare（稀少）、absent（没有）、few/little（很少，注：few/little 也可以用作代词）、exlusive of（无……）、short of（缺少……）。

> **例一：** At a median follow-up of 22 months (range, 1 to 43 months), 87 patients (92%) were **free of ES** and 63 patients (66%) were **free of VT recurrence**.
> 在中位数为 22 个月的随访期（1～43 个月）内，有 87 例患者（92%）无 ES，63 例患者（66%）无 VT 复发。

> **例二：** **Little is known about the factors** that the rate of appendiceal rupture and negative appendectomy in children remain high despite efforts to reduce them.
> 即使做了努力，儿童阑尾穿孔和阴性阑尾切除术的发生率依然居高不下，但对此因素还知之甚少。

4. 介词或介词短语

带有含蓄否定的介词或介词短语包括 above（超出）、beyond（超出）、instead of（而不是）、out of（脱离）、without（没有）、except（除……之外）、regardless of（不管，不顾）、out of（缺乏，丧失，脱离）等。

> **例一：** It remains to be determined whether the combination of a fibrate plus statin reduces the risk **beyond** that achieved with a statin alone.

联合应用二者是否会比单独应用他汀类药物可额外降低心血管病风险还没有定论。

例二：When only never smokers **without diabetes** were assessed, the age-, lipid level- and sex adjusted OR was 0.40.

当仅评估未患糖尿病的非吸烟者时，经年龄、血脂水平及性别校正后的 OR 为 0.40。

5. 副词或副词短语

带有含蓄否定的副词或副词短语有 hardly（几乎不）、scarcely（稀少）、never（从不）、barely（几乎不）、rarely（罕见）、seldom（不常）、instead of（而不是）。

例一：Earlier studies also **rarely addressed** whether the association between a psychologic variable and MI was specific and independent of other psychosocial correlates.

此外，早期研究很少涉及心理变量和心肌梗死之间是否有特异性关联，以及是否独立于其他心理相关因素。

例二：The causes of death occurring in clinical trials of myocardial infarction (MI) are **scarcely reported** in the literature.

急性心肌梗死临床试验中死亡原因的研究较少。

例三：Insulin therapy is most effective if dosage titrations are done regularly and frequently, which is **seldom** practical for most clinicians.

如果定期做剂量滴定，胰岛素治疗是最有效的，但大多数临床医生不太习惯这么做。

6. 具有否定意义的前缀和后缀构成的词

这类词在英语中占很大比例，如何充分、正确、恰当使用这类词，需要我们在阅读文献过程中慢慢积累，并运用到写作实践。例如：

例一：Human epidermal growth factor receptor 2 (HER2) genetic heterogeneity (GH) is an **infrequent** event.

人表皮生长因子受体 2（HER2）遗传异质性（GH）是一种罕见的疾病。

【析】infrequent 由否定意义的前缀 "in-" 构成否定。

例二：All abnormal findings **disappeared** 1 month after the cessation of treatment.

所有异常症状在停止治疗 1 个月后消失。

【析】由前缀 "dis-" 构成的动词表示否定。

七、离散与集合

对于我国作者来说，基本上较好地掌握了英语语法概念。但是，由于英文和中文语言的较大差异，通常会对名词的数量取舍踌躇不定。从词的形式看，英文名词分为可数名词与不可数名词。可数名词有单复数之分，而不可数名词主要由物质名词、抽象名词等组成，一般没有复数形式。然而，这类名词在实际使用中，常可见其复数形式表达，其词义的概念范畴也随之发生变化，这就是不可数名词的离散与集合。离散在数学概念上是指不连续的一组数值，集合则是一组具有某种共同性质的数学元素。以此类推，英文的不可数名词在使用中所产生的复数形式属于同样的道理，如 feeling 做抽象名词时意义为"感觉"，当出现 feelings 时则意为"情感"。常识告诉我们，人类的情感是复杂多样的，这就是为什么抽象名词可以转化为普通名词，从而出现复数形式。医学论文英文摘要写作中，如果抽象名词代表的是个体概念，写作时取其单数形式；若在语境中表示个体状态或行为等频数累积，就需要取其复数形式。

例一：Patients range **from age five to eighty-one years** and typically awake with severe bilateral visual loss.

患者的年龄从 5 岁至 81 岁不等，表现为典型的苏醒后伴有严重双眼视力丧失。

【析】age 用的是单数形式，强调个体。本句可以理解为"Patients range from age 5, 6, 7, 8, 9, 10…to 81…"。

例二：For the Society of Thoracic Surgeons coronary artery bypass graft surgery population studied, the **median age** was 66 years, with 37.2% of patients administrator ≥70 years old.

在 STS 数据库中，行 CABG 的患者中位年龄为 66 岁，其中 37.2% 的患者年龄≥70 岁。

【析】"median age"，因为平均年龄只有一个，所以用单数。

例三：For **ages** younger than 60 years, 60 to 79, and 80 years and older, respectively, control rates were 38%, 36%, and 38% in men (P= 0.30) and 38%, 28%, and 23% in women (P<0.001).

小于 60 岁、60～79 岁和大于 80 岁组男性的控制率分别为 38%、36% 和 38%（P=0.30）；女性的控制率分别为 38%、28% 和 23%（P<0.001）。

【析】借助句中语境可知，这是一个集合表达，小于 60 岁，即 60 岁以下的人群，以此类推，60～79 岁，80 岁以上均指年龄段，而年龄段必然是不同年龄数目的集合。故此，用复数形式。

例四：The association of murine asthma with adiposity may be mediated by adiponectin, an anti-inflammatory adipokine with reduced serum **concentrations** in the obese.

鼠哮喘模型与肥胖相关可能因脂联素介导作用。脂联素是一种抗炎症脂肪激素，其在肥胖者血清中浓度降低。

【析】concentration 意为"the amount of a specified substance in a unit amount of another substance"（浓度：在某一单位物质中另一特定物质的含量）。例如：体内无机阳离子之一的钾，其正常血清钾浓度为 3.5～5.5 mmol/L，这是一个集合数目。血清钾浓度若低于 3.5 mmol/L 就会导致低钾血症，即参照点为 3.5 mmol/L，指向点为个体数目。

例五： Perioperative mortality decreased steadily over time and accounted for 68.4% of all **deaths.**

围手术期死亡率随着时间稳定下降，占全部死亡患者的 68.4%。

【析】句中 deaths 指死亡人数，故用复数。

医学英语中类似的情况非常多见，如 vomiting（呕吐），vomitings 则是"呕吐的（次数）"或指"呕吐物"；diarrhea（腹泻），而 diarrheas 却是集合数目，指"腹泻（次数）"；在"Our aim was to investigate whether acute **infections** transiently increase the risk of venous thromboemoblism."（本研究目的是确定急性感染是否会短暂增加静脉血栓栓塞的风险。）中的 infecitons 就是集合数目，即"反复感染"。为此，作者在写作过程中，若涉及此类问题，不必拘泥于语法上的某些规则限制，而应从专业知识及语境方面考虑离散与集合数目的取舍。

例六： We assessed whether a mild regimen using lower doses of topical CS and a shorter duration could improve the outcome of BP patients even more.

评估短疗程内采用低剂量局部皮质类固醇（CS）是否能更好地改善大疱性类天疱疮（BP）患者的症状。

【析】显而易见，句中的 doses 是指在该疗程内反复使用 CS。

八、摘要写作常用比较结构

有比较才有鉴别，比较是人类认识客观事物的重要方法之一，也是人类进行思维活动、交流经验、传递信息的有效方式。比较结构可以用来表达事物的属性或特征的不同程度。因此，医学论文英文摘要写作，常涉及有关比较内容的描述。虽然汉语中也有比较表达方式，但中英文表达习惯和方式却有诸多差异，且英文表达更为灵活多样。

1. 等同/不等比较

等同比较结构表示被比较的双方在性质、程度、数量等方面相等或近似相等，常用"as…as…"结构。在这个结构中，第一个 as 是副词，其后只能跟形容词或副词；第二个 as 为连词，引导出一个完整的或省略的比较状语从句，表示比较对象。此外，还可以使用"the same…as…"结构。不等比较结构常用"not so(as)…as"句式。

例一： Non-HDL-C and the ratio of total cholesterol to HDL-C were **as good as** or better than apolipoprotein fractions in the prediction of future cardiovascular events.

非高密度脂蛋白胆固醇（non-HDL-C）及总胆固醇（TC）与高密度脂蛋白胆固醇（HDL-C）比值对预测心血管疾病发生率的预测效果与载脂蛋白相同或者更好。

【析】"as+形容词+as"结构。

例二： The benefit of intensive therapy in carriers was significant **as early as** day 30 of therapy.

携带者强化（降脂）治疗效果在第 30 天已开始明显显现出来。

【析】"as+副词+as"结构。

例三： Adult family members with this type of *H. pylori* had **the same strain as** currently noncohabiting adult family members in 68% cases, implying acquisition during childhood from each other or a common source.

感染此型幽门螺旋杆菌的成年家族成员中，68%与目前独立生活的成年家族成员有着相同的菌株，提示该菌为幼年时期相互感染或通过公共源感染。

例四： An oral vitamin D dose of 400 IU/d is **not so（as） sufficient as** that of supplementation between 700 to 800 IU/d for fracture prevention in elderly persons.

每天口服 400 IU 维生素 D 预防老年人骨折，其效果不及日剂量 700～800 IU/d。

2. 差等比较

差等比较结构表示比较的双方具有性质、特征、程度上的差异，前者优于或劣于后者。英语中此类比较的构成有两种方式，即在形容词或副词原级形式的词尾加上后缀-er（综合式）或在其之前另外加上 more/less（分析式）。构成 more/less…than…结构。More/less 代表形容词或副词的比较级形式，than 是专门用来表示不同等的连接词，后接从句，表明比较的客体（被比较对象）。为了突出比较的内容，than 后面的结构通常采用省略形式，即省去与主句中相同的部分。More/less 用作定语时，一般置于被其修饰的名词之前。

例一： Adverse events and serious adverse events were generally similar among the groups, although severe hypoglycemia was **more frequent** in the insulin-provision group (9.2%) **than** (severe hypoglycemia) in the insulin-sensitization group (5.9%, *P*=0.003).

虽然胰岛素增敏组的严重低血糖发生频率高于胰岛素供应组（9.2% *vs*.5.9%，*P*=0.003），但治疗组间的不良反应和严重不良反应基本接近。

例二： We report rates for cardiopulmonary resuscitation and mortality that are **more favorable than** those previously reported.

就心肺复苏率和死亡率而言，我们所得的结论优于以往的报道。

【析】those 替代 "rates for cardiopulmonary resuscitation and mortality"。

引自：*Paediatr Anaesth*, 2010, 20(1): 28

例三： There were **more patients** with adverse events after SrR (70%) **than** teriparatide (41%) treatment (*P*= 0.013).

口服雷尼酸锶（SrR）治疗组患者（70%）不良反应高于特立帕肽组（41%，*P*= 0.013）。

【析】more 修饰名词 patients。

引自：*J Bone Miner Res*, 2009, 24(8): 1358

例四： The proportion of responders was **significantly greater** in the psyllium group **than** in the placebo group during the first month (57% *vs*.35%; relative risk 1.60, 95% confidence interval 1.13 to 2.26) and the second month of treatment (59% *vs*.41%; 1.44, 1.02 to 2.06).

在治疗第一个月（57% *vs*.35%；相对危险度 1.60，95%可信区间 1.13～2.26）和第二个月（59% *vs*.41%；相对危险度 1.44，95%可信区间 1.02～2.06）期间，蚤草组治疗有效的患者比例明显高于安慰剂组。

引自：*BMJ*, 2009, 339: b3154

例五： Respiratory failure after extubation was **less frequent** in patients assigned non-invasive ventilation **than** in those allocated conventional oxygen therapy.

无创通气组发生气管拔管后呼吸衰竭的概率低于常规通气组。

引自：*Lancet*, 2009, 374(9695): 1082

例六： The hospital mortality rate was 18%, **lower than** that reported previously for pediatric acute lung injury.

医院死亡率为 18%，这一结果低于前期报道的儿科急性肺损伤的医院死亡率。

引自：*Pediatrics*, 2009, 124(1): 87

3. 累进比较

英语形容词或副词的比较有时既不表示差等比较，也不表示选择比较，而是表示两件事物在程度、数量上同等增加或等量减少。在实际语言应用中，表示累进比较的说法有两种，一种是"对应增加"或"平行增加"；另一种是"渐进增加"或"逐次增加"。前者表示双方具有相互依存的关系，即"甲增乙亦增"；后者表示某一事物随时间的变化而不断增强其程度，即"渐渐……"或"更加……"。句型采用综合形式："the +形容词或副词比较级"，或："more…more…""more and more…"。

例一： The more recent the era of operation, the more pronounced was the discrepancy between expected and observed mortalities.

进行手术的年代越接近现在，预期死亡率和观察死亡率之间的差异越明显。

【析】采用的是 the more…the more 式。

引自：*Eur Heart J*, 2009, 30(1)：74

例二： For individuals with no cardiovascular risk factors as well as for those with 1 or more risk factors, those who are obese in middle age have a higher risk of hospitalization and mortality from CHD, cardiovascular disease, and diabetes in older age than those who are normal weight.

对没有心血管危险因素的人群和有 1 个或 1 个以上危险因素的人群而言，中年时肥胖者老年后因 CHD、心血管疾病或糖尿病住院、死亡的风险高于中年时体重正常者。

【析】采用 "more…more" 结构："more risk factors…higher risk of…"。

引自：*JAMA*, 2006, 295: 190

例三： Fewer hypoglycemic episodes and less weight gain occurred in patients adding basal insulin.

在加用基础胰岛素治疗的病人中，低血糖的发作次数和体重增加都随之降低。

【析】采用 "more and more" 形式："Fewer hypoglycemic…less weight gain…"。

引自：*N Engl J Med*, 2009, 361(18): 1736

例四： Significant correlations were found between levels of haemoglobin and amplitude of all ERP components; the lower the haemoglobin, the more pronounced the ERPs amplitude.

血红蛋白水平与所有 ERP 成分的振幅之间存在显著的相关性；血红蛋白越低，ERPs 振幅越明显。

【析】递进比较："the lower the haemoglobin, the more pronounced the ERPs amplitude"。

引自：*Br J Haematol*, 2019, doi: 10.1111/bjh.15957.

4. 含蓄比较

英语中有一种句子结构，其文字表达虽然没有使用 more、most 之类的语法比较形式，但就其意义而言，两者关系密切，而且彼此相反，从而形成某种对比。这种比较是借助于词汇手段或蓄意于特定的语境中表示比较之意。因此，英语中凡是表示意义对比或转折的句子结构实际上都可看作含蓄比较。可用于表达此类意义的词包括连词（but、nevertheless、while、whereas 等）、副词（yet、however、instead、rather 等）、介词（above、below、beyond 等）及短语 [on the other hand、in the meantime、in opposition to、(in)contrast to/with, compare with/to 等]。这类比较形式虽然普遍，但我国作者在英文摘要写作中却不太善于运用。

例一： Following the task, only the upper trapezius had higher mean activation levels (mean difference 10.79% MVIC), while the serratus anterior/lower trapezius activation ratio was altered (mean difference–0.3).

试验还显示，当上部斜方肌存在较高的活化水平（平均 MVIC 差异为10.79%）时，前锯肌/下斜方肌激活化比发生改变（平均差–0.3）。

【析】借助具有对比意义的词 while 表示比较。

引自: *Med Biol Eng Comput*, 2009, 47(5): 487

例二：Mast cell-released mediators up-regulate the expression of IL-17 by macrophages, whereas IL-10 down-regulates IL-17 expression.

肥大细胞释放的介质通过巨噬细胞上调IL-17的表达，而IL-10下调IL-17的表达。

【析】借助具有对比意义的词 whereas 表示比较。

引自: *J Immunol*, 2008, 181(9): 6117

例三：Contrary to what would be expected for a caustic chemical injury, we found that reflux esophagitis started at postoperative day 3 as a lymphocytic infiltration in the submucosa that later progressed to the epithelial surface.

与预期的腐蚀性化学性损伤相反，我们发现，反流性食管炎发生于术后第 3 天，此时黏膜下层有淋巴细胞浸润，且随后罹及到黏膜上皮。

【析】借助形容词 contrary 实现比较。

引自: *Gastroenterology*, 2009, 137(5): 1776

例四：However, the available evidence suggests that use of CSS and minocycline-rifampicin CVCs are useful if the incidence of CRBSI is above institutional goals despite full implementation of infection prevention interventions.

但现有证据表明，如果在全面实施了感染预防干预措施的情况下，导管相关性血流感染（CRBSI）发生率仍高于设立的目标值，使用氯己定-磺胺嘧啶银（CSS）和米诺环素-利福平中心静脉导管（CVCs）是有效的。

【析】使用介词 above 提示对比意义。

引自: *Lancet Infect Dis*, 2008, 8(12) : 763

例五：Patients with unprotected left main coronary artery(ULMCA)disease treated with PCI had favorable early outcomes in comparison with the coronary artery bypass grafting (CABG) group.

ULMCA 患者 PCI 治疗早期结果优于 CABG。

【析】通过语境及短语"in comparison with"提示比较关系。

引自: *J Am Coll Cardiol*, 2008, 51(5): 538

例六：Hospital admission favorably influenced syncope short term prognosis. Instead, 1-year mortality was unaffected by hospital admission and related to comorbidity.

住院治疗对晕厥短期预后有利，但不影响一年死亡率，并与合并症有关。

【析】用 instead 表示前后对比。

引自: *J Am Coll Cardiol*, 2008, 51(3): 276

5. 独立比较

这是英文摘要写作中常使用的一种比较形式。其特点是，被比较对象不出现在句子中，且没有"比"（more、-er、than）之类的词汇出现，而要通过语境才能想象出来。事实上，它提示出一种特殊的比较含义。

例一： A total of 172 men (80%) receiving tolterodine ER plus tamsulosin reported treatment benefit by week 12.

服用托特罗定缓释片＋坦索罗辛12周后，共有172位（80%）男性患者认为治疗有效。

【析】句中 benefit 为主体。众所周知，"疗效"效果如何，必须有参照对象，即与被比对象比较后才可确认，而被比对象却未在句中出现。

引自：*JAMA*, 2006, 296: 2319

例二： Much progress has been made in defining gene defects in pancreatic cancer, but a full accounting of its molecular pathogenesis remains to be provided.

尽管在确定胰腺癌基因缺陷方面的研究已经取得了很大进展，但是胰腺癌的分子机制仍需进一步探索。

【析】同上例一样，句中"much progress"为独立比较。此外，医学写作中某些概念短语表达同属此类比较。例如："very low-protein diet"极低蛋白饮食；"very little research"很少有人研究等。

引自：*Cancer Cell*, 2009, 15(3): 207

6. 拉丁比较

这类比较主要决定于词的本身意义，所用词汇为英语外来形容词（拉丁语）。典型特征是以"-or"结尾。常见的有"superior to…"（优于…）；"inferior to…"（劣于…）；"senior to…"（超过…）；"junior to…"（比……低）；"anterior to…"（早于…，较……之前）；"posterior to…"（迟于…，较……之后）；"prior to…"（比……早）。借助此类词表达比较意义时，不能与 than 连用，更多见于书面语。

例一： There is no evidence that either of the two treatments was **superior to** the other in the prevention of recurrent stroke.

没有证据表明这两种治疗措施在预防卒中复发中均优于另一种疗法。

引自：*N Engl J Med*, 2008, 359(12)：1238

例二： Episodic use of antiretroviral therapy guided by $CD4^+$ cell counts is **inferior to** continuous antiretroviral therapy.

按 $CD4^+$ 细胞计数采取间断抗逆转录病毒治疗，其疗效不及连续抗逆转录病毒治疗。

引自：*Ann Intern Med*, 2008, 149(5)：289

例三： One quarter of patients had demonstrable HLA alloimmunization **prior to** the initiation of granulocyte therapy.

1/4 的患者在粒细胞治疗开始前出现 HLA 异源免疫。

引自：Haematologica, 2009, 94(12) : 1661

7. 强调比较

形容词或副词比较级之前，常与某些特定的修饰语（通常为状语成分）连用，从而使比较意义在程度上有所增强或减弱。此类比较结构称为强调比较（emphatic comparison）。与之连用的常见状语修饰语有：①表示增强意义（just、exactly、altogether、entirely、even、much、still、far、considerably、a good/great deal 等）；②表示消弱意义（almost、nearly、quite、somewhat、slightly、a little、a bit 等）。

例一： A statistically significant difference was found only for structural brain anomalies, which were **somewhat** more common in male patients.

仅有脑部结构异常存在统计学显著性差异，而脑部结构异常在男性患者中较为常见。

引自：J Am Acad Dermatol, 2008, 58(1): 81

例二： The mortality benefit from lung cancer screening by LDCT might be **far smaller than** anticipated.

低剂量螺旋计算机断层摄影术（LDCT）筛查可降低肺癌死亡率，然而，其结果可能远远低于预期。

引自：Am J Respir Crit Care Med, 2009, 180(5) : 445

例三： It seems, thus, that any excess mortality conferred by older RBCs in the combined Swedish and Danish transfusion recipient population is likely less than 5%, which is **considerably smaller than** in the hitherto largest investigation.

因此，在瑞士和丹麦所有接受红细胞输入的患者中，因输入陈旧红细胞所引起的死亡率升高可能低于 5%，而这一数值远远低于目前所有大型研究所提示的结果。

引自：Transfusion, 2010, 50(6): 1185

例四： Anti-VEGF agents may be able to improve survival of patients with glioblastoma, **even** without inhibiting tumor growth.

即便不能抑制肿瘤的生长，抗 VEGF 剂仍有可能延长胶质母细胞瘤患者的生存期。

引自：J Clin Oncol, 2009, 27(5): 438

例五： Haemophagocytic lymphohistiocytosis (HLH) is a severe, **even fatal,** inflammatory condition.

噬血细胞性淋巴组织细胞增多症（HLH）是一种严重的，甚至是致命的炎症。

引自：Br J Haematol, 2019, doi: 10.1111/bjh.15988.

8. 数量比较

数量比较在英文摘要"Result"写作中十分常见。其构成方式：一个有明确数字意义的词语充当修饰语，表示数学意义上的增加或减少。通常用于由"as...as..."或"more than..."结构构成的比较句。

例一： We found that fibromyalgia patients had significantly less total gray matter volume and showed a 3.3 times greater age-associated decrease in gray matter than healthy controls.

我们发现，纤维肌痛患者总灰质量明显减少，其减少量为健康同龄对照组的 3.3 倍。

引自：*J Neurosci*, 2007, 27(15): 4004

例二： The prevalence of PCOS in SGA women was twice as high as in AGA women in our study population.

本研究人群中，新生女婴小于胎龄的女性多囊卵巢综合征的发生率是适龄出生女性的两倍。

引自：*Hum Reprod*, 2010, 25(8): 2124

例三： This is the first time that a hydrogel has been used to produce proteins. The efficiency was about 300 times higher than current, solution-based systems.

这是水凝胶首次用于生产蛋白质，其效率比现用的溶液中的系统高 300 多倍。

引自：*Nat Mater*, 2009, 8(5): 432

例四： AC2 and SDA were far superior to culture for the detection of CT or GC from the oropharynx and rectum with AC2 detecting twice as many infections as culture.

从口咽和直肠检测沙眼衣原体(CT)或淋球菌(GC)时，AC2(Gen-Probe's APTIMA Combo2)和贝特-迪金逊探针技术（SDA）的敏感度远优于培养样本，其中 AC2 检测到的感染是培养样本的两倍。

引自：*Sex Transm Dis*, 2008, 35(7)：637

9. 终极比较

终极比较即形容词或副词的最高级表达形式。应注意的是，这类比较应在三类以上的事物中才可使用，同时可有增强型或削弱型。

例一： DNA damage was **highest** in newly diagnosed untreated patients.

未经治疗的新诊断类风湿关节炎（RA）患者 DNA 损伤程度最高。

引自：*J Exp Med*, 2009, 206(6)：1435

例二： In a large, hospital-based cohort study, we identified serial BUN measurement as **the most** valuable single routine laboratory test for predicting mortality in AP.

　　在这项大型、以医院为基础的队列研究中，我们确认了血尿素氮（BUN）的变化是最有价值的实验室常规检测，并可用来预测急性胰腺炎（AP）的死亡率。

引自：*Gastroenterology*, 2009, 137(1): 129

例三：In the 1990s, uncontrolled hypertension in women increased **the most** in Idaho and Oregon (by 6 percentage points) and **the least** in the District of Columbia and Mississippi (by 3 percentage points).

　　在 20 世纪 90 年代，女性未控制的高血压在爱达荷州和俄勒冈州增加最多（6 个百分点），在哥伦比亚和密西西比增加最少（3 个百分点）。

引自：*Circulation*, 2008, 117(7): 905

例四：The efficiency of the algorithm was **highest** during the first trimester of pregnancy and lowest during the third trimester.

　　该算法在妊娠初 3 个月效率最高，在妊娠晚期效率最低。

引自：*N Engl J Med*, 2019, 380: 1139

九、写作基本句型及其扩展

　　句子是相对完整而又独立的、最高一层的语言单位。若要表达完整的思想，起到真正的交流作用，离不开结构正确、逻辑严谨的句子。英文句子的核心构成为主语和谓语。用作主语的名词、代词等相对稳定，但因构成谓语的英语动词或动词词组多样性，于是产生出不同的英语句型结构。英语基本句型可归纳为五种类型，而任何看起来较长，有时显得复杂的句子都是借助一定的语法手段扩展出来的。

　　1. 基本句型

　　（1）"主语+谓语"结构：构成此类结构的谓语动词为不及物动词，动词后无须跟宾语，但可跟副词修饰成分。

　　例：Sixty deaths occurred.
　　　　死亡 60 人。
　　　　【析】此例还可改写为" Sixty deaths occurred at the early stage of the trials."。

　　（2）"主语+谓语+宾语"结构：构成此类结构的动词为单宾语及物动词，即动词后必须跟一个直接宾语，句义才完整。

　　例：Aspirin failed to suppress platelet aggregation.
　　　　阿司匹林无法抑制血小板聚集。

　　（3）"主语+谓语+补足语"结构：构成该结构中的谓语为联系动词。因联系动词本身不能单独作谓语，只能与名词、代词、形容词、副词、非谓语动词、介词短语或句子搭配使用才能表达完整的概念意义。

例：The average hospital stay was 7 days.

平均住院日为 7 天。

（4）"主语+谓语+宾语 1+宾语 2" 结构：该结构中宾语 1 为间接宾语，代表人，故用表示人的名词或人称代词充当，间或用指物的名词表示。宾语 2 为直接宾语，代表物，故用表示物的名词担任。

例：We gave the patient adivce orally.

我们予以患者口头医嘱。

（5）"主语+谓语+宾语+宾补" 结构：构成这一结构的谓语动词只限于某些能带复杂宾语的及物动词。

例：We kept him awake during operation.

手术中，我们让他处于清醒状态。

2. 句型扩展

英语中，无论是陈述句、肯定句、主动句、被动句还是疑问句，千变万化的英语句型都是由基本结构演变而来的。即借助一定的语法手段，通过增加修饰语使句子加以扩展，使之成为表达更为复杂、意义多样的语言。增加修饰语的方法多种多样，但有一点需要注意的是，增加的修饰语必须合乎语法规范。例如：若想扩展主语，可以在主语前增加前位修饰词或短语或用后位修饰法，也可用名词从句等。总之，必须在大脑中具备完整的语法框架概念。

例一：A systematic review of all the relevant randomized controlled trials (RCTs) on topical tacrolimus for atopic dermatitis was performed according to International Cochrane Collaboration.

应用国际 Cochrane 协作网系统评价方法对外用他克莫司治疗异位性皮炎的随机对照试验（RCT）进行系统评价。

【析】这是一个 "主语+谓语" 的结构句型。主干部分为 "Review was performed."。名词中心词 review 前后分别增加了不同修饰语，谓语后也增加了修饰语。

例二：Surgical neonates admitted to a tertiary cardiac unit between March 1999 and February 2002 were retrospectively reviewed with analysis of risk factors for outcome.

对 1999 年 3 月至 2002 年 2 月间入住一所三级心脏中心行心脏手术的新生儿进行回顾性分析，确定影响其预后的危险因素。

【析】主干为 "Neonates were reviewed."。

例三：The aim of this study was to determine what baseline and post-treatment factors affect treatment response.

本研究的目的是明确影响治疗反应的基线及治疗后因素。

【析】该句为"主语+谓语+宾语"结构。主干成分为"Aim was to determine what..."。主语中心名词增加了后位修饰，宾语采用了名词性从句，从而包含更多信息。

例四： For clinical trials in functional bowel disorders (FBD), the definition of a responder, one who meets the predefined criteria for a clinical response, is needed.

为了进行功能性肠紊乱（FBD）的临床试验，必须弄清楚对治疗有反应者的定义，即符合临床反应的预定义标准。

【析】此为"主语+谓语+补足语"结构。主干为"Definition is needed."。前面增加了介词短语"For"，作为状语修饰全句。Definition 后增加了后位修饰。"One who meets"为插入语，起主语同位语作用。

例五： Whether a pregnancy-adapted algorithm could be used to safely avoid diagnostic imaging in pregnant women with suspected pulmonary embolism is unknown.

是否可以使用一种适合妊娠的算法来安全地避免疑似肺栓塞孕妇的诊断成像尚不清楚。

【析】本句借助名词性从句"Whether a pregnancy-adapted algorithm could be used to safely avoid diagnostic imaging in pregnant women with suspected pulmonary embolism"扩展主语。

例六： We conclude that increased adiposity without a concomitant increase in IHTG content does not cause additional abnormalities in adipose tissue, skeletal muscle, and hepatic insulin sensitivity, or VLDL metabolism.

我们的研究结果表明，不伴有肝内甘油三酯（IHTG）含量增多的肥胖加重不会引起额外的脂肪组织、骨骼肌、肝脏胰岛素敏感性或极低密度脂蛋白（VLDL）代谢的异常。

【析】这是"主语+谓语+宾语"结构（We conclude that...）。借助宾语从句扩展全句，从而包含更多信息。

例七： Homocysteinuria is a genetic disease whose manifestations include severe hyperhomocysteinemia and decreased bone strength.

高半胱氨酸尿是一种遗传性疾病，其表现形式包括严重高同型半胱氨酸血症和骨强度降低。

【析】本句在其表语中心名词后接了一个形容词从句，后位修饰 disease。

例八： Pulmonary embolism was ruled out if none of the three criteria were met and the D-dimer level was less than 1000 ng per milliliter or if one or more of the three criteria were met and the D-dimer level was less than 500 ng per milliliter.

如果三个标准中没有一个被满足，并且 D-二聚体水平低于每毫升 1000 ng 或如果三个标准中的一个或多个被满足，并且 D-二聚体水平低于每毫升 500 ng，则排除肺栓塞。

【析】本句的主干结构为 "Pulmonary embolism was ruled out"，后面采用由 if 引导的两个条件句做状语扩展。

例九： The results of the study clearly indicate that there is an underestimation of nightmare frequency in the parents' ratings compared to the children's data and the closeness between influencing factors and nightmare frequency is considerably higher for the data based on the children's responses; the proportion of explained variance was twice as high.

研究结果清楚地表明，与儿童的数据相比，父母低估了儿童的噩梦频率，基于儿童反应的数据，其影响因素和噩梦频率之间的接近度较高；解释方差的比例是原来的两倍。

【析】这是一个长句，其主干结构为 "主语（The results）+谓语（indicate）+宾语（从句）（that）"。动词 "indicate" 后跟两个并列宾语从句（indicate that…; and （that） and nightmare frequency is considerably…）。从句内部还有其他修饰语。需要注意的是，我们使用修饰语对某个词或句子成分进行修饰时，一定要符合语法规范。

十、倒装结构及其应用

英语句子通常有两种语序。语序属于语法结构，是指句子中各语言单位排列的顺序。英语句子按结构分为自然语序和倒装语序。自然语序为主语在前，谓语在其后。倒装语序则相反，谓语在前，主语在后。同时，倒装语序又分为两类：全部倒装和部分倒装。英语中使用倒装语序的语义功能，一是强调、突出信息中心，二是出于篇章结构上的需要，包括实现语篇的黏着，意义的连贯，句子结构上的平衡等。尽管倒装结构的使用在科技文体中远不及文学文体，但仍然是科技文章写作中不可或缺的修辞手段。

例一： In critically ill patients was increased use of the PAC.(=Use of the PAC was increased in critically ill patients.)

对于重症患者而言，肺动脉导管（PAC）的使用次数增加。

【析】主谓倒装。结构为：状语（介词短语）+谓语动词+主语。

例二： Interestingly, not only was this protection mediated by CD4$^+$ T cells, but IL-22-expressing natural killer (NK) cells also conferred protection.

重要的是，这种保护作用不仅是由 CD4$^+$ T 细胞介导，表达 IL-22 的自然杀伤（NK）细胞也具有保护作用。

【析】连词短语 "not only…but（also）"，当 "not only" 置于句首时，主

谓倒装，但"but（also）"后面的主谓部分则不倒装。

引自: *Immunity*, 2008, 29(6) : 947

例三： Then calculated summary risk ratios (RRs) for mortality.

计算总风险率（RRs）以估计死亡率。

【析】状语倒装，即将状语提至句首。

例四： Mean fat-free mass decreased in the placebo group but increased in the MK-677 group (change, –0.5 kg [95% CI, –1.1 to 0.2 kg] *vs.* 1.1 kg [95%CI, 0.7 to 1.5 kg], respectively; $P<0.001$), as did body cell mass, as reflected by intracellular water (change, –1.0 kg [95%CI, –2.1 to 0.2 kg] *vs.* 0.8 kg [95%CI, –0.1 to 1.6 kg], respectively; $P=0.021$）.

安慰剂组的平均无脂组织减少，MK-677 组则增加[前者减少（–0.5 kg, 95%CI, –1.1～0.2 kg）; 后者增加（1.1 kg, 95%CI, 0.7～1.5 kg）; P<0 .001]。从细胞内水含量可以看出，身体细胞量也有相似趋势[前者减少(–1.0 kg, 95% CI, –2.1～0.2 kg）; 后者增加（0.8 kg, 95% CI, –0.1～1.6 kg）; P=0 .021]。

【析】本句后半部分"as did body cell mass, as reflected by …"为 as 引导的方式状语从句。谓语倒装。在正式文体中，若使用如 hardly、scarcely、rarely、never、seldom 带有否定意义的副词或状语置于句首时，均需要主谓倒装。如例五。

引自: *Ann Intern Med*, 2008, 149(9): 601

例五： Rarely seen is bilateral adrenal neuroblastoma.

双侧肾上腺成神经细胞瘤极为罕见。

例六： Cross-sectional data from 4181 male individuals who underwent general health screening were analyzed.

对来自 4181 名健康普查的男性横断层面资料进行了分析。

【析】本句主语后接一个含有形容词从句修饰的介词短语，主语部分显得太长，给人一种头重脚轻的感觉，如果采用部分倒装，即调整定语位置，则能更好地平衡句子结构。修改为"Cross-sectional data were analyzed from 4181 male individuals who underwent general health screening."。

例七： Data on patients admitted to a hospital through 2003 with a first episode of heart failure in the absence of congenital heart disease were collected.

数据收集自 2003 年医院确诊的心力衰竭首次发作且无先天性心脏病的患者。

【析】同例六，本句应修改为"Data were collected on patients admitted to a hospital through 2003 with a first episode of heart failure in the absence of congenital heart disease."。

例八： Procedural data from 252 consecutive patients who underwent left atrial ablation (166 [66%] persistent, 86 [34%] for paroxysmal AF) were analyzed.

对 252 例接受左心房消融术的患者[166 例（66%）持续性心房颤动患者，86 例（34%）阵发性心房颤动患者]的手术数据进行了分析。

【析】本句主语过长，显得不平衡，因此，可以改写为倒装结构："Analyzed were procedural data from 252 consecutive patients who underwent left atrial ablation (166 [66%] persistent, 86 [34%] for paroxysmal AF).";或将定语置后，修改为"Procedural data were analyzed from 252 consecutive patients who underwent left atrial ablation (166 [66%] persistent, 86 [34%] for paroxysmal AF). "。

十一、语态与人称

撰写医学论文英文摘要时，该采用何种人称及语态，中外期刊存在较大差异。导致这种差异主要有两个方面的原因。一是某些期刊在其投稿要求中做出了明确规定，要求用第三人称来写作；二是国标《文摘编写规则》（GB 6447—86）的硬性规定。该规则在6.7条款中明文规定"要用第三人称的写法。应采用'对……进行了研究'、'报告了……现状'、'进行了……调查'等记述方法标明一次文献的性质和文献主题，不必使用'本文'、'作者'等作为主语"。至于国外医学期刊，尽管只有为数不多的期刊在'读者须知'中要求使用非第一人称和被动语态，对于人称和语态的使用，绝大多数未作强制规定。无论是何种原因，差异客观存在。

例一：【Abastract】Objective To investigate the risk factors of worsening renal function(WRF) in patients with chronic heart failure(CHF) and WRF influence on prognosis. Methods A case-control study was undertaken to analyze the independent risk factor statistically related to the incidence of WRF, and to assess the influence of WRF on prognosis. Results Renal function deterioration occurred in 31% of the hospitalized patients with heart failure.The independent predictors of WRF were creatinine level at admission (OR 2.248, 95% CI 1.088-4.647, P=0.029) and NYHA class on admission (OR 2.485, 95% CI 1.385-4.459, P=0.002). The mortality of patient with WRF was obviously higher than that of control group during hospitalization (OR 3.824, 95% CI 2.452-5.137, P<0.015). Conclusions WRF is a common complication among patients hospitalized for CHF, and is obviously associated with mortality during hospitalization. Higher creatinine level and weak heart function are independent risk factors for incidence of WRF of patients with CHF.

【摘要】目的 研究慢性心力衰竭（心衰）患者肾功能恶化的危险因素及其对预后的影响。方法 采用病例对照研究方法，分析与肾功能恶化发生有统计学关联的独立危险因素，同时观察肾功能恶化对预后的影响。结果 住院心衰患者肾功能恶化发生率 31%，入院肌酐水平及心功能分级与肾功能恶化的发生独立相关，OR 值分别为 2.248（95%CI，1.088～

4.647，*P*=0.029）和 2.485（95%CI，1.385～4.459，*P*=0.002）。发生肾功能恶化的患者住院期间病死率明显高于对照组（16.7% 比 2.1%，*P*=0.000），调整混杂因素后，肾功能恶化是死亡的独立危险因素，OR值 3.824（95%CI，2.452～5.137，*P*<0.015）。**结论** 肾功能恶化在住院心衰患者中发生率较高，与住院期间病死率明显相关。入院肌酐水平偏高及心功能差为发生肾功能恶化的独立危险因素。

引自:《中华内科学杂志》, 2011, 50(7): 568

例二：【Abastract】**Objective** To investigate the long-term effects of contrast medium on renal function in a rat contrast-induced nephropathy(CIN)model. **Methods** Forty-eight SD rats were pretreated intravenously with L-NG-nitroarginine methyl ester(L-NAME 10 mg/kg) and indomethacin (10 mg/kg). Then 30 minutes later diatrizoate (DTZ 8 ml/kg)was administrated in test group(n=24)to establish contrast-induced acute renal injury models, and saline (8 ml/kg)was injectd in control group (n=24). Renal function and histopathological changes were monitored at 24 hours,and at the end of 1st, 2nd and 3rd month after the administration. **Results** There was no significant difference of serum creatinine baseline value between test and control group. Twenty-four hours after DTZ injection, serurn creatinine in test group increased significantly from(48.02±5.53) μmol/L to (112.7±45.35) μmol/L(*P*<0.001). Meanwhile, the pathological changes were characterized by extensive cytoplasmic disruption, interstitial congestion and edema, especially in the outer medulla. Although serum creatinine dropped back to the baseline 3 months after DTZ injection in test group, focal interstitial inflamation still existed, and rave lesions of the tubulointerstitium were partly replaced by fibrous tissues. **Conclusions** Renal function of the SD rats may not recover completely 3 months after DTZ administration as the maintenance of chronic tubulointerstitial lesions.

【摘要】**目的** 观察造影剂所致大鼠急性肾损伤的远期影响。**方法** 48 只雄性 SD 大鼠经静脉注射消炎痛（10 mg/kg）和 L-NG-硝基精氨酸甲酯（L-NAME 10 mg/kg）预处理，30 min 后实验组大鼠（n=24）静脉注入复方泛影葡胺（DTZ 8 ml/kg）建立大鼠造影剂所致的急性肾损伤模型，对照组大鼠（n=24）缓慢推注生理盐水 8 ml/kg。给药后 24 h、1、2、3 个月观察大鼠肾功能、肾组织病理学变化。**结果** 对照组和实验组血肌酐基线值无明显差异。实验组注射 DTZ 24 h 后，血肌酐与基线值相比明显升高［（48.02±5.53）μmol/L *vs.*（112.7±45.35）μmol/L，*P*<0.001］，肾组织病理改变以片状小管坏死和间质充血为主，尤以外髓明显；注射 DTZ 3 个月后，尽管血肌酐与基线值及对照组相比差异无显著统计学意义，但实验组仍存在明显的肾间质局灶性炎症细胞浸润，部分早期损害严重

的小管被纤维组织所取代。**结论** 造影剂对大鼠肾脏造成的急性肾损伤并未完全恢复，而留下长期的慢性肾小管间质损伤。

引自：《复旦学报(医学版)》, 2011, 38(1): 24

例三： **Background: We** evaluated the efficacy of a maternal triple-drug antiretroviral regimen or infant nevirapine prophylaxis for 28 weeks during breast-feeding to reduce postnatal transmission of human immunodeficiency virus type 1 (HIV-1) in Malawi. **Methods:** We randomly assigned 2369 HIV-1-positive, breast-feeding mothers with a CD4$^+$ lymphocyte count of at least 250 cells per cubic millimeter and their infants to receive a maternal antiretroviral regimen, infant nevirapine, or no extended postnatal antiretroviral regimen (control group). All mothers and infants received perinatal prophylaxis with single-dose nevirapine and 1 week of zidovudine plus lamivudine. We used the Kaplan-Meier method to estimate the cumulative risk of HIV-1 transmission or death by 28 weeks among infants who were HIV-1-negative 2 weeks after birth. Rates were compared with the use of the log-rank test. **Results:** Among mother-infant pairs, 5.0% of infants were HIV-1-positive at 2 weeks of life. The estimated risk of HIV-1 transmission between 2 and 28 weeks was higher in the control group (5.7%) than in either the maternal-regimen group (2.9%, $P=0.009$) or the infant-regimen group (1.7%, $P<0.001$). The estimated risk of infant HIV-1 infection or death between 2 and 28 weeks was 7.0% in the control group, 4.1% in the maternal-regimen group ($P=0.02$), and 2.6% in the infant-regimen group ($P<0.001$). The proportion of women with neutropenia was higher among those receiving the antiretroviral regimen (6.2%) than among those in either the nevirapine group (2.6%) or the control group (2.3%). Among infants receiving nevirapine, 1.9% had a hypersensitivity reaction. **CONCLUSIONS:** The use of either a maternal antiretroviral regimen or infant nevirapine for 28 weeks was effective in reducing HIV-1 transmission during breast-feeding.

背景： 在马拉维（Malawi）对哺乳期母亲予以三联抗逆转录病毒药物或婴儿使用奈韦拉平（nevirapine）连续治疗 28 周，随后评估该治疗方案对于减少母乳喂养期间 1 型人类免疫缺陷病毒（HIV-1）在婴儿出生后母婴传播的疗效。**方法：** 将 2369 名 HIV-1 阳性、每立方毫米外周血 CD4+ 淋巴细胞计数在 250 个以上的哺乳期母亲及其婴儿随机分组：母亲接受抗逆转录病毒疗法；婴儿接受奈韦拉平治疗；不延长产后抗逆转录病毒疗法（对照组）。所有母亲和婴儿均接受单剂量奈韦拉平围产期预防治疗，并联用齐多夫定（zidovudine）和拉米夫定（lamivudine）治疗 1 周。采用 Kaplan-Meier 法以评估出生 2 周后 HIV-1 阴性婴儿 HIV-1 传播累积风险或 28 周的死亡情况。采用对数秩检验计算概率。**结果：** 母-婴配对（结果显示），5.0%的婴儿出生 2 周时 HIV-1 呈阳性。对照组在 2 至 28 周 HIV-1 传播的估计风险（5.7%）高于母亲治疗组（2.9%，P=0.009）和婴儿治疗组（1.7%，P<0.001）。2 至 28 周婴儿 HIV-1 感染或死亡的估计风险如下：对照组为 7.0%；母亲治疗组为 4.1%（P=0.02）；婴儿治疗组为 2.6%（P<0.001）。中性粒细胞减少症在接受抗逆转录病毒治疗的妇女发生率为 6.2%，高于奈韦拉平组（2.6%）和对照组（2.3%）。接受奈韦拉平治疗的婴儿中，有 1.9%出现过敏反应。**结论**：无论是母亲接受抗逆转录病毒疗法还是婴儿使用奈韦拉平联系治疗 28 周，两种方案均能有效减少母乳喂养期间 HIV-1 的传播。

引自：*N Engl J Med*, 2010, 362(24): 2271

例四： **Context:** Guidelines recommend antibiotic therapy for acute exacerbations of chronic obstructive pulmonary disease (COPD), but the evidence is based on small, heterogeneous trials, few of which include hospitalized patients. **Objective:** To compare the outcomes of patients treated with antibiotics in the first 2 hospital days with those treated later or not at all. **Design, Setting, And Patients:** Retrospective cohort of patients aged 40 years or older who were hospitalized from January 1, 2006, through December 31, 2007, for acute exacerbations of COPD at 413 acute care facilities throughout the United States. **Main Outcome Measures:** A composite measure of treatment failure, defined as the initiation of mechanical ventilation after the second hospital day, inpatient mortality, or readmission for acute exacerbations of COPD within 30 days of discharge; length of stay, and hospital costs. **Results:** Of 84 621 patients, 79% received at least 2 consecutive days of antibiotic treatment. Treated patients were less likely than nontreated patients to receive mechanical ventilation after the second hospital day (1.07%; 95% confidence interval [CI], 1.06% -1.08% *vs.* 1.80%; 95% CI, 1.78% -1.82%), had lower rates of inpatient mortality (1.04%; 95% CI, 1.03%-1.05% *vs.* 1.59%; 95% CI, 1.57%-1.61%), and had lower rates of readmission for acute exacerbations of COPD (7.91%; 95% CI, 7.89%-7.94% *vs.* 8.79%; 95% CI, 8.74%-8.83%). Patients treated with antibiotic agents had a higher rate of readmissions for *Clostridium difficile* (0.19%; 95% CI, 0.187%-0.193%) than those who were not treated (0.09%; 95% CI, 0.086%-0.094%). After multivariable adjustment, including the propensity for antibiotic treatment, the risk of treatment failure was lower in antibiotic-treated patients (odds ratio, 0.87; 95% CI, 0.82-0.92). A grouped treatment approach and hierarchical modeling to account for potential confounding of hospital effects yielded similar results. Analysis stratified by risk of treatment failure found similar magnitudes of benefit across all subgroups. **Conclusion:** Early antibiotic administration was associated with improved outcomes among patients hospitalized for acute exacerbations of COPD regardless of the risk of treatment failure.

背景：《治疗指南》建议对慢性阻塞性肺疾病（COPD）急性加重期予以抗生素治疗，然而，其依据仅来源于几个规模较小，不同类型的试验，而且，这些试验未能囊括住院患者。**目的**：对入院两天内应用抗生素治疗的患者、入院两天后应用抗生素治疗或不用抗生素治疗的患者治疗结果进行比较。**设计、地点和病人**：回顾性队列研究。研究对象为美国各地的 413 家急救医疗机构于 2006 年 1 月 1 日至 2007 年 12 月 31 日期间收治的 40 岁或 40 岁以上的因 COPD 急性发作而住院的患者。**主要观察指标**：治疗无效的综合补救措施（定义为第二个住院日之后开始机械通气）；住院死亡率；或出院后 30 天内因 COPD 急性发作再次入院情况；住院时间和住院费用。**结果**：84 621 例患者中，79%接受了至少连续两天的抗生素治疗。与未用抗生素治疗的患者相比，抗生素治疗后的患者在第二个住院日接受机械通气的可能性较少（1.07%; 95% CI，1.06%～1.08% *vs.*1.80%; 95% CI，1.78%～1.82%），有较低的住院死亡率（1.04%；95% CI，1.03%～1.05% *vs.* 1.59%；95% CI，1.57%～1.61%），并有较低的 COPD 急性发作的再入院率（7.91%；95% CI，7.89%～7.94% *vs.* 8.79%；95% CI，8.74%～8.83%）。与未用抗生素治疗的患者（0.09%；95% CI，0.086%～0.094%）相比，接受抗生素制剂治疗的患者中因艰难梭菌感染所致的再入院率较高（0.19%；95% CI，0.187%～0.193%）。经过多变量调整后（包括抗生素治疗倾向选择，抗生素治疗失败），各风险在接受抗生素治疗患者中明显降低（优势比，0.87；95% CI，0.82～0.92）。分组治疗方法和证明医院影响潜在混杂影响的分层建模提示了相似结果。对所有亚组的治疗失败风险的分层分析也显示出相似程度的益处。**结论**：如果不考虑治疗失败，抗生素的早期应用与 COPD 急性发作的住院患者治疗结果的改善有一定的关联。

引自：*JAMA*, 2010, 303(20): 2035

上述 4 个完整摘要分别选自中外具有代表性的学术刊物。例一来自我国中华医学会旗下的核心期刊，例二为学院派的代表，例三为国际顶级刊物，例四则为美国医学会所主办。从以上四个例证可以看出，摘要写作中，在人称和语态方面，不仅中外学术刊物存在较大差异，而且，国外刊物也有较大不同。尽管不能以一概全，但差异确实存在。例如，对"方法"的描述，例一、例二均使用的是被动结构，例四使用的是非完整结构，例三中的"方法"总共 4 个句子，有 3 个主动结构，且使用了第一人称代词 we。

摘要是浓缩的语篇，其话语功能主要有介绍研究的背景，提出研究目的，简述论文所做的工作，得出研究结果、结论并分析该研究的意义。因此，摘要中的语态与人称该如何取舍，首先要考虑的是行文的流畅性和语篇的逻辑性。在此基础上，采用多样化句式表达。不应受到某些不合理的规约限制。语态方面，尽可能使用主动结构，因为主动语态更能突出话语中心，保持句子的结构平衡。人称方面，建议避免使用第一人称单数。人称代词的使用一定要合理、恰到好处，否则会导致表达缺乏精练，甚至造成阅读障碍。例如，例三中的"All mothers and infants received perinatal prophylaxis with single-dose nevirapine and 1 week of zidovudine plus lamivudine. **We** used the Kaplan-Meier method to estimate the cumulative risk of HIV-1 transmission or death by 28 weeks among infants who were HIV-1-negative 2 weeks after birth."，从句子内部连贯一致性考虑，后一句用了人称代词，读者在阅读时会有较大停顿。若将后一句改为被动式，整个语篇反而更流畅一些。同样，若将例一"方法"中的"A case-control study was undertaken to analyze the independent risk factor statistically related to the incidence of WRF, and to assess the influence of WRF on prognosis."改写为"We undertook a case-control study to analyze the independent risk factor statistically related to the incidence of WRF and assess the influence of WRF on prognosis."会更通顺。关于人称代词，写作时可有多种选择，如"Our diagnostic strategy proved useful and sensitive for BCNE workup."（我们的诊断策略对于 BCNE 诊断既有效又灵敏）。

十二、中英文标点符号

标点符号是辅助文字记录语言的符号，是现代书面语言中不可或缺的有机组成部分。一方面，书面语中若无标点符号，则无法准确传递信息，造成读者阅读困难；另一方面，若错误使用标点符号，则会导致读者理解障碍，甚至错误解读语言信息。

标点符号具有三大辅助修辞功能：①表示停顿；②表示语气（陈述、疑问、感叹）；③表示句中某些词句的性质。

（一）英语与汉语标点符号在书写、用法等方面异同比较，如下表所示

标点符号名称	中文书写形式	英文书写形式	说明
句号（full stop/period）	。	.	英文中不可使用中文句号"。"；中英混排时，请参考 CY/T 154—2017《中文出版物夹用英文的编辑规范》
逗号（comma）	，	,	使用于分句与分句之间，表示信息未终止。例如：In this study, we investigated the effects of…；或 Periodontitis, which is caused by…
分号（semicolon）	；	;	使用场合见下节（二）标点符号使用实例分析相关例证
冒号（colon）	：	:	使用场合见下节（二）标点符号使用实例分析相关例证
问号（interrogation mark/queston mark）	？	?	仅用于表示疑问
感叹号（exclamation mark）	！	!	医学论文，包括摘要中罕用，甚至禁用
顿号（caesura sign）	、	无	仅用于中文，英文中无顿号
破折号（dash）	——	—	上下居中

标点符号名称	中文书写形式	英文书写形式	说明
连字符或连接号（hyphen）	– — ~	-	英文中连字符常用"-"，约为半个英文字母的宽度，也可用于汉语；另外，汉语中的连接号还可以有长横"——"（约占两个字的长度）或波浪"～"（占一个字的长度）
引号（quotation marks）	"" ' '	" " ' '	表示引用，摘要中罕用，除非表示特殊概念，如"…was facilitated through supervision only 'rarely' or 'sometimes'."
括号（brackets/marks of parenthesis）	（ ） [ ]	( ) [ ]	除前两者外，汉语中还有六角括号"〔 〕"和方头括号"【 】"
省略号（dots/ellipsis）	……	…	汉语中省略号常用6个小圆点表示；英语中常用3个小圆点表示
斜线号（slash/virgule）	/	/	科技写作中也有使用斜线号的情况。斜线号用于表示两组对立或两者择一的概念意义，如：（31±12）g/L；21.6%（27/125）。
撇号（apostrophe）	无	'	汉语中无撇号，英文中主要表示属格关系，如：patient's body weight.
书名号（book title mark）	《 》 < >	无	英文中无书名号。若表示书名时可用斜体字表示。如《新英汉词典》，英语则写成：A New English Chinese Dictionary.
间隔号（dividing mark）	·	无	英语中无间隔号。汉语中主要用于外国人和少数民族人名内各部分的分界，如"马克·雷登"

（二）标点符号使用实例分析

对于标点符号的使用，一般来说不是十分困难，具体使用及在文本录入时，可参考上表说明即可。本节就一些特殊使用符号的场合进行实例分析讲解，以便为大家提供参考模板。

例一：Twenty-six patients with BRVO-ME were prospectively enrolled, and underwent intravitreous injection with 0.05 ml conbercept (10 mg/ml) using "1+PRN" protocol. All eyes were observed at week 1, month 1 and 3 for BCVA, central macula thickness (CMT), macular volume and the rupture length of ellipsoid zone before and after treatment to assess the related factors affecting BCVA after medication.

方法：前瞻性研究。纳入 26 例 BRVO-ME 患者，"1+PRN"方案康柏西普（10 mg/ml）0.05 ml 玻璃体腔注射，观察 1 周、1 个月、3 个月，了解 BCVA、黄斑中心凹厚度、黄斑区容积、黄斑区椭圆体带断裂长度变化情况；评估 BCVA、黄斑中心凹厚度、黄斑区容积、黄斑区椭圆体带断裂长度与视力预后的相关性。

【析】① "…conbercept （10 mg/ml）"：补充信息可以放入括号。补充信息放入括号内，在摘要写作中比较常见，如缩写词"central macula thickness（CMT）"；说明试剂、软件、器械设备产地/制造商"A bio-informatics software package（CLC Genomics Workbench 12.0）"；分组样本信息"…randomized into sham operation group（*n*=10）"。② "…using '1+PRN' protocol"："1+PRN"为治疗方案，放入引号内防止误读。③ "…at week 1, month 1 and 3 for BCVA, central macula thickness（CMT），macular volume and the rupture length of ellipsoid zone"："at week 1, month 1" 分属不同的时间段，用 "，" 分隔，而 "month 1 and 3" 具有同类时间属性，故用 and 连接，不用符号分隔。此外，本句介词 for 的后面为并列关系，不同概念之间用 "，" 分隔。必须注意的是，汉语中用 "、" 分隔，而英文用 "，" 替代汉语中的 "、"。④英文中使用的括号有 "（ ）" 和 "[ ]" 两种形式。当多个信息组合，需要选用上述两种括号表示时，国内外期刊使用习惯是有区别的，如 "…in the analysis segment（0.68 [0.60] *vs.* 1.0 [0.61] mm; *P*<0.001）"（国外期刊首先用半圆括号 "（ ）"，再用方括号和 "[ ]"，而国内期刊则表示为："…stent group [（10±3）d *vs.*（13±4）d, RR, 1.5（95% CI, 1.0-2.2）；*P*=0 .07]"。

例二： This review considers areas of key educational need, including the clinical characteristics of COPD; factors that contribute to the disease, effective diagnosis, and clinical management of patients; and the implementation of treatment guidelines.

本综述关注的是重点培训需求，包括 COPD 的临床特征；导致该疾病的因素、有效诊断和患者的临床治疗，以及如何贯彻治疗指南。

【析】本句中 "the clinical characteristics of COPD; factors that contribute to the disease, effective diagnosis, and clinical management of patients; and the implementation of treatment guidelines" 为 including 的并列宾语成分，所以用分号 "；" 表示并列关系。英文摘要中使用 "；" 表示并列关系的其他场合：①表示并列关系的统计结果，如 "hazard ratio, 0.82；95% CI, 0.68 to 0.98；*P*=0.03"；②表示组间同一指标比较，如 "pressure of less than 140 mm Hg (usual control; *n*=553) or less than 130 mm Hg (tight control; *n*=558)."。

例三： Patients were divided into 4 groups based on stent type and self-reported clopidogrel use: DES with clopidogrel, DES without clopidogrel, BMS with clopidogrel, and BMS without clopidogrel.

根据支架类型和自行报告的氯吡格雷使用情况，将患者分为 4 组：DES 与氯吡格雷、DES 无氯吡格雷、BMS 与氯吡格雷、BMS 无氯吡格雷。

【析】本句 "clopidogrel use" 后使用冒号 "："，对前文 "4 groups" 做出列举，为同位关系，又如 "Lifestyle modification advice by health care providers included: Increase physical activity/exercise, reduce dietary fat/calories, control/lose weight, and all of the above." 及 "confidence interval: 21 to 28"。另外，主标题和副标题之间也应使用冒号 "："，如 "Treatment of Chronic

Obstructive Pulmonary Disease in the Primary Care Setting: How Can We Achieve More for Our Patients?"

另外需要注意的是，使用逗号"，"时，如果句子中遇有数字，如"As of September 1257 people were discharged."，这样书写会因标点符号位置不当导致错误理解，因此，主句中的数字应采用完整表达。本句可改写为 "As of September 1, two hundred and fifty-seven people were discharged."。

十三、量、单位与符号

为了统一规范，准确传递信息，医学论文写作中所使用的量、单位与符号必须正确书写，符合相关标准和规定。在我国，法定单位由两部分组成，一是国际单位制（The International System of Units，SI）；二是我国选定的非 SI 单位。量是指用尺、容器或其他作为标准的东西来确定事物的长短、大小、多少或其他性质，如时间、速度、长度、温度、浓度、热量、波长、面积等；所谓单位，是指计量事物的标准量的名称，如厘米为计算长度的单位，克为计算质量的单位；符号则为标记。本节 SI 基本单位等引用自《国际单位制及其应用》（GB 3100—93），主要罗列了与医学密切相关的单位表示法。超出本文引用的其他表示法，读者可参考该标准执行。

（一）SI 基本单位

SI 基本单位见表 9-1。

表 9-1 SI 基本单位

量的名称	单位名称	单位符号
长度	米	m
质量	千克（公斤）	kg
时间	秒	s
电流	安［培］	A
热力学温度	开［尔文］	K
物质的量	摩［尔］	mol
发光强度	坎［德拉］	cd

资料来源：节选自《国际单位制及其应用》（GB 3100—93）。

注：本表中圆括号表示同义关系，即括号内的名称与前面的名称可以互换；方括号表示省略关系，即：书写时可以省略方括号内的词。下表同。

（二）具有专门名称的 SI 导出单位

具有专门名称的 SI 导出单位见表 9-2。

表 9-2　具有专门名称的 SI 导出单位

量的名称	单位名称	单位符号	用 SI 导出单位式例
［平面］角	弧度	rad	
立体角	球面度	sr	
频率	赫［兹］	Hz	s^{-1}
力	牛［顿］	N	$Kg \cdot m/s^2$
压力，压强，应力	帕［斯卡］	Pa	N/m^2
能［量］，功，热量	焦［耳］	J	$N \cdot m$
功［率］，辐［射能］通量	瓦［特］	W	J/s
电荷［量］	库［仑］	C	$A \cdot s$
电压，电动势，电位（电势）	伏［特］	V	W/A
电容	法［拉］	F	C/A
电阻	欧［姆］	Ω	V/A
电导	西［门子］	S	A/V
磁通［量］	韦［伯］	Wb	$V \cdot s$
磁通［量］密度，磁感应强度	特［斯拉］	T	Wb/m^2
电感	亨［利］	H	Wb/A
摄氏温度	摄氏度	℃	K
光通量	流［明］	lm	$cd \cdot sr$
［光］照度	勒［克斯］	lx	Lm/m^2
［放射性］活度	贝可［勒尔］	Bq	s^{-1}
吸收剂量，比授［予］能，比释动能	戈［瑞］	Gy	J/kg
剂量当量	希［沃特］	Sv	J/kg

资料来源：节选自《国际单位制及其应用》（GB 3100—93）。

（三）GB 3100—93 选定的与国际单位制并用的非 SI 单位

GB 3100—93 选定的与国际单位制并用的非 SI 单位见表 9-3。

表 9-3　GB 3100—93 选定的与国际单位制并用的非 SI 单位

量的名称	单位名称	单位符号	与 SI 单位的关系
时间	分	min	1 min = 60 s
	［小］时	h	1 h = 60 min = 3 600 s
	日，（天）	d	1 d = 24 h = 86 400 s
［平面］角	［角］秒	″	$1'' = (\pi/648\,000)rad$
	［角］分	′	$1' = 60'' = (\pi/10\,8000)rad$
	度	°	$1° = 60' = (\pi/180)rad$

续表

量的名称	单位名称	单位符号	与 SI 单位的关系
旋转速度	转每分	r/min	1 r/min = (1/60) s^{-1}
质量	吨 质子质量单位	t u	1 t =10^{3}kg 1 u ≈ 1.660 540×10^{-27}kg
体积	升	l, L	1L=1 dm^3 = 10^{-3} m^3
级差	分贝	dB	

注:《国际单位制及其应用》(GB 3100—93)共规定了 16 个非 SI 单位。本表仅选用的是与医学写作相关的单位。

(四)常用单位、量符号的书写

1. 斜体字母

量的符号必须使用斜体字母,只有 pH 例外。此外,符号后不加缩写点,句末例外。如 m(质量)、t(时间)、V(体积)。同时还应注意某些希腊字母与拉丁字母(或英文)的区别。

2. 正体字母

单位符号应采用正体字母书写,但要注意区分单位符号的大小写。总体上,一般单位符号采用小写体,来源于人名的单位,首字母应大写。例如:m(米),kg(千克);J(焦),Wb(韦)等。此外,SI 的词头符号也用正体,它与单位之间不留空隙。词头符号与与之紧紧相连的单个符号就构成了一个新的单位符号。

3. 统计学符号的使用

按国家标准《统计学名词及符号》(GB3358—82)的规定,样本的算术平均数用小写 $\bar{x}$,不用大写 X 或 M。标准差用 s,不用 SD。标准误用 $S\bar{x}$,不用 SE;t 检验用小写 t;F 检验用大写 F;卡方检验用希腊文小写 χ^2;相关系数用英文小写 r;自由度用希腊文小写 υ;样本数用英文小写 n;相对危险度用 OR;概率用大写 P。

4. 组合单位的符号

每一组合单位符号中,斜线不得多于 1 条。例如,每天每公斤体重用药剂量 20 mg 应写成 20 mg/(kg·d),不能写作 20 mg/kg/d,否则会引起歧义。

5. 下标符号

量符号下标的书写形式需要注意两点。一是使用标准化的下标符号,如 E_R(辐射能),切不可写成 $E_辐$。二是注意下标符号的正体或斜体书写。通常遵循的原则:表示物理量时用斜体下标,如 R_m(磁阻),其他则用正体下标,如 C_p(p:压力)。另外,写作时,还有可能使用复合下标,如 $R_{m, max}$,(m 代表 magnetic,max 为 maximum 的缩写)。因为复合下标至少表示两个内容，所以容易引起混淆。对于这个问题，没有相关标准做出特殊规定，而且也不便于规定。作者若遇到此类情况，建议参阅拟投稿杂志的编辑体例。

6. 数值（量值）范围符号

按国标相关规定，表示数值范围时采用波纹线"～"。需要注意的是，中文文本中可以采用波纹线，而英文文本中则应采用短破折号（–en dash），如 CI: 7.9 – 9.8。

7. 参量与其公差

表达参量与其公差时，均应附带单位说明。当参量与其公差的单位相同时，单位符号可以只写 1 次，如 10.0 mm ± 0.3 mm 可以写作 (10.0 ± 0.3) mm，但不能表示为 10.0 ± 0.3 mm。但如果附带单位的量值相乘表示面积或体积时，应一一标出每个量值的单位。如表示（移植）皮瓣的面积 6 × 4 cm 或 6 × 4 cm^2，则为错误的书写方法，正确的写法是 6 cm × 4 cm。

8. 部分废弃的量名称

对于无法确定的或部分废弃的量名称的表示（规范标注），请参考国家标准 GB3100—3102-93 或参考投稿期刊要求执行。

9. 其他书写问题

常用量和单位的书写，不仅要符合标准规范，同时也要满足期刊编辑体例，如表示"5 天"，无论是在图表还是在数字叙述中，标准书写为 5 d，非标准往往写为 5 days. 但在正文文字或句首中应写作 five/Five days. 类似的写法还包括年、月、周等。

十四、练　习

9-1　按照要求完成下列练习

1. 用 it 作形式主语改写

To consider LIS in the diagnosis of developmental delay as many patients may be diagnosed as cerebral palsy is important.

2. 用分词改写画线部分，并注意逻辑结构

Lissencephaly ("smooth brain," from "lissos, " meaning smooth, and "encephalos, " meaning brain) is a severe developmental disorder in which neuronal migration is impaired, <u>and leads to a thickened cerebral cortex whose normally folded contour is simplified and smooth.</u>

3. 找出句子中错用的分词形式，并改正

One-year-old boy, presenting to Pediatric Neurology Clinic of a tertiary care hospital with myoclonic seizures from 4-month of age, 10-40 episodes/day with gross developmental delay, hearing impairment and excessive weight gain.

4. 找出句子中主谓不一致，并改正

These results, together with our earlier observations (40), indicates that Bid is activated during renal ischemia-reperfusion.

5. 找出句子中误用的关系代词，并改正

Most authorities consider hyperuricemia in metabolic syndrome to be the consequence of elevated serum insulin levels, what have been shown to stimulate renal reabsorption of uric acid.

6. 用平行结构改写

For two years, IMPACT patients were less depressed, they functioned better physically and they enjoyed a better quality of life, and were more satisfied with their depression care.

7. 找出错误并改正

It is known that approximately two thirds of the DMD cases is familial and only one third are sporadic.

8. 找出错误并改正

The number of instances in which the warning from the case report were incorporated into the product information.

9. 找出错误并改正

Data from controlled studies that supported the postulated link between the drug and the adverse event was available in only three cases.

10. 找出错误并改正

To determine what individual case reports fulfilled their role as early warning signals that stimulated more detailed studies we used two methods to establish whether such additional validation studies had been carried out.

11. 略去句子中的冗词，使之简洁

This study is for the purpose to aim at representing the experience of a tertiary care center in Saudi Arabia on non-cystic fibrosis bronchiectasis.

12. 利用多数值表达法改写句子中相关结构，使之成为平行结构

A total of 151 cases were diagnosed as Non-CF bronchiectasis. Seventy-five were males and they accounted for 49.7%, 76 were females, which was 50.3%. One hundred forty-eight, the percentage bei ng 98%, are alive and 3 died with a percentage of 2%.

13. 按平行结构改写

The result of vitamin D supplement was good in mere 12%, satisfactory in 38%, and 50% had the unsatisfactory result of it.

14. 修改该句，使之结构平衡

A 8-year follow-up investigation on a case of chronic myeloid leukemia diagnosed in 2002 in a man of 18 years of age is reported.

15. 修改该句，使之结构平衡

Data which suggest that sudden-death ischemic heart disease may be due to hypomagnesaemia in and around the coronary arterial and arteriolar vessels will be presented.

9-2　将下列句子加上标点符号

1. The most common presentation comprised cough suppurative bronchitis and hemoptysis with one case of massive hemoptysis in all cases the delay between appearance of symptoms discovery of the cyst and operation varied from a few hours to 6 years mean 2 years and 2 months

2. In the first case calcified hydatid cyst of left-lower lobe was erroneously reported Figure-1

3. Ten patients recovered neurologically within 2 weeks to 8 months but others continued to have residual weakness or cerebral symptoms

4. The patients were divided into three groups normal weight mildly obese and markedly obsess

5. The median age of the patients was 54 years 61 patients were females

6. 45 306 men aged 45-79 years and without a history of cancer completed a food-frequency questionnaire in 1997

9-3　根据语境，在下列句子中填上适当的名词形式（单、复数）

1. _____(level) of interleukin (IL)-6 in the bronchoalveolar lavage (BAL) fluid were an independent predictor of mortality. Thus, IL-6 _____(level) in BAL fluid and serum CRP _____(level) may be used to guide appropriate management of pulmonary problems in immunocompromised patients.

2. This inhibitory response was sustained at higher dose _____(level) of 50-100 $\mu g \cdot kg^{-1} \cdot day^{-1}$.

3. For example, while _____(death) from respiratory disease accounted for 13% of all deaths in England and Wales in 2002, funding for respiratory research claimed only 2.8%.

4. Based on the symptoms and ECG_____(finding) a diagnosis of LQTS was made and the child was started on oral propranolol.

5. _____at referral to our center was 6.3 ± 4 years.

6. The commonly used formulation is a racemic mixture that contains equal_____(amount) of both R and S isomers.

7. These results suggest that 0.31 mg LEV should be the starting_____(dose) in children 4-11 years as compared to adults

8. It has been shown to improve_____(survival) when given continuously and there are strict guidelines for its use.

9. If the subject's tidal volume fell below 8 ml/kg or rose above 15 ml/kg body_____(weight), he/she was asked to increase or decrease the tidal volume respectively.

10. Low birth _____(weight) was an important risk factor for the development of ARF.

11. Higher＿＿＿＿＿＿＿＿＿＿(dose) of JB3 produced no further reduction in kidney wet weight demonstrating that 10 μg•kg^{-1}•day^{-1} was a maximal＿＿＿＿＿＿＿＿＿＿(dose).

12. In males from other strains and all female mice, body＿＿＿＿＿＿＿＿＿＿(weight) increased during the course of the experiments and were similar between diabetic and control animals.

13. However, since depression is chronic and recurrent, and many patients experience residual symptoms and＿＿＿＿＿＿＿＿＿＿(relapse), understanding the long term effects of collaborative care is important.

14. DQs were used in comparing patient＿＿＿＿＿＿＿＿＿＿(group) with and without a given MRI abnormality.

15. The mean lactate＿＿＿＿＿＿＿＿＿＿(concentration) confirm that subjects had a moderately high intensity of muscle effort.

9-4　请英译下列短语

1. 血管经皮冠状动脉介入治疗
2. 住院死亡率
3. 早期肾功能不全
4. 前瞻性病例对照研究
5. 血清总胆红素水平
6. 冠脉旁路移植手术
7. 左室舒张末期压
8. 内镜黏膜下层剥离术
9. 口服葡萄糖耐量
10. 高血清脂联素浓度
11. 直肠癌筛检计划
12. 肠易激综合征
13. 获得性免疫缺陷综合征患者
14. 慢性乙型肝炎患者
15. 血小板反应性
16. 五年存活率
17. 平均动脉压
18. 空腹胰岛素水平
19. 手术并发症发生率
20. 癌胚抗原

第十章 英文摘要汉译英的原则与方法

一、医学论文英文摘要的文体特征

所谓文体（style），是指"the typical way that someone uses words to express ideas, tell stories, etc."。与其他科技英语一样，医学论文英文摘要作为科技论文的一个重要组成部分，亦有其自身文体上的典型特征，即学术性、科学性、客观性；格式规范；所使用的语言要清晰、准确、精练、严密、客观。

二、翻译的实质

翻译就是转换承载信息的语言，将一种语言所承载的信息用另一种语言表达出来。通过两种语言的转换达到信息交流的目的。翻译在社会、经济、文化和科技的发展中起着重要的作用。但是，要做好翻译工作并非一件容易的事情。我国英文学习者通常总误以为，只要掌握了源语和译语两种语言的语法规则和足够的词汇量，就能从事翻译工作，然而事实并非如此。因为科技内容的翻译不仅涉及专业知识，还需要精通语法知识，同时还应具备较好的修辞和逻辑基础知识。

翻译过程改变的只是语言体系，保持不变的应是话语信息内容。翻译又有别于创作。鉴于原文和译文两种语言体系之间客观存在的差异因素，虽难以达到绝对等值，但翻译过程中应摆脱原作语言结构的约束，依靠语言环境，寻求最佳方案，避免差异过大，尽可能等值地传递原文话语信息，即不随意删改和增减原文信息内容。

三、英文摘要翻译标准

翻译是原著的再现。原著是意义内容、话语风格和语言表达的统一体，译文要如实地再现这个完整的统一体。医学是与人类健康最为密切的一门科学，文字表达具有较强的严密性，翻译过程中若稍有差池，必会对人类健康造成严重影响，甚至威胁人类生命安全。因此，医学翻译，包括医学论文摘要翻译必须遵循"忠实明确、简练通畅"的原则。"忠实明确"就是要求译者明白无误地表达原文的含义，不能随意增、减原文内容；

"简练通畅"则是满足"摘要"语篇要求。因为"摘要"不仅是一篇高度浓缩、独立的短文，同时还应通畅地传递完整信息。因此，译文语言表达应该通顺易懂，符合语言规范。例如：

【结果】手术时间 90～246 min，平均 135 min。切除前列腺重量平均 63.6 g。术后平均留置管时间 4.5 d，术后平均住院时间 5 d。术后 3 个月随访，最大尿流率（Q_{max}）由术前（6.3±1.6）ml/s 显著上升为（16.1±5.0）ml/s，国际前列腺症状评分（IPSS）由术前（29.8±1.2）分降至（7.3±1.0）分，生活质量评分（QOL）由术前（5.2±0.8）分降至（1.8±0.5）分，剩余尿（RUV）由术前（150.0±68.0）ml 降至（40.0±20.6）ml（$P < 0.01$）。"

【Results】Duration of the procedure ranged from 90 to 246 min with an average of 135 min, and the prostate removed measured 63.6 g averagely. Postoperative catheter maintenance was 4.5 d on average and hospital stay 5 d. Three consecutive months of follow-up suggested that Q_{max} was elevated from （6.3±1.6） ml/s to （16.1±5.0）ml/s, whereas scores for IPSS, and QOL were reduced（29.8±1.2 *vs.* 7.3±1.0 for the former; 5.2±0.8 *vs.* 1.8±0.5 for the latter, respectively），and RUV was also decreased from 150.0±68.0 ml to 40.0±20.6 ml, which had significantly statistical difference （$P<0.01$）.

英文完整、流畅地再现了原文信息。

四、英文摘要翻译方法

翻译方法是由于采用不同的翻译单位，侧重于不同的翻译标准而形成的处理译文的方法。对于医学论文摘要的英译，在上述翻译原则框架内，大体上可采用直译和意译两类方法，综合两类翻译方法的优点就形成等值翻译。

1. 直译

汉语是分析型语言，语序固定，句子的语法关系完全通过词汇、词序、句法手段来表达。因此，直译在翻译单位方面是在较低层次上的翻译，以语言形式共性为基础，在保持原文表达形式及内容的同时，将原文内容依据其表达形式用英文对应表述出来。这里所指的表达形式包括词序、语序、语气、结构、修辞等。例如：

例一：MRI 是诊断肝脏血管平滑肌脂肪瘤的主要方法。

MRI is the main diagnostic means of hepatic angiomyolipoma.

例二：在 8 年随访中，3069 例慢性肾病患者仅有 38 例进展为终末期肾病。

During the eight year follow-up, only 38 of the 3069 patients with chronic kidney disease progressed to end stage renal disease.

例三：胃十二指肠溃疡或上消化道出血发生风险在使用螺内酯的患者中明显增加。

The risk of gastroduodenal ulcers or upper gastrointestinal bleeding is significantly increased in patients using spironolactone.

例四：探讨对伴有乳头溢液的乳腺癌采取保乳手术治疗的可行性。

To investigate the feasibility of breast conserving treatment in breast cancer patients with nipple discharge.

例五： 雌螨，体卵圆形，淡黄色。躯体长（颚体前端至躯体后缘）约 278.3μm，宽约 169.3μm。颚体小，几乎为前足体覆盖，但颚体结构可见。

The female body looks nearly ovoid in pale yellow, and measures (from the anterior gnathosoma to the posterior margin of the body) about 278.3 μm in length and 169.3 μm in width. Gnathosoma is small, and mostly fused with the propodosoma, yet the contour of gnathosoma is still identifiable.

直译之所以成为可能，是因为中文的基本句型框架结构和英文的基本句型基本对应。直译的过程可以分为理解中文和表达英文两大步骤。所谓理解中文，是指理解汉语句子的框架结构；表达过程就是利用源语和译入语之间的语序"形似"，用译语再现出来。然而，我国学习者中有相当一部分人在汉语和英语语法知识方面基础非常薄弱，通常在翻译时无所适从。其实，建议将复杂问题简洁化，因为，无论是汉语还是英语，其主干结构上势必存在一定的相似性，如中文基本框架"谁做/怎么了？"＝主语（谁）＋谓语（做）＝英文句型"S+V"（主+谓）；"谁？做什么"＝主语（谁）＋谓语动词（做）＋宾语（什么）＝英文句型"S+V+O"；"谁让某人做某事"＝主语（谁）＋谓语动词（让）＋宾语（某人）＋宾语补语（某事）＝英文句型"S+V（cause）+O（sb）+C（to do sth.）"。例如：

例一： 5 例死亡。

Five patients died.

【析】中文句的结构为"谁（5 例），怎么了（死亡）？"，采用对应的英文结构"S（Five patients）+V（died）（英语使用不及物动词）"。

例二： 咬肌中肌细胞凋亡数量显著增加。

The number of apoptotic myocytes was significantly increased in masseter muscle.

【析】中文句"谁（肌细胞凋亡数量），怎么了（增加）？"，采用对应的英文结构"S（The number of apoptotic myocytes）+V（was significantly increased）（英语使用 be 动词）"。

例三： 4 例有实性组织病变者均行病理检查。

Four patients with solid tissue lesion received pathological examination.

【析】中文结构为"谁？做什么"，等同英文结构"S（Four patients with solid tissue lesion）+V（received）+O（pathological examination）"。

例四： 子宫肌瘤挖除术对患者卵巢功能无影响。

Myomectomy doesn't influence the ovary function.

【析】该结构同上，其对应关系为"S（Myomectomy）+V（doesn't influence）+O（the ovary function）"。

然而，语言是有民族特点的。两种语言单位不可能一一对应，如修饰语等。过分追求形式一致，则会忽略信息的等值。例如：本组患者年龄为 25 至 50 周岁。"The ages in this group ranged from 25 to 50 years of age."，应改为："The ages in this group ranged from 25 to 50. "。

2. 意译

意译在翻译单位方面是在较高层次上的翻译。所谓意译，是将原文所表达的内容采用释义手段，通过译语将其意义表达出来。它通常把句子、话语作为翻译单位，而不考虑词序、词语、语序、语法结构等方面的对应。这是因为，汉语和英语属于两种不同的语系，在语言结构上存在诸多差异，如汉语词序比较固定，而英语则相对自由；汉语较少使用被动结构，而英语为了突出客观事物，则广泛使用被动结构；无论修饰语多长，汉语采用前位修饰，而英语则采用后位修饰；在时间表示上，汉语无动词形态变化，仅通过时间副词呈现，而英语则采用不同的动词形式体现时间关系等。总而言之，意译侧重于译语通顺，用译语的习惯表达方式将原文的真实内容和话语风格翻译出来。因为，在某些情况下，如果将中文摘要逐字硬性对译为英文，必会造成英文摘要措辞累赘冗长、重复，甚至费解。试比较下述例句。

例一：男性包皮环切术有手术切除和器械切除两种。

译文一：Male circumcision has two methods—surgery and device.

译文二：Male circumcision is available either by conventional surgery or circumcision device.

【析】显然，译文一采用对等直译，结果导致重要信息丧失。而译文二采用意译，将原文的意义忠实、通顺地表达出来。

例二：病理诊断为血管外皮细胞瘤。

译文一：The pathologic diagnosis was hemangiopericytoma.

译文二：Hemangiopericytoma was diagnosed pathologically.

【析】上述两种译文中，译文一采用直译，导致逻辑不通。译文二使用意译，完全脱离了原文限制。即结构上，原文为主动式，译文为被动式；词语上，原文"病理诊断"为偏正结构的名词词组，译文中改为了动词表达。

例三：按年级进行分层后，整群抽取某医学院在校大一、大二、大三学生共 3738 名。本次问卷调查量表包括网络成瘾量表，抑郁量表（SDS）和焦虑量表（SAS）。

译文一：After stratified sampling by grades, a total of 3738 students from the first, second and third year of students in a medical college were recruited. The questioonnair consisted of Internet Addiction Scale, Self-rating Depression Scale (SDS) and Self-rating Anxiety Scale (SAS).

译文二：By stratified sampling method, a total of 3738 subjects were recruited from the first, second and third year of students in a medical college, and subjected to the questionnaire survey using Internet Addiction Scale, Self-rating

Depression Scale (SDS) and Self-rating Anxiety Scale (SAS).

【析】上述两种译文中，译文一完全按照对等法，虽然能呈现对等信息，但译文逻辑关系松散；而译文二，突破了原文的结构，采用意译，实现了动态等值信息传递，译文也更流畅，逻辑更严谨。

例四：虽然有报道证明耐力训练（ET）能保持心功能，但有证据表明，ET 由于白蛋白诱导的血浆容量扩张而增加左心室（LV）内径增大。

译文：Although endurance training (ET) has been reported to preserve cardiac function, evidence suggests that Et increases left ventricle (LV) interior dimensions as a result of albumin-induced plasma expansion.

【析】本句采用的是意译，完整再现原文信息。①英文中省略了"但是"。虽然汉语"虽然…但是…"为连用的连接词语，但英语"although 和 but"不可连用；②"虽然有报道证明耐力训练（ET）能保持心功能"为主动结构，英译时采用的是被动结构。

无论是直译还是意译，均有其优劣。最佳的翻译方法是糅合两者的优点，寻求等值翻译。所谓等值（equivalent），就是翻译时根据需要，灵活采用各个层次的翻译单位，全面达到翻译标准，动态地再现原文信息和话语风格，使译文语言表达既能内顾词语对应，又能外顾话语协调，从而实现准确的信息传递、保持原文风格、语言通畅自然，合乎译语规范，最终满足医学论文英文摘要的专业性、客观性和精练性要求。

3. 词汇的选择

用词要忠实于原文，弄懂汉语词汇和所用英文词汇的真正、准确含义。翻译时，要注意汉英词汇在其广义、狭义、具体意义、抽象意义等方面的差异，尤其在特定语境中，词的搭配意义。

例一：5 个月后，患者出现眼眶及眼睑水肿。

After 5 months the patient **appeared** orbital and eyelid edema.

【析】本例中，"出现"使用了"appear"。尽管 "appear"在英文中有"to become visible；come into existence"之意，但使用"appear"，语义关系不当，应改为"After 5 months the patient **developed** orbital and eyelid edema. "。

例二：为了评价两位医师读片的变异性，采用 Kappa 统计评价两位医师之间判定的一致性。

To determine the film **reading** difference between the two radiologists, we conducted the measurement of inter-rater agreement with the Cohen's kappa statistics.

【析】"Reading"在英文中的意思是"The act or activity of one that reads"。按本句语境，句中的"读片"所提示的意义为"对某种客观存在的事实做出诠释"。故应改为"To determine the film **interpretation** differences between the two radiologists, we conducted the measurement of inter-rater agreement with the Cohen's kappa statistics."。

汉语和英语的语言中，一词多义的现象较多。翻译时，若逐字硬译，不考虑英文的真正含义，势必造成读者无法理解你的译文。因此，在满足特定语境前提下，有时候可有更灵活的选择。例如：

例三：活检组织结果表明这是一种罕见的恶性病变。

The results of a biopsy indicated a rare malignant condition/lesion/case.

【析】中文"病变"对应的英文可选词有 condition, lesion 或 case。

例四：采用免疫法测定血清 cystatin C。

Plasma cystatin C was measured/determined/detected using an immunonephelometry method.

【析】中文"测定"对应的可选词：measure、determine 或 detect。

例五：评价慢性阻塞性肺疾病急性加重期部分生物标志物在抗菌治疗中的表达。

To observe the expression of biomarkers in antimicrobial treatment of chronic obstructive pulmonary disease(COPD) during acute exacerbation.

【析】原句中的动词"评价"所搭配的概念是"表达"，如果我们直接使用对等英文动词 evaluate 或 assess，显然违背概念意义，因此，选择动词 observe 或 investigate 就更为妥当。这种情况在结构式摘要中的"目的"句十分常见。

例六：探讨超声内镜引导下细针穿刺活检术（EUS-FNA）鉴别胰腺囊性病变良恶性的价值。

To assess the value of endoscopic ultrasound guided-fine needle aspiration (EUS-FNA) in differential diagnosis of benign or malignant pancreatic cystic lesions.

【析】该句中"探讨"搭配的概念名词是"价值"，如果对等选择相应的英语动词，如"investigate、explore"等，即会导致概念搭配不当。

4. 词义的引申

语言的意义总分为词汇意义、语法意义和修辞意义三大类。词汇意义是表示客体的理性意义，语法意义表示客体之间、词语之间关系的意义。修辞意义则表示主体对客体的感情评价意义。这三种意义相互关系密切，构成整个语言的语义体系。一方面，词汇意义有其客观性、概括性和相关性等。无论是何种语言，日常所使用的词，大部分都有几个，甚至几十个意义，如"疾病"，就高度概括了与之相关的各种身体任何部分、器官和（或）系统的结构或功能的偏离正常或停止，表现为颇具特征性的症状及体征，可以表示普通感冒、精神性障碍、机体器官的恶性病变等。而英语中与疾病相关的词汇有 disease、sickness、illness、disorder、suffering、condition、malady、ailment 等。另一方面，词义的任务是表达事物，而每一事物又有其特点，这些特点就通常反映在本义中。本义有了这些特点，即产生出不同的引申义（extended meaning of words）。这犹如一个车轮，轮毂代表本义，引申义就是轮辐。

众所周知，翻译就是把原来用甲语言表达的信息改用乙语言来表达，使不懂甲语言者也能获得同样的信息，为了实现信息传递达到等效的效果，英译时，对某些词的处理，不应拘泥于词的字面意义或词典提供的语义、释义，而应按具体语境对特定的词进行引申，翻译出其隐含意义，从而使词义更加具体化。

（1）抽象化引申（**from specific to general/abstract**）：将比较具体形象的词译成该形象所代表的属性或概念的词。这种引申手段应用于汉译英时，是为了使译文更"雅"，使译文增色，因而亦可称为修辞性引申。例如：

例一：短期效果评价指标为完整的程序电刺激和住院结果。

> Short-term efficacy was defined by a complete **protocol** of programmed electric stimulation and by in-hospital outcome.

【析】中文词"结果"用具有概括意义的 protocol 代表。

例二：对 110 名最佳矫正视力≥20/40 的戴镜矫正老视患者进行横断面调查，所采用的为标准有效的时间权衡效用分析调查问卷。

> One hundred and ten patients with spectacle-corrected presbyopia and a best-corrected visual acuity of 20/40 or better were interviewed in a cross-sectional fashion using a standardized, validated, time trade-off utility analysis questionnaire.

【析】中文词"调查"用比较笼统的词 fashion 代表。

例三：160 例平均年龄为（50±5）岁的男性患者，在心肌梗死后 3～18 周进行了一系列的运动试验。

> One hundred and sixty men with a mean age of （50±5）years underwent serial exercise testing 3 to 18 weeks after myocardial fraction.

【析】"男性患者"为比较具体的词，用比较概括性的词 men 替代。

例四：60 例患者因感染性心内膜炎并发症而接受心脏瓣膜置换术。

> Sixty candidates underwent cardiac valve replacement because of complications of infective endocarditis.

【析】用比较概括的词 candidate 表达汉语中具体的词"患者"。

例五：本研究旨观察在人狭窄的主动脉瓣上植入开伞支架的效果。

> This study was designed to study the behavior of a stent deployed inside human stenotic aortic valves.

【析】用比较虚的词 behavior 表示汉语中比较实的词"效果"。

例六：急性病毒性传染病中，狂犬病是第一位致死性疾病。

> Rabies is the first killer of the acute virus infectious disease.

【析】用 killer 代表汉语词"致死性疾病"实现修辞效果。

例七：全直肠系膜切除术治疗老年直肠癌既有利，又有弊。

> Total mesorectal excision for rectal cancer in elderly patients is another mixed blessing.

【析】用"mixed blessing"表示"既有利，又有弊"，具有高度概括性，从而使得表达更为精练。

（2）**具体化引申（from general to specification）**：有时候，原文中用代表抽象概念或属性的词来表示一种具体事物，这些词在特定的语境中，含义是清楚的，但译成英文时，还需要做具体化引申，从而避免译文概念不清或过于笼统。例如：

例一：观察急性心肌缺血再灌注后 VCAM-1 在心肌组织中表达的规律，探讨急性心性猝死的诊断指标。

To **establish the diagnostic criteria** for sudden cardiac death by examining the regular pattern of VCAM-1 expression in acute ischemia-reperfusion myocardium.

【析】"探讨"在本句特定语境中与其宾语搭配后，具有明确的概念，应用具体的词 establish，而不能使用 investigate。这种引申方式在摘要"目的"句中尤为多见。

例二：探讨唑来膦酸联合化疗治疗肿瘤骨转移性疼痛的近期疗效及安全性。

To **observe** the short-term effect and safety of combined zoledronic acid with chemotherapy in treatment of cancer patients with pain resulted from bone metastasis.

【析】"探讨"隐含意义为 observe 或 evaluate。

例三：编码 CYP 酶的蛋白具有多态性。

The **genes** encoding CYP enzymes are polymorphic.

【析】用更具体的词 gene。

例四：细菌菌群构成失衡——生态失调——被认为是导致人类疾病如炎症性肠病的主要因素。

Imbalances in the composition of the bacterial microbiota, known as dysbiosis, are postulated to be a major factor in human **disorders** such as inflammatory bowel disease.

【析】用 disorders 表达更加具体的概念，同时也符合语境所隐含的含义。

例五：我们认为，在非炎症性和动脉硬化病变中，趋化因子介导的信号能精密地确定血液及骨髓中单核细胞的频率。

We show that chemokine-mediated signals critically determine the frequency of monocytes in the blood and bone marrow under both noninflammatory and atherosclerotic **conditions**.

【析】根据语境，本句中的"病变"显然提示的是一种状态，用 condition 更加具体。

5. 词性转换

汉语和英语不仅在语言结构与表达方式方面不同，在词性方面也存在较大差异。为了使译文流畅、通顺自然，符合英文表达习惯，汉译英时，可根据句法结构需要，对某些词类进行适当的转换，即将汉语中的某一词类转换成英语的另一词类。

（1）名词转译为动词

例一：按组织学定义我们将宿主表型分为生理性食管炎，或 Barrett's 食管（肠上皮化生）。

Host phenotypes **were** histologically **defined as** normal, esophagitis, or Barrett's esophagus (intestinal metaplasia).

【析】汉语名词"定义"转译为英语动词 define。

例二：金色葡萄球菌是感染性心内膜炎（IE）最常见的病原菌，具有形成心脏瓣膜血栓及引起远端器官栓塞的特点。

Staphylococcus aureus is the most frequent causative organism of infective endocarditis (IE) and is **characterized** by thrombus formation on a cardiac valve that can embolize to a distant site.

【析】汉语名词"特点"转译为英语动词 characterize。

例三：奥氮平组和安慰剂组均有显著改善，但终点时两组改善幅度没有差异。

Both olanzapine and placebo groups showed significant improvements but did not **differ** in magnitude at end-point.

【析】汉语名词"差异"转译为英语动词 differ。

（2）动词转译为名词

例一：脊柱手术，其他外科手术及各种诊断措施后，患者的疼痛/不适感明显减轻。

The greatest **improvements** after spine surgery, other surgical procedures, and different diagnoses were in the pain/discomfort domain.

【析】汉语动词"减轻"译为英语名词 improvement。

例二：我们观察到 TSC2 和 mTOR 信号通路的频繁缺失证明血管上皮样细胞肿瘤的癌基因谱系（作为一个独特的 TSC2 连接肿瘤）与血管平滑肌脂肪瘤的癌基因谱系相类似。

Our **observations** of frequent deletion of TSC2 and the mTOR signalling pathway provide evidence that the oncogenetic lineage of PEComa, as a distinct TSC2-linked neoplasm, is similar to that of angiomyolipoma.

【析】汉语动词"观察"译为英语名词 observation。

例三：校准多元模型基线特征后，MSCT 成为相对 MPI 具有增量性预后价值的一项独立的（不良）事件预测因子。

After **correction** for baseline characteristics in a multivariate model, MSCT emerged as an independent predictor of events with an incremental prognostic value to MPI.

【析】将汉语动词"校准"转译为英语名词"correction"。

例四：有必要进一步弄清最佳治疗方法。

Further **knowledge** for optimal management are needed.

【析】汉语动词"弄清"译为英语名词 knowledge。

（3）动词转译为形容词

例一： 一旦进入体内，疫苗立即与微金粉分离并被激活。

Once inside the body, the vaccine separates from the gold particles and becomes **active**.

【析】汉语动词"激活"译为英语形容词 active。对于本句，主干部分如果英文采用对应的动词翻译，则会有两种形式，①…the vaccine….and is activated；②…the vaccine…and activates。然而，这两种形式都有问题。"…the vaccine spearates…and is activated"前后语态不一致；"…the vaccine….and activates"，虽然语态一致，但逻辑意义上（即疫苗的免疫机制）出现差错，而采用形容词 active 则完美地再现原文意义。

例二： 与窦律队列患者相比，易发生术后心房颤动的患者能量代谢产物调控失调。

Compared with the SR cohort, the group **susceptible** to post-operative atrial fibrillation showed a discordant regulation of energy metabolites.

【析】汉语动词"发生"译为英语形容词 susceptible。

例三： 夜间给予羟丁酸钠可改善帕金森病患者白天睡眠过多及疲劳症状。

Nocturnally administered sodium oxybate is **conductive** to excessive daytime sleepiness and fatigue in Parkinson disease.

【析】汉语动词"改善"译为英语形容词 conductive。

例四： 研究表明，Kir3.1 通道中的 Phe137 在特非那定介导的抑制中起重要作用。

Our findings suggested that Phe137 in Kir3.1 is **responsible for** the terfenadine-mediated inhibition.

【析】汉语动词"起作用"译为英语形容词 responsible (for)。

（4）动词转译为介词：英语中的介词在古英语中曾是动词。不仅如此，英语中的介词具有极强的搭配能力，所构成的介词短语功能多样，具有极其丰富的表达能力。因此，灵活运用介词可使译文更为简洁。

例一： 使用高分辨率的回波多普勒超声检查测量血管内皮依赖性舒张（功能的改变）。

Endothelium-dependent flow-mediated dilatation was measured **by** high-resolution echo-doppler ultrasonography.

【析】汉语动词"使用"译为英语介词 by。

例二： 现在还没有确切的抗纤维化的方法治疗肝硬化。

There are currently no approved antifibrotic therapies **for** liver cirrhosis.

【析】汉语动词"治疗"译为英语介词 for。

例三： 虽然可以应用抗生素活性对抗肺炎链球菌，但因流行性感冒后继发感染所导致的肺炎仍是发病和死亡率过高的一项主要原因。

Pneumonia occurring as a secondary infection after influenza is a major cause of excess morbidity and mortality, despite the availability and use of antibiotics active **against** Streptococcus pneumoniae.

【析】汉语动词"对抗"译为英语介词 against。

（5）名词转译为形容词

例一：接受这3种治疗方案的患者，如我们所预料，除更多患者在基线时接受的是英夫利昔单抗联合治疗外，其他基线特征没有显著差异。

The baseline characteristics of the patients assigned to the 3 strategies were not significantly **different**, except that, as expected, more patients were receiving combination therapy with infliximab.

【析】汉语名词"差异"译为英语形容词 different。

例二：本文旨在分析最近提出的分类法，并测定何种分类法在临床上有使用价值。

The purpose of this study was to analyze the newly proposed classification and determining which classification was clinically **useful**.

【析】汉语名词短语"使用价值"译为英语形容词 useful。

例三：虽然在对照组 RCA 的血流量收缩期与舒张相似，pH 组收缩期血流存在障碍，并且与右心室压力和体积成正比。

Although in controls, RCA flow is similar in systole and diastole, in PH there is systolic flow impediment, which is **proportional** to right ventricular pressure and mass.

【析】汉语名词"正比"译为英语形容词 proportional。

（6）副词转译为名词

例一：尽管已努力地做了大量研究工作，但该病的病因学和发病机制仍不清楚。

Despite considerable research **effort**, the aetiology and pathogenesis of this condition remains enigmatic.

【析】汉语副词"努力地"译为英语名词 effort。

例二：医生在诊断先天性代谢病时应非常谨慎。

The **diagnosis** of inborn errors of metabolism requires meticulous care on the part of the physicians.

【析】汉语副词"在诊断时"译为英语名词 diagnosis。

（7）副词转译为形容词

例一：突然停药后仍可观察到血压持续降低、血浆肾素活性持续受抑。

After **abrupt** withdrawal, persistent BP reduction and prolonged suppression of plasma renin activity is observed.

【析】汉语副词"突然（地）"译为英语形容词 abrupt。

例二： 共有 2078 例患者纳入本试验，治疗周期平均为 33 个月。

A total of 2078 patients were recruited, and **mean** treatment duration was 33 months.

【析】汉语副词"平均"译为英语形容词 mean。

例三： 患者极其良好地恢复了健康。

The patient made an **excellent** recovery.

【析】汉语副词"极其良好地"译为英语形容词 excellent。

（8）形容词转译为副词

例一： RCA 的收缩期/舒张期流量比，每克右心室组织平均流量与右心室质量呈负相关。

The systolic-to-diastolic flow ratio in the RCA, and mean flow per gram RV tissue, were **inversely related to** RV mass.

【析】汉语形容词"负"修辞名词"相关"，译为英语副词 inversely。需要注意的是，采用此类转译方式时，汉语的名词也应相应地转译为动词。

例二： 转移肿瘤抗原 1 和肝细胞癌患者术后复发、生存率差密切相关。

Metastatic tumor antigen 1 is **closely** associated with frequent postoperative recurrence and poor survival in patients with hepatocellular carcinoma.

【析】汉语形容词"密切"修饰名词"相关"，译为英语副词 closely，同时转译名词"相关"为动词。

例三： 多发性硬化症的主要特征为既有局限也有弥散、不均匀的脊髓损害病灶，造成 MRI 检查结果难与临床相联系。

Multiple sclerosis is **chiefly characterized by** both focal and spatially diffuse spinal cord lesions with heterogeneous pathologies that have limited attempts at linking MRI and behaviour.

【析】汉语形容词"主要"修饰名词"特征"，译为英语副词 chiefly，同时转译名词"特征"为动词。

（9）副词转译为动词

例一： 许多情况下，术后早期心律失常可能与心包炎和儿茶酚胺水平升高有关，且常自行缓解而无须进一步治疗。

In many cases, the arrhythmias that occur early in the postoperative course may be related to pericardial inflammation or increased catecholamine levels and **tend** to resolve without further therapy.

【析】汉语副词"常常"译为英语动词 tend。

例二： 分子仍然紧密地聚集在一起，但不再继续保持有规则的固定排列形式。

The molecules **continue** to stay close together, but do not continue to retain a regular fixed arrangement.

【析】汉语副词"仍然"译为英语动词 continue。

　　从上述各词类转译实例中可以看出，不同词类之间相互转译现象十分普遍，且多种多样。至于一种词类能否转译为另一种词类，关键要注意：①转译后是否满足目的语，即译语的表达规范；②转译后的语言表达是否能满足专业技术的理解；③处理方法不同，也可能有不同的转译方法，翻译时可灵活使用。

　　6. 词的增译

　　汉语是分析型的语言，单音单字。其特点是词基本上无专门表示语法意义的附加成分，没有词形变化，语法关系靠词序和虚词来表示。
　　在翻译中，增译与省译是一对相互排斥的概念。它们在翻译手段的范畴中是两种技巧，互为补充、相辅相成。由于汉英语言在词法、句法和修辞上的差异，在翻译时，若照搬到译文中，就会影响到译文的简洁、忠实、通顺、逻辑关系等。增译就是增加原语中无此类表达的或省略了的词语，使译文更符合目的语的表达规范。

例一：青霉素的作用是不让细菌制造细胞壁。
　　　Penicillin works by not allowing a bacterium to build **its** cell wall.
　　　【析】增加了限定词"its"来限定属性关系。
例二：在为期 12 个月中（止于 2008 年 11 月），围产期死亡率从 3.2%降至了零。
　　　The perinatal mortality rate was reduced from 3.2% to zero in **a** 12 month period ending in November, 2008.
　　　【析】增加了冠词"the"和"a"。汉语中无冠词，而英语却不同。
例三：针对儿童心肌病引的发心衰发生率和后果进行了首次前瞻性、国际性、多中心的研究。
　　　We undertook the first prospective, national, multicenter study to describe the incidence and outcome of heart muscle disease-induced heart failure in children.
　　　【析】增加了代词"we"，达到强调动作实施者的目的。
例四：多数神经循环无力患者不愿接受这种精神疗法。
　　　Most of the patients **with** neuron circulatory asthenia are unwilling to accept psychotherapy as such.
　　　【析】增译了介词"with"。大量使用介词是英语的一大特点，因此，英译时，应按英语句法结构，增加适当的介词。
例五：排除肺栓塞的患者不予抗凝治疗，均随访 3 个月。
　　　Anticoagulants were withheld from patients classified as excluded, **and all patients** were followed up for 3 months.
　　　【析】增译了连词"and"和前置限定词"all"及名词"patients"，从而使得句法结构内部达到连贯一致。
例六：《黄帝内经》确立了中医学的独特理论体系，成为中医学发展的基础。

Yellow Emperor's Canon of Medicine, a collection of the medical achievements and clinical experience before the Spring-Autumn Period and Warring States, has established the unique theory of traditional Chinese medicine and laid the foundation for its development.

【析】增加了说明性的解释语 "a collection of the medical achievements and clinical experience before the Spring-Autumn Period and Warring States"。这种增加说明性词语或表达在中医翻译中十分必要。如果按字面直译，势必会造成外国读者理解上的困难。

例七：本研究系统回顾了贫血类型和促红细胞生成素的治疗作用。

This study **provides** a systematic review of the type of anemia and the effects of erythropoietin therapy.

【析】增译了动词 "provide"。

例八：为了评价两位医师读片的变异性，采用 Kappa 统计评价两位医师之间判定一致性。

To determine the film interpretation differences between the two radiologists, **we** conducted the measurement of inter-rater agreement with the Cohen's kappa statistics.

【析】增译人称代词作主语，使得整个句子具备完整的逻辑结构。

除上述增译实例外，汉译英时，如在名词性从句中增加引导词（that，what 等），或者为了体现英语动词的 "时" 和 "体"，通常采用不同的动词形式（如 have/has/had been/doing 等）来表达目的语的语法概念，这都属于增译手段。

7. 词的省译

例一：采用 Wells 临床评定标准二分法将患者分为 "肺栓塞可能性小" 和 "肺栓塞可能性大" 两组。

Patients were categorized as "pulmonary embolism unlikely" or "pulmonary embolism likely" using a dichotomized version of the Wells clinical decision rule.

【析】省略了汉语词 "两组"。若按对等直译，将 "两组" 用英语 two groups 表示出来，结果就造成重复，这不符合英语简洁原则。

例二：这导致血小板表面 beta-1 和 beta-3 整合素由低亲和状态向高亲和状态变化。

These events lead to the shift of beta-1 and beta-3 integrins on the platelet surface from a low to a high affinity.

【析】省略了汉语名词 "状态"。对于抽象名词，在汉语中，通常与相应的表示其内涵意义的词连用，如作用、过程、现象、状态、能力、方法、形式、术语等，从而使抽象名词具体化，但译成英语时，这些描述性的词均可省略不译，如下例。

例三：甲氨蝶呤和抗肿瘤坏死因子治疗对 19 562 例类风湿关节炎病人患淋巴瘤

风险的影响：89 710 位病人年随访期的观察结果。

The effect of methotrexate and anti-tumor necrosis factor therapy on the risk of lymphoma in rheumatoid arthritis in 19,562 patients during 89,710 person-years of observation.

【析】这是一个标题，英文中省略了汉语名词"结果"。

例四：虽然联合治疗比单一疗法能更大程度地减少蛋白尿，但总的来说它使得主要肾脏后果更为恶化。

Although combination therapy reduces proteinuria to a greater extent than monotherapy, overall it worsens major renal outcomes.

【析】省略翻译连词"但…"。汉语的逻辑关系一般依靠连词来连接，而英语通常借助于句子内部的关联。

例五：（目前）尚不清楚在多大程度上地中海饮食与炎症的相关性是由于遗传或其他家族因素所造成的。

It is unknown to what extent the association between the Mediterranean diet and inflammation is due to genetic or other familial factors.

【析】省略了汉语动词"造成"。

省译的前提是根据英文表达方式和语法修辞习惯，将原语中的某些词省略，如并列结构中的动词，或英文词本身暗含了此类意义，在不改变原意、不会造成读者理解困难的基础上所做出的删减。

8. 数词、量词的译法

医学英语中，数词使用的频率较高，翻译数词本身并不难。但当数字在句子中表达各种概念时，翻译那些表示数量概念的句型结构时，英语和汉语在表达方式上存在一定的差异。若翻译不当，则会造成信息传递出现错误。

（1）小数字直译、大数字换算

例一：作者对 180 例乳腺囊肿患者的 320 例囊液标本做了细胞学检查，结果仅 1 例找到了癌细胞。

A series of 180 patients with breast cysts has provided 320 specimens of cyst fluid for cytological diagnosis. Only one of these specimens was reported positive for malignant cells.

【析】直接用对应的英文表达。

例二：据估计，2003 年因性接触而引发的新病例至少有 330 000 000 起。

It is estimated that at least 330 million new cases of sexually transmitted diseases occurred in 2003.

【析】大数字借助英语中表示大数字的词 thousand、million、billion 来表达。

（2）不定量数字的译法：不定量数字是指那些表示若干、许多、大量、不少、成千上万等概念的词组，如 tens/decades of（数十、几十）等。

例一：心脏介入术后缺血性脑卒中尽管不普遍，但每年可导致成千上万患者死
亡和致残。

Ischemic strokes after cardiac catheterization procedures, although uncommon, lead to the morbidity and mortality of **thousands of** patients each year.

【析】用 thousands of…表达"成千上万"这样不定量数字。

例二：肥胖是世界范围内的普遍现象，它使千百万人变得虚弱，并且在健康花
费上给社会带来上百亿的负担。

Obesity, a global pandemic that debilitates **millions of** people and burdens society with **tens of billions of** dollars in health care costs, is deterred by exercise.

【析】用 millions of…和 tens of billions of…表示"千百万"和"上百亿"。

例三：克罗恩病活动指数（CDAI）低于 150 分的患者随机接受 ω-3 游离脂肪
酸 4 g/d 或安慰剂治疗，为期 58 周。

Patients with a Crohn's Disease Activity Index (CDAI) score of **less than** 150 were randomly assigned to receive either 4 g/d of omega-3 free fatty acids or placebo for **up to** 58 weeks.

【析】表达"超过"、"以上"、"多达"等不定量数字时，在数字前可加英
语词 above、more than、over、up to 或 as…as 结构等来表示。

例四：本研究的目的是调查城市卫生项目对不足 3 岁儿童的腹泻发病率的流行
病学影响。

This study aims to investigate the epidemiological effect of this city-wide sanitation programme on diarrhoea morbidity in children **less than** 3 years of age.

【析】表达"低于"、"以下"、"不足"等不定量数字时，在数字前可加英
语词 below、less than、fewer than、under、within 等来表示。

例五：工作压力对冠心病发病的效应大约有 32%因不健康的生活方式和代谢综
合症所导致。

Around 32% of the effect of work stress on CHD was attributable to its effect on health behaviours and the metabolic syndrome.

【析】表示"大约"、"左右"、"将近"、"接近"等不定量概念时，可用英
语词 about、around、close to、nearly、or so、some、towards、approximately、roughly、more or less、in the neighborhood of 等表示。

（3）量词的翻译：汉语表示人或事物的单位，各有独特的名量词。表示动作的次数，
也各有独特的动量词。而量词经常与数词一起使用。①汉语中表示人和事物单位的名量
词，如果后跟可数名词，用英语表示时无须译出。仅在英语名词前加上不定冠词或数词，
即可表示出汉语的数词和名量词两层意思，如 "一位患者"（a patient），"两个观察组"

（two observational groups）。②汉语中表示人或事物的种类或集体单位时，各有独特的名量词，如种、类、双、套、组、对、群等。在英语中均有表示名量词的可数名词，如"每对股骨"（each pair of femur），"一种手术方式"（a type of operative procedure），"一系列研究"（a series of studies）。③汉语有些名词（如物质名词或抽象名词）译成英语时成为不可数名词。其量词在英语中也有独特的表示方法，如"一个证据"（a piece of evidence）；"两种不同的中间宿主钉螺"（two species of intermediate host snails）。④汉语表示动作单位用动量词（如"次、回、遍、阵"），而英语却没有对应的动量词。英语可用名词化方法表示动量的概念。如"当疾病恶化次数为 3 次及以上时"（when deterioration occurs 3 times or more）；"每周进行三次"（exercises performed three times a week）。

（4）倍数增减的译法："增加"是在原来的基础上加多，具体指数目（如人数、件数）、数额、数值、数量、度量及百分数和分数的增多、增长、增高、上升和提高，与减少、减小、减缩和下降是相对的。英语可用 to increase、rise、be raised、go up、shoot up 等动词表示"增加"的意思。"增加"的概念涉及"增加了"、"增加到"、"达到"和"高达"四个方面。①增加了：increasing by；②增加到：increasing to；③表示百分数、分数增加到：to increase/rise to；④多达、长达、高达：as many/much as，as tall/high as，as long as 等。相反，"减少"是从总量中减除一部分，如同增加一样，英语可用动词 to decrease、reduce、be reduced、go down、fall、drop、dwindle，名词 decrease、reduction、fall 等表示"减少"的意思。"减少"的概念涉及"减少了"和"减少到"两个方面。①减少了：decreasing by；②减少到：decreasing to。百分数由汉语译成英语，常用结构有：①增减意义的动词+by+n%；②表示减少的动词+to+n%；③n%+比较级+than；④n%+比较级+名词；⑤a n%+increase；⑥n%+（of）名词或代词。

例一：结果显示预期寿命增加了 6.8 个月。

The results suggested that the life expectancy **increased by** 6.8 months.

例二：患者平均住院时间缩短了 1/4。

The mean hospital stay for the patients was **reduced to** four time.

例三：同时，婴儿死亡率比 2008 年降低了 40%。

At the same time, the infant mortality was **40 percent lower than** that of the 2008.

9. 句子构成要素及其译法

汉语句子的特点是分句较短，结构紧凑，承上启下，频繁地使用动词。汉语有单句和复句之分，要表达一个相同的意思时，通常采用不同的表现手法。汉语常用"意合法"（parataxis），即主要借助词序及词与短语之间的内在逻辑关系连接，构成联合复句、偏正复句、多重复句。而英语在采用"形合法"（hypotaxis），即使用各种连词、关系代词或关系副词来表示分句及主句与从句之间的各种逻辑关系，因此，英语的句子有长有短，简单结构与汉语的单句基本一致，但并列句及复合句就显得较为复杂。构成英语句子的要素包括主语、谓语、表语、宾语、定语、状语和补足语。鉴于汉英两种语言在句子构成要素上的差异，翻译时切不可死译、硬译。这就需要在认真分析和理解原语的基础上，按目的语表达规范对原句的成分要素进行适当的转换，从而使译文连贯、通顺。

（1）"意""形"转译

例一： 哺乳动物线粒体内含有约 1100 个蛋白质。

Mammalian mitochondria contain about 1100 proteins.

【析】汉语单句转译为英语简单句。

例二： 从全国各地招募的研究对象中有许多是南方人。

There are participants from all over the country and many of them are from the south.

【析】汉语单句转译为英语并列句。

例三： 我们必须考虑所有这些致病因素。

It is necessary **that we should take all these etiological factors into consideration**.

【析】汉语单句转译为英语主从句。

例四： 上述结果提示托特罗定缓释片＋坦索罗辛联合治疗对有中、重度下尿路症状的男性患者有益。

These results suggest **that treatment with tolterodine ER plus tamsulosin provides benefit for men with moderate to severe lower urinary tract symptoms.**

【析】汉语单句转译为英语宾语从句。

例五： 肿瘤生物学的一个根本问题就是潜在的肿瘤起始细胞是人肿瘤内常见的还是罕见的细胞。

A fundamental question in cancer biology is **whether cells with tumorigenic potential are common or rare within human cancers.**

【析】汉语单句转译为英语表语从句。

例六： 人们应该熟悉那些提示肿瘤的症状和体征。

People should be familiar with those symptoms and signs **which may be indicative of tumors**.

【析】汉语单句转译为英语定语从句。

例七： 指南公布后所有年龄段患者血管重建率无明显变化。

There were no differences in the rates of change in revascularization rates based on the date **when the guidelines were released regardless of patient age**.

【析】汉语单句转译为英语状语从句。

例八： 只需要再经过几次失败，就能造出价格低廉的人工心脏了。

The development of an economical artificial heart is only a few transient failures away.

【析】汉语偏正复句转译为英语简单句。

例九：骨具有内分泌器官的特性，可产生骨钙素。

Bone has recently been described as exhibiting properties of an endocrine organ by producing osteocalcin.

【析】汉语并列复句转译为英语简单句。

例十：大疱性类天疱疮是最常见的威胁生命的自身免疫性疾病，常累及中老年人，其中循环性自身抗体 IgG 是针对 XⅦ表皮型胶原的抗体（COL17）。

Bullous pemphigoid is the most common life-threatening autoimmune blistering skin disease that affects the elderly, **in which circulating IgG autoAbs are directed against epidermal type ⅩⅦ collagen** （COL17）.

【析】汉语并列复句转译为英语主从复合句。

例十一：治疗药物无特殊规定，但是不鼓励使用影响心肌收缩力的药物（inotrope）。

Medications were not specified, but inotrope use was explicitly discouraged.

【析】汉语并列复句转译为英语并列复合句。

例十二：幼年呼吸道感染对呼吸系统的影响可能不仅持续到成年，而且影响成年呼吸系统疾病的发展和持续。

The impact of childhood respiratory infections on the respiratory system may not only last into adulthood but also influence development and persistence of adult respiratory morbidity.

【析】汉语联合复句转译为英语并列句。

例十三：出生前先天性房室传导阻滞的电生理特性尚未得到广泛研究，但是该病死亡率却较高。

The electrophysiological characteristics of congenital atrioventricular block before birth have not been extensively studied, yet the mortality from this disease is substantial.

【析】汉语偏正复句转译为英语并列句。

（2）语态的转译：汉英两种语言中，其句子均有主动语态和被动语态。汉语中较少使用被动语态，而英语，尤其是医学英语，被动语态使用较为普遍。有些句子，汉语用被动语态（标记性词：被、受、为……所；遭、把、使、由、以、将、予以等），译成英语时同样使用被动语态。而另一些汉语句不一定要使用被动语态，也无标记被动意义的词语，译为英语时却要使用被动语态，特别是那些无主语句和表示泛指意义的句子。因此，由汉语句译为英语句时应注意语态的转换。

例一：眼科医师在会诊围手术期视力丧失的病例时，如果患者眼部自身原因不明显，应立即行神经影像学检查以排除颅内病变。

If, when an ophthalmologist **is consulted** for a patient with perioperative visual loss, an obvious ocular cause is not apparent, urgent neuroimaging should be obtained to rule out intracranial pathology.

【析】主动句"眼科医师在会诊围手术期视力丧失的病例时"，无被动标记词，译为被动结构。

例二：评估肺动脉导管的随机临床试验一直受到研究样本量较小的限制。

Randomized clinical trials (RCTs) evaluating the pulmonary artery catheter (PAC) **have been limited** by small sample size.

【析】有被动标记词"受到"，对等翻译为英语被动句。

例三：肾功能受损的定义为低肾小球滤过率[< 60 ml/（min·1.73 m²）]和浸渍片尿液分析为蛋白尿（≥1+蛋白）。

Impaired kidney function **was defined** as low glomerular filtration rate [< 60 ml/(min·1.73 m²)] and proteinuria (≥1+protein) on dipstick urinalysis.

【析】有被动标记词"为"，对等翻译为英语被动句。

例四：必须保证足够的机械通气。

Mechanical ventilation **must be properly guaranteed**.

【析】汉语句为无主语句，译为英语被动句。

例五：目前有几种射频消融方法治疗心房颤动。

Several approaches **have been developed** for radiofrequency catheter ablation of atrial fibrillation.

【析】汉语有主语，但原句中未提及主动者，译为英语时，多用被动语态。又如下例。

例六：我们尚需开展远期研究来评价限制热量能否延缓人类衰老过程。

Studies of longer duration **are required** to determine if calorie restriction attenuates the aging process in humans.

例七：人们认为未诊断出的心肌梗死是构成冠心病潜在致命性危险因素之一。

Unrecognized myocardial infarction (UMI) **is known** to constitute a substantial portion of potentially lethal coronary heart disease.

【析】汉语中，主语为泛指的人，译为英语时多用被动语态。此类主语标记词包括"人们""有人""大家""我们"等。此外，还有习语"据…."构成的句子。包括"有人主张……(It is asserted that…)"；"据推测……(It is supposed that…)"等。又如下例。

例八：普遍认为，单独服用抗胆碱能药或α-受体拮抗剂对有下尿路症状及膀胱过度活动症的男性患者可能无效。

It is widely acknowledged that men with overactive bladder and other lower urinary tract symptoms may not respond to monotherapy with antimuscarinic agents or alpha-receptor antagonists.

例九：人类疟疾是由顶复门属5种疟原虫属寄生虫引起的。

Malaria in humans **is caused by** apicomplexan parasites belonging to 5 species of the genus *Plasmodium*.

【析】汉语句中，为了强调话语中心，即为了突出接受动作的人或事的重要性时，此类汉语句多数情况下均转译为英语被动句。又如下例。

例十：采用 Duke 心肌危险分数对病人进行分组后，亦得到类似结果。

Similar results **were obtained** after grouping patients by Duke Myocardial Jeopardy Score.

例十一：镰刀形红细胞病以脉管阻塞性危象疼痛为特征，在脉管阻塞过程中红细胞黏附分子和血管壁蛋白异常相互作用扮演了一个重要的角色。

Sickle-cell disease plays a critical role in abnormal interactions between erythroid adhesion molecules and vessel-wall proteins and **is characterized by** painful vaso-occlusive crises.

【析】有时候，为了在同一个句子中保持上下文的连贯一致，避免变化主语，可将其中的一部分译为英语的被动结构，这种转译手段有助于保持译文的流畅性。

例十二：手术清除的重要性在本次评估中得以证实。多次复发的预后指标与首次复发相类似。

It confirms the overwhelming importance of surgical clearance. Prognostic indicators after recurrences **resemble** those known from first recurrence.

例十三：细胞蛋白酶体功能抑制剂的临床进展表明，将泛素-蛋白酶体系统的其他成分作为目标的复合物被证明治疗人类恶性肿瘤有效。

The clinical development of an inhibitor of cellular proteasome function suggests that compounds targeting other components of the ubiquitin-proteasome system might **prove** useful for the treatment of human malignancies.

【析】例十二、例十三汉语句均为汉语被动句，译为英语后用主动句。这是英语词性所决定的。英语中有：①表示状态的动词，如"fit、resemble、have、lack、suit"；②某些连系动词，如"feel、prove、wear、sound"等；③某些实义动词，如"act、clean、read、wash"等，常用主动语态表示被动意义。因此，涉及此类情况时，英语句用主动式来进行转译。

10. 否定的转译

汉语和英语一样，在表达形式上有肯定和否定两种形式。虽然在翻译时，形式可保持对应，但汉英两种语言在表达否定概念时，所使用的词汇手段、语法手段，甚至语言逻辑却有较大差异。若采用完全对等直译，则会导致译文不畅，不符合英语表达规范，甚至出现翻译错误。因此，将汉语的否定转译为英语的否定时，应注意适当的成分转换。

例一：在仔细进行临床评估的基础上加用肺动脉导管可增加预期不良事件的发生，但对总死亡率和住院率没有影响。

Addition of the pulmonary artery catheters to careful clinical assessment increased anticipated adverse events, but **did not** affect overall mortality and hospitalization.

【析】在不影响表达，不会导致歧义的情况下，汉语的否定可直接转译为英语的否定。又如下例。

例二： 未见到与 PAC 使用相关的死亡事件，住院和 30 天总死亡率没有差异。

There were **no deaths** related to PAC use, and **no difference** for in-hospital plus 30-day mortality.

【析】上述两例均为全部否定，转译为英语时，可借助英语中具有全部否定意义的词，如 not、no、none、never、neither、nothing、nobody 等来实现。

例三： 应用植入式心脏复律除颤器（ICD）治疗先天性心脏病，在法乐（氏）四联症患者中最常见。然而，对于 ICD 在这种患者中的应用价值尚不清楚。

Tetralogy of Fallot is the most common form of congenital heart disease in implantable cardioverter-defibrillator (ICD) recipients, yet **little is known** about the value of ICDs in this patient population.

【析】汉语的否定式翻译成英语的肯定式。这种表达，从形式上看为肯定，事实上却有否定意义。这是由英语某些词的词性所决定的。英语中有一类词或词组，形式为肯定，但表示的意义为否定，包括 little、seldom、hardly、absent、absence、failure、far from、unless 等形容词、副词、动词、名词、连词、介词及短语。又如下例：

例四： Kaplan-Meier 分析显示患者如果不进行肝移植的一年生存率为 55%，6 年生存率为 14%。

Kaplan-Meier indicated a survival **free of** liver transplantation of 55% after 1 year, and only 14% after 6 years.

【析】用形容词短语 free of 肯定式表示否定意义。

例五： IFN-β 是多发性硬化的主要治疗手段。然而，这种治疗并不总是有效的。

Interferon-beta (IFN-beta) is the major treatment for multiple sclerosis. However, this treatment is **not always** effective.

例六： 研究结果证明并非两种药物都有效。

The findings suggested that **both** drugs could **not** produce therapeutic outcomes.

【析】例五、例六为部分否定句。部分否定是指非全部否定，仅否定句子的部分意思，而另一部分则为肯定。汉语中的标记词为"并非所有、并非每个、未必都、不全是、不都是、不总是、不是都、不多、不常"等。此类否定转译为英语时，可以用英语否定词 not 与 all、always、some、both、every、many、much、well、often 等词搭配来实现。

例七： 如不进行均质化，合成则不可能实现。

Synthesis **cannot** take place **without** homogeneization.

【析】这是双重否定句的转译方法。汉语中，使用双重否定是为了达到强调意义的目的，实则为肯定意义。对于此类话语结构，转译为英语时可有两种方法，一是直接转译为英语的双重否定；二是汉语句意义是肯定的，为了达到修辞效果，英语可以用否定形式来表示。如下例。

例八：口服抗生素时，病人务必遵守医嘱。

By oral antibiotics, a patient shall **not fail to** observe physician's orders.

【析】英语用 not fail to...的否定形式。

例九：无论是 R3 区还是接受密集化疗患者，都没有改善无病生存率并且没有改变预后指标。

Neither R3 **nor** adaptation of chemotherapy intensity was capable of improving probabilities of event-free survival or of overcoming prognostic factors.

【析】本例中，汉语否定在谓语，译成英语时，否定转移至主语。

例十：我们发现依托咪酯和医院死亡之间并没有联系。

We found **no association** between etomidate and dying in hospital.

【析】本例中，汉语句否定在谓语，译成英语时，否定转移至宾语。通过例九、例十可见，汉英两种语言在表达否定时，所采用的句法结构存在一定的差异。汉语中有些句子否定的是谓语，英语中否定的却是主语或宾语。此外，汉语否定偏句中的谓语或兼语是第二谓语，翻译成英语时涉及英语中某些特定的词，如 believe、consider、expect 等，译成英语时否定位置却要转移至英语主句，否定主句的谓语。因此，翻译时要特别注意此类差异，在正确理解原文的基础上，结合英语表达习惯，以期达到译文通顺，合乎规范。

汉英翻译是一个复杂的过程，总体概括起来为：①理解过程。只有正确理解原文，才能准确无误地表达出原文所应有的含义。②表达过程。在理解的基础上，结合目的语表达规范，将原文明白无误、流畅通顺地表达出来。这一过程还包括对长句、难句的逻辑关系剖析。③校核过程。我国唐朝诗人贾岛做过一首诗，其中的"鸟宿池边树，僧敲月下门"，是历来传诵的名句。由此而衍生出的词语"推敲"人人皆知。所以，校核就是对译文的斟酌、推敲过程，是翻译过程中不可或缺的阶段。

如前所述，医学英语有其自身的语言特点和规律。同时，翻译又是一种创造性实践活动，掌握并了解一些翻译理论知识和技巧固然重要，但仅有这些知识是远远不够的。更重要的是"兼修内外"，即通过大量的阅读并仔细体会英语语言特点，提高对英语语言的感知能力，同时提升母语的素养，通过反复翻译实践，才能最终成为"达人"。

五、练　　习

10-1：将下列摘要翻译成英文

A

【摘要】目的　评价吞水磁共振食管造影的临床应用能力。

方法　经术后或内镜活检病理证实的胸段食管癌 30 例和正常食管的健康志愿者 10 例均分别经历了常规 MRI 和吞水磁共振食管造影检查。其中放疗的 4 例还进行了放疗后第二次吞水磁共振食管造影检查。评价吞水磁共振食管造影图像效果；与常规 MRI 相比，对其在食管癌瘤体上端和下端显示清晰度、瘤体定位准确性、瘤体长度测量准确性、大体病理分型符合率及肿瘤分期准确性等方面进行评价；另通过放疗前与放疗后吞水磁共振食管造影比较，对食管癌放疗疗效进行评价。

结果　40 例共 44 次吞水磁共振食管造影中矢状位和横断位的优级图像分别为 97.7%（43/44）和 81.8%（36/44）。30 例食管癌治疗前吞水磁共振食管造影瘤体端显示清晰率 93.3%（56/60），而常规 MRI 为 11.7%（7/60），二者差异有统计学意义（$P < 0.005$）。25 例进行了根治性手术，其术前常规 MRI 对 22 例瘤体长度测量、5 例中下段交界区分段及 19 例肿瘤大体病理分型均不能明确；吞水磁共振食管造影对瘤体长度测量（优级）、瘤体定位分段及大体病理分型诊断准确性分别为 88%（22/25）、100%（25/25）和 68%（17/25）。吞水磁共振食管造影对肿瘤分期准确性为 80.8%（21/26），而常规 MRI 为 92.3%（24/26）。4 例食管癌放疗均获得好的疗效。

结论　吞水磁共振食管造影具有食管腔造影能力。吞水磁共振食管造影在胸段食管癌术前诊断和胸段食管癌放疗疗效评价方面具有较高价值，是常规 MRI 的补充。

B

【摘要】中国新感染 HIV 者中异性性传播的比例逐年快速上升，2007 年已达 44.7%。为了减少 HIV 通过异性传播，改善国民的生殖健康水平，本文介绍了国际上有关包皮环切能够预防 HIV 异性传播的流行病学研究证据，病毒经包皮感染的分子细胞生物学机制，以及在非洲取得的大规模随机对照的包皮环切预防艾滋病临床试验的最新研究成果。1997～2007 年，发表的 4 份调查报告表明，在中国不同地区 15 109 名儿童和青少年中，包皮过长者和包茎的比例分别为 43.90% 和 11.55%，但是包皮环切率只有 2.66%。鉴于包皮环切是高效、简单和价廉的预防艾滋病的新措施，我们呼吁国家有关部门，如同推动其他预防艾滋病的多种措施一样，尽快制订推广包皮环切的实施计划，大力普及男性生殖健康的知识，把新生儿包皮环切、未成年人和成年人包皮环切列入医疗保险范围，尽早对 HIV 感染的高危成年男人及妻子为 HIV 阳性而丈夫为阴性者实行免费包皮环切，开展有关包皮环切的流行病学和社会文化的科学研究，以及安全、简单和价廉的新技术研究。

第十一章 英文摘要写作中常见错误分析

医学论文英文摘要写作，作为科技论文写作的一个分支，在遣词造句方面有其独特的风格特点，即其体裁有别于其他文体。所谓体裁，指的是以鲜明的风格、形式或内容为标志的表现手法（a category of artistic composition marked by a distinctive style，form，or content）。语言不仅是信息的载体，满足各民族的交际需要，同时也是文化的载体。交际中的语言无法独立于其赖以存在的文化背景，这就造成了各民族语言间的"异"、"同"共存。汉语和英语是两种截然不同的语言，有着迥异的语法、词汇、规则变化，从中也反映出中西方文化的巨大差异。因此，中、英语言的对等与不对等是相对的而非绝对的。英语语言的表现力在相当程度上依赖于它的丰富词汇，正因为这样，医学论文英文摘要写作中，对于国内长期受到汉语习惯干扰的学习者和作者来说，最明显的干扰体现在具备典型汉语句子结构的英语和纯汉语式的词的搭配及汉语意念的简单化，即词义选择的完全对等，这就是我们常说的"中式英语"（Chinglish），导致语用失误。另外，在较高的层面可能更为突出，即语篇层面。本章就常见的一些失误表达错误做一归类分析。在前面的相关章节中已经重点提及过的有关用法问题，为避免重复，本章不再赘述。

一、词法、词义类错误

1. 用于列举的词：like 和 such as

like 和 such as 使用频率较高，尽管这两个词均可用来列举事物，但所表示的语义关系却有所差异。Like（如……；像……；）其实际意义为"for example"。而 such as 的真实含义为" of this kind；of such quality（这样的）"。由此可以看出，两者是有区别的。

例一： Pituitary tumor transforming gene (PTTG) is a newly discovered oncogene, and serves as a marker of malignancy grades in several forms of cancer, particularly endocrine malignancies **like** pituitary adenomas.

垂体癌转移基因（PTTY）为新近发现的致癌基因，可以作为几种癌症恶性程度的分级标志，尤其是内分泌恶性肿瘤如垂体腺瘤。

【析】句子中 like 要改成 such as 更为恰当。因为整句都讲的是恶性肿瘤，垂体腺瘤属于此类。

例二：The occurrence of continuous blood pressure (BP) fluctuations is an intrinsic feature of the cardiovascular system and is related to complex cardiovascular mechanisms and environmental stimulations or daily habits **such as** coffee drinking.

持续性血压波动是心血管系统的一个固有特征，血压波动与复杂的心血管机制、环境刺激或日常生活习惯有关，如饮用咖啡。

【析】如果将句中的 such as 改成 like，所表示的意义就有所差异。即可能是与此类似的饮料，不一定就是具有较强刺激性作用的咖啡。

2. relation 和 relationship

这是两个同根名词，relation 意为 "a logical or natural association between two or more things; relevance of one to another"（关系），特指两个或更多的事物之间逻辑或自然的联系，相互的关联。而 relationship 的意思是 "The condition or fact of being related; connection or association."（关系），特指有关系的事实或状态。其后缀-ship 来自古德语词，意为条件、性质、本质（condition、nature、quality）。据此可知，relation 尽管是名词，强调的是动态的关系或关联，而 relationship 强调的是静态关系。

例一：The **relationship** between the type of feeding, circumcision and urinary tract infection (UTI) was significant ($P<0.05$).

喂养类型、包皮环切和尿路感染之间的关系非常明显。

【析】从本句所表达的意思可知，句中"喂养""包皮环切""尿路感染"明显提示的为动态关系，即一件事物为另一件事物变化的诱发动因。因此，该句中的 relationship 应改为 relation。

例二：This **relation** persisted after adjustment for baseline characteristics.

基线特征调整后仍然持续存在这种关联。

【析】本句中 relation 应改用 relationship，因为，语境提示这是一种状态，而非相互之间的作用。

3. 易混淆的 in vitro 和 in vivo

从拼写上看，这两个词很容易混淆，但意义却不相同。in vitro 和 in vivo 都可用作形容词或副词。in vitro 意为 "in an artificial environment outside the living organism"（体外的），指"在生物体外的人工环境中"；in vivo 意指 "within a living organism"，体内的，在生物体内。

例一：…the adverse effect, this included **in vitro** laboratory studies and **in vivo** tests in patients exposed to the drug.

……药物的副反应，这包括对服用这类药物的病人所做的活体外实验研究和活体研究。

【析】做形容词使用，位置关系恰当。

例二： At a molecular level, we found that PDGF-CC both ***in vitro*** regulated glycogen synthase kinase (GSK)-3β phosphorylation and ***in vivo*** expression.

在分子水平上，我们发现 PDGF-CC 可调控糖原合成酶激酶（GSK）3β 磷酸化，且可在体外和体内表达。

【析】从本句句法结构看，*in vitro* 和 *in vivo* 为副词性质，因此，应修改为"…that PDGF-CC regulated glycogen synthase kinase (GSK)-3β phosphorylation and expression both *in vitro* and *in vivo*"。另外，按照 MeSH 公布的 2015 年新旧医学概念变化使用规定，*in vitro* 和 *in vivo* 后增加说明词 technique。

4. effective 和 efficacious

英文摘要写作中，作者通常会用这两个词来表示效果。虽然同为形容词，汉语均指"有效的"，但意义不同。effective 的意思是"having an intended or expected effect"（有效的；具有预期或先见效果的）；efficacious 则指"producing or capable of producing a desired effect"（灵验的；能产生或产生所期的效果的）。effective 通常用于描述某种干预方法所产生的效果，efficacious 则与药物疗效有关。

例一： A newer anticonvulsant, levetiracetam, can be more **effective**.

左乙拉西坦作为一种较新的抗惊厥药，其疗效更好。

【析】effective 在本句中貌似正确无误，但搭配的概念是药物，故使用 efficacious 更合理。

例二： As far as prenatal lung maturation is concerned, antenatal steroids remain the single most **efficacious** intervention thus far.

就促进胎儿期肺功能发育成熟而言，迄今为止，妊娠期补充类固醇类药物仍然是唯一最有效的干预手段。

【析】本句中修饰的概念是"干预手段"，故用 effective 更恰当。

5. normal 和 healthy

英文摘要中常涉及对"异常"或"正常"对象、某种结果的描述，措辞时要注意 normal 和 healthy 的意义差异。normal 意为"the usual or expected state, form, amount, or degree"（正常状态）；healthy 指"possessing good health"（健康的；拥有良好健康状况的）。如我们可以说"normal body temperature"（正常体温），不可以说"a normal appearance"（健康的外表）。因此，下列表达中就存在措辞不当的问题。

例一： All **normal** subjects were allocated to control group.

所有正常对象作为控制组。

【析】该句应该为"All healthy subjects were allocated to control group."

例二： Reference values of C1r, C2, C5, C7, Properdin, and factors D, H, and I and C3a and C5a have been determined in cord blood samples from **healthy** term newborns.

测定正常足月产新生儿脐血标本中的 C1r、C2、C5、C7 和备解素参考值及 D、H、I、C3a 和 C5a 因子。

【析】句中的 healthy 不能用 normal 代替，描述正常的人，意即拥有良好的健康状况，如 "a normal child" 则指 "智力正常的儿童" 而非 "健康儿童"。若表示某种检测结果 "正常" 也要谨慎，如 "患者 X 线检测正常"，不能表达为 "X-ray examination of the patient was normal"，而应表达为 "The results from X-ray examination of the patient was normal"。因为，前一句表示的意思是 "正常" 的 X 线，即说明 X 线是无害的，或设备完好，能进行正常检查。那么，由此推断 "异常" 的 X 线应是 abnormal，即表示对人体是有害的，或设备出现问题，无法执行检查。

6. admit 和 hospitalize

这两个词均有 "住院" 之意，但所表达的概念不同。admit 的含义是 "to permit to enter"（允许进入），表示患者的身份地位的确定 "to permit to exercise the rights, functions, or privileges of"（允许行使……的权利，作用或特权）；而 hospitalize 指 "to place in a hospital for treatment, care, or observation"（进入医院进行治疗、照顾或观察），常有作者误用这两个词。

例：The present prospective randomized controlled parallel study was conducted on 93 children up to 12 years admitted in our hospital between May 2002 and April 2004 with clinical presentation of typhoid fever.
前瞻性随机控制平行研究，研究对象为我院从 2002 年 5 月至 2004 年 4 月收治的 93 例具有典型伤寒症临床症状的 12 岁儿童。

【析】句中的 admit 仅仅表示患者作为患者身份的确定，并不表示 "住院" 治疗。这是一个很重要的界线问题。如若将本句该写成 "The present prospective randomized controlled parallel study was conducted on 93 children up to 12 years **hospitalized** in our hospital between May 2002 and April 2004 with clinical presentation of typhoid fever."。那么，其意思就是 "这些儿童的住院时间为 2002 年 5 月至 2004 年 4 月"。这显然有悖于常态。

7. case、patient 和 subject

表示 "病例" 时，作者通常难以把握这三个词的选择，从而导致概念表达失误，甚至 "非人化"。case 指 "an occurrence of a disease or disorder"（某种疾病的案例），patient 指 "one who receives medical attention, care, or treatment"（接受治疗的人），而 subject 则指 "one that experiences or is subjected to something or the object of clinical study"（在医学研究、调查中特殊的人、动物或微生物）。

例一：**Case** I was treated for 8 weeks with synthetic drugs.
第一例患者用合成药物治疗 8 周。

【析】此句中 case 应该为 patient，因为指的是接受治疗的患者。又如，"Management of pulmonary disease in patients with cystic fibrosis."（伴囊肿性纤维化肺病患者的治疗）。

例二：In the current **case** series family history was positive in only one-third number of **cases**.

目前病例系列中，仅 1/3 的家族史呈阳性。

【析】句中指的是某种疾病的案例，故 case 不能换成 patient。

例三：The telephone disease management (TDM) program consisted of regular contacts with each **subject** by a behavioral health specialist (BHS) to assist in assessment, education, support, and treatment planning.

电话指导疾病治疗方案包括：由一名行为健康专家定期帮助评估、指导、支持和安排治疗计划。

【析】句中的 subject 指的是特定的研究对象，故不可以用其他词代替。

8. middle、medium 和 moderate

上述三个词均含有"中等"之意，意义比较接近，因而作者在使用时常出问题。middle 常表示位置关系，但可用于表示年龄，如"middle age"（中年）。medium 常表示药物的剂量，如"medium dosage"（中等剂量）。moderate 表示疾病或症状的严重程度，如"moderate pain"（中度疼痛）。

例一：Obesity in **midium** age and future risk of dementia: a 27 year longitudinal population based study

中年肥胖与未来患痴呆症的风险：一项基于人群的 27 年纵向研究。

【析】句中的 medium 应改为 middle。

例二：These results suggest that treatment with tolterodine ER plus tamsulosin for 12 weeks provides benefit for men with **moderate** to severe lower urinary tract symptoms including overactive bladder.

上述结果提示，托特罗定缓释片＋坦索罗辛联合治疗（为期 12 周）对有中、重度下尿路症状（其中包括膀胱过度活动症）的男性患者有益。

【析】显而易见，句中 moderate 表示程度，不可使用其他词替换。

9. diseased people 和 very old patient

表达某些与人有关的特定概念时，应注意体现出以人为本的思想。diseased people 实属贬义，即"病态的人"而非"病人"。受汉语思维习惯的影响，中国作者在表达上述概念时通常出现语用失误，从而导致"非人化"。类似的例子还很多，如将"艾滋病人"表示成"HIV patients"；将"有残疾的病人"说成"disabled patients"；"年老的病人"写成"very old patients"；这不仅常见于中国作者，韩国作者也有此类表达失误。例如，韩国作者将"老年病人"写成"senior patients"或"senile patients"，而英、美作者却罕用这类表达。在英语中 senile 暗示"年老体衰"等。那么，要表达上述有关的概念时，该如何表达？用较为具体的表达方式即可。上述概念我们可以改写成如下表述：

"**HIV patients**"改为"patients infected with HIV"或"HIV-infected patients"。

"**Disabled patients**"改为"patients with disabilities""physically disabled patients""developmentally disabled patients""patients with physical disabilities""patients with learning disabilities"等。

10. death rate 和 mortality 有关的"率"

摘要写作中少不了描述各种各样的"率"。同样受汉语思维的影响，作者通常将各种"率"生搬硬套，于是出现了"positive detectable rate; positive rate; negative rate; detection rate; cured rate; improved rate; successful rate"等的"率"。英语中的"率"和汉语中的"率"有对等与不对等表示之分。有些"率"在英语中有对应的词表示，而另一些则要用具体描述来表达。例如"死亡率"，英文可以是 death rate 或 mortality，但两者还有区别。前者表示病死率或动物的实验性死亡率，后者指在大样本调查中的死亡比例。

例一：Echocardiographic measures of EF and diastolic function, measurement of blood levels of BNP, and 6-month **mortality**.
超声心动图测得的 EF 值和舒张功能、血 BNP 水平及 6 个月的死亡率。

例二：The **death rate** of the experimental animals accounted for 49%.
实验动物的死亡率为 49%。

例三：Heart failure with preserved EF is associated with a high **mortality rate**, comparable to that of patients with reduced EF.
与 EF 降低的心力衰竭患者相似，EF 正常的心力衰竭患者死亡率也较高。

例四：Between 25 and 55 years of age, the age-sex-adjusted **death rate** from natural causes was 15.4 deaths per 1000 person-years.
在 25 至 55 岁之间，按自然性别进行年龄调整后的死亡率为每 1000 人中每年 15.4 例死亡。

例五：...antigen was found positive in 30% of the patients.
患者中抗原阳性率为 30%。

【析】通过大量检索以英语为母语的作者写成的摘要，我们发现，他们在表达如例四、例五中所涉及的"率"时，均采用具体概念的表示方法。

11. however、but、whereas 和 while

话语表达离不开意义转折，however、but、whereas、while 常用来表达转折关系，它们之间意义的区别如下所述。① however："...in spite of that..."；nevertheless；yet（尽管；然而；还是）。②but：on the contrary（而是；相反的）。③ whereas："It being the fact that...""...in as much as..."（出于……事实，鉴于；相反）。④while：whereas；and（然

而；而且）。从其英文释义不难看出，它们连接的分句之间具有不同的逻辑关系。

例一： Acute lower respiratory tract infection is the most common condition treated in primary care. Many physicians still prescribe antibiotics; **however**, systematic reviews of the use of antibiotics are small and have diverse conclusions.

在初级医疗机构治疗的疾病中，急性下呼吸道感染最为常见。尽管有关抗生素应用的系统综述很少，且得出的结论各有不同，但仍有许多内科医生开处抗生素。

【析】后一分句 "systematic reviews of the use of antibiotics are small and have diverse conclusion" 是前一分句 "many physicians still prescribe antibiotics" 的补充说明，前后分句之间存在让步关系。

例二： Several investigations as well as prospective studies have shown a significant correlation between glucose metabolism and atherosclerosis in patients without diabetes, **but** differences in parameters of glucose metabolism among the various degrees of coronary disease in such patients have not been specifically evaluated.

一些临床观察和前瞻性研究表明，非糖尿病病人葡萄糖代谢与动脉粥样硬化显著相关，但是尚未在该组病人中对不同程度冠心病病变葡萄糖代谢参数的差异进行专门评估。

【析】but 连接的前后分句之间所表达的意义完全不对应，即分属两个不同的意义。

例三： Prevalence of hypertension and drug treatment increased with advancing age, **whereas** control rates were markedly lower in older women (systolic <140 and diastolic <90 mmHg).

高血压的患病率和药物治疗率随着年龄增加而升高，但是在老年女性控制率（收缩压<140 mmHg，舒张压<90 mmHg）显著降低。

【析】从本句语境可知，whereas 连接的分句之间所暗含的逻辑关系为对比关系。

例四： **While** studies of relatively short duration have suggested that thiazolidinediones such as pioglitazone might reduce progression of CIMT in persons with diabetes, the results of longer studies have been less clear.

尽管相对短期的研究显示，噻唑烷二酮类药物（如匹格列酮）可以减缓 CIMT 的进展，但是长期研究结果目前尚不明确。

【析】国内作者在表示转折时常用 while 代替 whereas。尽管英文释义中也用了 whereas，但 while 强调的是让步或递进关系，而非纯粹转折。

12. district 和 region

这两个词均与"区域"有关。district 意为 "a division of an area, as for administrative purposes"（地区；行政区；一个地域的分支，如为了管理的目的），region 虽有"地区"

之意，但更强调的是 "a specified district or territory"（特定地区；特定领地）。在医学英语中，如指人体解剖部位时应用 region。

例一： At age 40-50, the nuclear **district** of advanced nuclear cataract lenses was found to be approximately 46 times harder than that of normal lenses of the same age.

在 40～50 岁年龄时,过熟核性白内障晶状体的核区域大约是相同年龄正常晶状体硬度的 46 倍。

【析】本句中 district 属明显误用。显而易见，句中所涉及的概念为解剖学上的部位, 因此, 应改写为 "At age 40-50, the nuclear **region** of advanced nuclear cataract lenses was found to be approximately 46 times harder than that of normal lenses of the same age."。然而，下列两例中的 region 同样不可被 district 替代，因为句子的语境告诉我们，指的是特定区域，而非广义的行政区域。又如：RNA coding regions（RNA 编码区）。

例二： ...in the West Midlands **region** of England from 1984-2002.

……（收集）1984～2002 年在英格兰 West Midland 地区的（病例）。

13. cycle、period 和 duration

首先注意本段文字的描述："In primates, the cycle is a menstrual **cycle**, and its most conspicuous feature is the periodic vaginal bleeding that occurs with shedding of the uterine mucosa（menstruation）. The length of the **cycle** is notoriously variable, but an average figure is 28 days from the start of one menstrual **period** to the start of the next."。由此可知，cycle 和 period 在表示"周期"时是有区别的。cycle 的意思是 "an interval of time during which a characteristic, often regularly repeated event or sequence of events occurs"（周期；循环期；一段时间间隔；即在这段时间里通常有规律重复的事件）；period 的意思是 "stretch of time"（一段时间）；duration 则指 " a period of existence or persistence"（持续时期）。

例一： 1650 women with regular menstrual **period** undergoing their first cycle of in-vitro fertilisation were enrolled from Aug 1, 2016, to June 3, 2017.

有规律月经周期的 1650 名妇女在 2016 年 8 月 1 日至 2017 年 6 月 3 日期间接受了第一周期体外受精。

【析】period 应改为 cycle。另注意对比观察下例正确表示法。

例二： Seventy percent of the patients was of chronic **duration**（11. 1±9.2） weeks.

70% 为慢性病程（11. 1±9.2）周。

例三： One patient died of renal failure during perioperative **period**.

一例患者在围手术期死于肾衰竭。

14. damage、injure、harm、hurt、wound 和 impair

这 6 个词都与"损伤、损害、伤害"有关，但意义各有差异。

例一：Despite adequate epicardial artery reperfusion, a number of patients with ST-segment elevation myocardial infarction (STEMI) have a poor prognosis because of microvascular **hurt**.

尽管有足够的心外膜动脉再灌注，但很多 STEMI 患者因为微循环受损预后差。

【析】hurt 应改为 damage。英语中具有"伤害"之意的词有 damage、injure（injury）、harm、hurt、wound 和 impair，但各自的语义不同。①damage 意为 "impairment of the usefulness or value of person or property；harm"（对有用或有价值的人或财产的破坏）。②injure 意为 "to cause physical harm to；hurt"（造成肉体上的伤害，injury 为其名词形式，可以指意外事故伤，也可用于微观的细胞损伤等）。③harm 意指 "physical or psychological injury or damage"（身体或心理上的损害或伤害）。由此可见，上述六个词所代表的意义是不同的。④hurt 意为 "to cause physical damage or pain to"（引起肉体或精神上的伤害或疼痛）。⑤wound 意为 "an injury, especially one in which the skin or other external surface is torn, pierced, cut, or otherwise broken."（创伤伤口，尤指由于皮肤或其他表层被撕裂、刺伤、割伤或其他形式破坏而造成的损伤）。⑥impair 意指 "to cause to diminish、as in strength、value, or quality"（削减，造成力量、价值或质量等的减少）。又如下例：

例二：Acute renal failure from both ischemia and contrast are postulated to occur from free-radical **injury**.

普遍认为，自由基损伤能导致缺血和造影剂引发的急性肾衰竭。

例三：After the second trimester, the bone marrow becomes the major hematopoietic organ. A variety of perinatal conditions can **impair** production and functional activity of neutrophils in neonates.

妊娠中期后，骨髓就成了主要造血器官。围产期各种疾病可能会抑制新生儿体内的中性粒细胞产生和功能活性。

15. fever 和 temperature

例一：In general examination, authors took note of general condition, level of consciousness, **fever**, pulse rate, pulse character, respiratory rate, blood pressure.

体检时，我们记录了患者的一般状况、意识状态、体温、脉速、脉相、呼吸频率及血压。

例二：**Temperature** was the main presenting symptom in all the cases.

所有病例中，主要症状为发热。

【析】上述两例主要错误为词义误解。fever 意指 "abnormally high body temperature"（不正常的高体温）；temperature 意指 "The degree of heat in the body of a living organism"（体温，有机生物体的热量程度）。若要表

示机体温度异常，需要用 "high temperature in…"。据此，第一例中的 fever 应改为 temperature；第二例中的 temperature 应是 fever 或 high temperature。

16. microscopy 和 microscope

例：Confocal **microscope** was used to define the interaction of milk proteins (100 μM each) and amoebas.

使用共焦显微镜检查牛乳蛋白质和阿米巴之间的相互作用关系。

【析】microscope 应改为 microscopy。很多作者在这类词的选择上常出现差错。microscope 的意思是 "optical instrument to magnify objects"（指仪器设备）；而 microscopy 则强调 "the use of microscopes"（显微镜的使用，即技术手段）。医学英语中类似的表达还有很多，如 gastroscopy（胃镜检查术）；gastroscope［胃镜（用以检查胃内部情形），胃窥器］；choledochoscope（胆道镜），胆道镜检查应表达为 choledochoscopy、choledochofiberscope（胆道纤维内窥镜）。由于词义不同，所以，使用时，搭配的动词也就有差异。例如：

用显微镜／胃镜检查或观察……：

　　　　"be examined /observed with/using…microscope/gastroscope"

在显微镜／胃镜下检查或观察……：

　　　　"be examined/observed under/in…microscope / gastroscope"

使用显微镜／胃镜技术检查或观察……：

　　　　"examined /observed by/using…microscopy / gastroscopy"

使用某……显微镜……：

　　　　　　　"…were observed under a light microscope"

　　　　"…was examined in a scanning electron microscope"

　　　"…was examined using a fluorescent light microscope"

17. professional 和 occupational

例：We aimed to evaluate the efficacy of this newly-marketed drug in treatment of **professional** diseases.

评价该新药对治疗职业病的疗效。

【析】这两个词的词义有着本质上的差异。professional 的意思是 "Engaging in a given activity as a source of livelihood or as a career"（从事某一特定活动作为职业或谋生手段或有专业特长的），而 occupational 为 "engagement in a particular occupation"（从事某一特定工作）。因此，句中 professional 应改为 occupational。又如："Eighty-one patients （72.3%）who screened positive for bipolar disorder sought **professional** help for their symptoms."

18. standard 和 criterion

例一： To compare resuscitation outcomes following out-of-hospital cardiac arrest when an automated LDB-CPR device was added to **criterion** emergency medical services (EMS) care with manual CPR.

比较增加使用自动化 LDB-CPR 装置的标准医疗急救服务（EMS）与人工 CPR 的院外心脏停搏复苏效果。

【析】句中 criterion 应用 standard 替代。虽然两个词都有"标准"之意，但 standard 指"an acknowledged measure of comparison for quantitative or qualitative value"（公认的衡量数量或者质量的标准），有"标准化"之意。criterion 为单数形式，复数为 criteria，意思是"a standard, rule, or test on which a judgment or decision can be based"（以做出判断或决定的标准、准则，特指自行设定的某种尺度，用于测试或衡量品质等）。试比较下例：

例二： Exclusion **criteria** were multiple birth delivery, mixed vaginal and caesarean delivery, and four or more deliveries.

排除标准为多胎分娩，混合阴道和剖宫产，四次或四次以上分娩史。

【析】本句中的 criteria 不可用 standard 代替。

19. marker、indicator 和 index

例： Our goal was to evaluate the role of myocardial nicotinamide adenine dinucleotide phosphate (NADPH) oxidase activity and plasma **index** of oxidative stress in the pathogenesis of post-operative atrial fibrillation (AF).

我们的研究目的是评价心肌辅酶Ⅱ（NADPH）氧化酶活性和血浆氧化应激标志物在术后心房颤动发病中的作用。

【析】index 需要改为 markers。这三个词的词义区别分别为：marker 指"标记或充当标志之物，尤指当某一生物标志物质在血清中异常大量增加或减少时，预示可能有疾病存在"，如"Pituitary tumor transforming gene（PTTG）is a newly discovered oncogene, and serves as a **marker** of malignancy grades in several forms of cancer, particularly endocrine malignancies such as pituitary adenomas."（垂体肿瘤转化基因（PTTG）是一种新发现的致癌基因，可作为几种肿瘤恶性程度分级标志，特别是内分泌恶性肿瘤，如垂体腺瘤）。anti-oxidant markers（抗氧化标志）。indicator 为"指示剂，指标或任何一个统计数值"之意，如"Brain natriuretic peptide（BNP）, left ventricular（LV）systolic function, and mitral filling pattern （MFP） are prognostic **indicators** in patients with heart failure （HF）."［脑钠肽（BNP）左心室（LV）收缩功能及二尖瓣灌注模式（MFP）是心力衰竭（HF）患者的预后因子。］；"Serum 25-hydroxyvitamin D is the generally accepted **indicator** of vitamin D status, but no universal reference level has been reached. "（血清 25 羟维生素

D 可反映机体维生素 D 水平，但尚无统一的参考标准。）；"Clinical Quality Indicators"（临床治疗指标）。index 意为 "an indicator or a pointer, as on a scientific instrument"（标记或指标符号，如在科学仪器上的刻度），如 "The systolic area **index** had a sensitivity of 97% and a predictive accuracy of 100% for the identification of patients with surgically proven CP."（外科证实的 CP 患者收缩面积指数敏感性为 97%，特异性为 100%。）；splenometric index（脾测定指数）；　body-mass index（体重指数）。

20. use 和 usage

例一：Oral prednisone for 6 days provided important relief, and she stayed on daily **usage** of steroids, refusing other forms of therapy.

口服泼尼松 6 天后，症状缓解明显，之后患者持续每日口服皮质激素，未使用其他治疗药物。

【析】usage 改为 use。use 既可用作动词，也可用作名词。use 当名词用时其意义为 "The condition or fact of being used"（使用的状态或事实），而 usage 则指 "The act, manner, or amount of using"（用法，用量）。又如下例。

例二：We sought to assess the association of amiodarone **use** with mortality during consecutive periods in patients with post-acute myocardial infarction with left ventricular systolic dysfunction and/or HF treated with a contemporary medical regimen.

研究胺碘酮的使用是否会增加经序贯治疗，伴有心力衰竭和（或）左心功能障碍的急性心肌梗死患者的死亡风险。

例三：antihypertensive medication **usage.**

抗高血压药物用量

21. whole 和 complete

例一：In patients with brain metastases, it is unclear whether adding up-front **complete-brain** radiation therapy (WBRT) to stereotactic radiosurgery (SRS) has beneficial effects on mortality or neurologic function compared with SRS alone.

尚不清楚在脑转移瘤患者中，预先全脑放射治疗（WBRT）联合立体定向放射外科（SRS）对死亡率和神经功能的疗效是否比单独 SRS 更好。

【析】whole 和 complete 均表示"全部的，完整的"。whole 在科技文体中表示 "Not divided or disjoined; in one unit"（完整的，未经分割或分离的，整体的）。complete 表示 "Absolute; total"（彻底的；全部的，所有必要的）。根据句意可知，"全脑"应是 "**whole-brain**"。为了更好地了解这两个词的词义区别，请仔细体会下例。

例二： After further adjustment for intake of meat, dairy, fruits and vegetables, refined grains, and **whole grains,** analysis of individual food groups revealed that meat, fried foods, and diet soda also were adversely associated with incident metabolic syndrome（MetSyn）.

进一步对肉食、牛奶、水果、蔬菜、精粮、全谷物摄取校正后，个体食物组分析显示肉食、油煎食品、苏打也与代谢综合征呈负相关。

例三： To evaluate the feasibility and the incidence of **complete** heart block (CHB) after non-surgical septal myocardial reduction by coil embolization in hypertrophic obstructive cardiomyopathy (HOCM).

评价使用非外科手术线圈栓塞消融法治疗肥厚型梗阻性心肌病（HOCM）的可行性及术后完全性心脏传导阻滞（CHB）的发病率。

更多正确使用如下：the complete drug reference（药物参考大全）; whole blood samples（全血样本）; whole genome linkage analysis（全基因组连锁分析）; bilateral whole-leg ultrasonography（双侧全腿超声检查）; complete response/ remission （完全反应/缓解）等。

22. 介词误用

英语介词是显示名词与名词、形容词及动词之间关系的辅助词，由于其使用灵活，因而很难被非英语为母语作者准确地把握和运用，英文摘要中虽然涉及的介词不多，但出错率较高。介词，是英语中活跃的词类，在有限的篇幅内是无法一一说清楚的。要想避免这类错误，只能依靠作者在阅读英文资料时细心体会并长期积累有关常用介词的搭配用法和意义。在写作中，使用介词失误主要表现在误用、多用、漏用三个方面。

例一： The difficulty **of** doing research related to dehydration is that there is no good standard **of** determining the level of dehydration.

有关脱水作用研究的困难在于没有确定脱水等级的标准。

【析】第一介词 of 应改为 in；第二个 of 应改为 for。这类错误为误用介词。误用介词主要在于介词的搭配方面。如 approach（es）for/to/in…, management of/for…。虽然其后的介词有可选余地，但除此之外，不可以用其他介词替代。

例二： Recent studies of drug-eluting intracoronary stents suggest that current antiplatelet regimens may not be sufficient **for** prevention of late stent thrombosis.

近来的冠状动脉内药物洗脱支架研究提示，现行的抗血小板治疗方案可能并不足以预防后期支架内血栓形成。

【析】for 应改为 to。

例三： To summarize current evidence on about how pregnancy reveals risk **of** chronic disease.

总结妊娠期慢性病发病风险证据

【析】句中 evidence 之后出现了两个介词 on 和 about。about 应删除。此类失误一般有两种情形，一是介词重叠使用，二是在及物动词之后添加了不必要的介词。例如："…respiratory distress syndrome **raised to** public concerns…"中 raise 本身就是及物动词，可以直接接宾语，to 就是多用的介词。产生此类错误的最大因素可能是受到母语的干扰，从而导致多用了介词。

例四： Patients referred dysplasia management or with prevalent adenocarcinoma were excluded.

发育不良但接受过治疗的及常见腺癌的患者被排除。

【析】本句中 patients referred 之后遗漏了介词 for。这是介词遗漏的情况。遗漏介词一般表现在使用及物动词或在定语从句中介词前置到关系代词之前等场合。例如，define 为及物动词，但使用时通常用作 "…defined as…"。又如："There is a high priority for introducing genetic testing for those genetic diseases **in** which a limited number of genes allow a high yield of successfully genotyped patients."。句中 which 之前的介词 in 很容易遗漏。

例五： The woman was successfully cured from ovarian cancer by chemotherapy.

通过化疗，这位妇女的卵巢癌终于治愈了。

【析】cure 应与介词 of 连用，构成 "cure somebody of…"，故上句应改写为 "The woman was successfully cured of her ovarian cancer by chemotherapy."。

例六： Of the 56 patients with placental presentation, one died of massive haemorrhage.

在 56 例胎盘早剥患者中，1 例因大出血而死亡。

【析】"one died of…" 应改为 "one died from…"，from 表示原因，即 "overeating, wounds, some unknown causes, unnatural causes" 等，表示"由于某种原因而死"；"of" 表示"有关……的"，如 "die of an illness, a disease, hungry, an overdose of sleeping pills"，由于……疾病而死。

23. 动词搭配错误

广泛使用中的英语语言不仅有其特定的域，而且有着非常活跃的各类搭配。从严格意义上说，搭配有广义和狭义之分。狭义上的搭配包括动词与介词、副词的连用，即我们常说的短语动词；形容词、名词与介词的连用；形容词与名词、名词与名词等。广义上的搭配包括词的所有搭配使用。鉴于医学英文摘要的特殊性，本节主要针对写作中使用频率较高的某些动词与名词的搭配错误做些提示，这也是写作中的一大难点。一旦搭配不当，极有可能导致语用失误，语言表达缺乏准确性。同掌握介词用法一样，动词与名词的搭配需要长期的语感和积累。医学摘要写作中常涉及的动词搭配有 undergo、receive、undertake、perform、conduct、determine、measure、examine、evaluate、develop、carry out 等。相关动词的用法在前面各个章节中已经有过讨论，恕不赘述。

例一： **The systolic pressure** of the patient **raised** after 24 hours.

24 小时后患者收缩压上升。

【析】raise 为及物动词，意为"提高、增加"，常识告诉我们，一个人的血压上升为外界因素或病理因素所致，没有人会主动提升血压。本句应改写成"**The systolic pressure** of the patient **elevated** after 24 hours."。

例二：**A double-blind, randomized, controlled trial was done** in 736 children aged 6-15 years of old.

对 736 名 6～15 岁儿童做了双盲随机控制试验。

【析】动词 done 与名词搭配不当，do 一般指做事，而该句中的动词与名词之间的关系是实施某种行为。根据意义搭配，应改写为"**A double-blind, randomized, controlled trial was performed** in 736 children aged 6-15 years of old."。

例三：Although the epidemic of obesity has been accompanied by an increase in the prevalence of the metabolic syndrome, not all obese **establish the syndrome** and even lean individuals can be insulin resistant.

尽管肥胖的流行伴随着代谢综合征的患病率增加，但并不是所有肥胖都会导致代谢综合征，甚至瘦人也可以存在胰岛素抵抗。

【析】句中 "establish the syndrome" 为动宾关系，从语境分析，应为词义搭配不当。establish 虽有 "To bring about; generate"（招致；引起）之意，但为褒义，如 "establish goodwill in the neighborhood"（给邻居带来美好的祝福）。establish 可以将其更改为"develop：to bring into being gradually"（逐渐形成）。显而易见，句中的语境提示的是因果关系，即肥胖导致机体内分泌失调。

例四：The aim of this study was to determine whether platelet reactivity on clopidogrel therapy, as **evaluated by a point-of-care platelet function assay,** is associated with thrombotic events after percutaneous coronary intervention (PCI) with drug-eluting stents (DESs).

本研究的目的是通过即时测定血小板功能，评价氯吡格雷治疗后的血小板反应性是否与用药物洗脱支架经皮冠状动脉介入治疗（PCI）后的血栓性形成相关。

【析】同样是词义搭配不当。evaluate 意指 "To ascertain or fix the value or worth of"（确定……的数值或价值），而 measure 则强调对某种物质含量的测定。故原句宜改为 "The aim of this study was to determine whether platelet reactivity on clopidogrel therapy, as **measured by a point-of-care platelet function assay,** is associated with thrombotic events after percutaneous coronary intervention (PCI) with drug-eluting stents (DESs)."。

更多正确概念常用搭配如下，供写作参考：

1）undergo/receive cardiac surgery/treatment（接受心脏手术；接受治疗）

2）undergo/receive primary angioplasty（原发性血管成形术）

3）randomised controlled trial was undertaken/conducted/carried in（在……地方进行的

随机控制试验）

  4）diagnostic manoeuvre to be undertaken（after/in）（进行诊断操作）

  5）CT enterography(CTE)was performed（行 CT 肠造影（CTE）

  6）liver biopsies were performed（进行肝脏活检）

  7）conducted a systematic search of（对……进行系统研究）

  8）develop cholestasis（发生胆汁淤积症）（该词与疾病搭配）

  例五： "...and mean survival days of the mice were improved ($P<0.05$)."

    ……，同时小鼠的平均存活天数延长了（$P<0.05$）

    【析】 谓语动词跟主语概念就搭配不当。时间是不能改善的（improved），只能讲时间"延长"或"缩短"，因此，应把句子中的谓语动词 improved 改为 prolonged.

24. -ic 和-ical 词尾问题

  英语中以-ic 或-ical 结尾的形容词随处可见，通常情况下，以-ic 或-ical 结尾的形容词在意义上没有多大差异，但也有例外情况。从严格意义上来说，后缀-ic 表示的意义为"属于……的，有……特性的"。例如，acidic（酸性的）；化学上意为"离子或酸处于两个氧化态中较高的那个状态"。后缀-ical 表示的意义是"……的"，"……似的"，如 chemical。更多的例子如下：

  例一： **systolic** blood pressure.

    收缩期血压

  例二： Underinvestigation and undertreatment of carotid disease in elderly patients with transient **ischaemic** attack and stroke:Comparative population based study

    短暂性脑缺血发作和卒中老龄患者中颈动脉疾病的检查和处理不足：基于人群的比较研究

  例三： How these or other yet identified factors come together to create the classic clinical and **pathologic** features is the subject of much research.

    这些因素或未确定的因素是如何协同作用而导致典型的临床和病理特征的，这已成为研究焦点。

  例四： Intraventricular hemorrhage (IVH) comprises a spectrum of **pathological** processes that result from blood filling in and around the ventricles.

    脑室内出血（IVH）包括一系列的病理过程，这些病理过程是由脑室及其周围的血液充盈引起的。

    【析】 上述例句均来自国外文献资料，由此可见，一般情况下用-ic 或-ical 结尾的词没有意义上的差异，这是由于英语单词词尾退化的缘故。但要注意例外，英语中某些单词以-ic 或-ical 结尾，其词义有所不同。例如，classic 和 classical，前者意为"经典的"；后者意为"古典的"；clinic（*n.* 临床），clinical（*adj.* 临床的）。

25. inner- 和 intra- 前缀

有些作者为了表达某一特定概念的需要，通常会凭借类推手段，自我创造一些词汇，英语构词中的常用前缀 inner-和 intra-就是其中之一。前缀 inner-和 intra-构词的意义是有区别的。作为前缀使用时，inner-表示 "located or occurring farther inside"（内部的；发生在或位于内部的）；intra-意为 "within"（在……内部）。

例一： Recent studies of drug-eluting **intracoronary** stents suggest that current antiplatelet regimens may not be sufficient to prevent late stent thrombosis.
近来对药物洗脱冠状动脉内支架的研究表明，现行的抗血小板治疗方案可能并不足以预防后期支架内血栓形成。

例二： Schizophrenia is a common major mental disorder. Inner-uterine nutritional deficiency may increase the risk of schizophrenia.
精神分裂症是一种常见的中度精神障碍。子宫内营养缺乏可增大患精神分裂症的危险。

【析】该句中 Inner-uterine 应改为 Intra-uterine。又如："an intra-aortic balloon"（主动脉内球囊）；"intra-population genetic variation"（群体内遗传变异）；"intra-operative grade I complications"（术中一级并发症）；"intra-abdominal pressure"（腹内压）；"inner-membrane"（内膜）等。

英语的前缀构成的词，某些情况下有其特殊意义，不可随意凭空造词，如 "inconceivable female patients"（未妊娠女患者）就是错误的。虽然该词是由前缀 in+conceivable 构成，而且 conceivable 来源于动词词根 conceive（妊娠），但 conceivable 意义为"impossible to image"（不能想象的；不可思议的）。因此，"未妊娠"应用 unpregnant。类似错误还有，如受到汉语影响主观臆断的中式英语，将 "自身免疫"（auto-immune）误表达为 self-immune。

对于我国作者来说，在英语词类使用上的差错不胜枚举，这与我国学者的语言学习习惯有关，即孤立地背诵记忆单词及其中文定义，而忽略词性、词义的内涵和外延等。例如："The alcohol acetylates easily." 应改写为 "The alcohol is acetylated easily."，因为 acetylate 是及物动词；又如："Urinalysis results were normal."（尿检结果正常），正确的说法是 "Urinalysis was normal."，因为 urinalysis 本身就表示 "尿分析（法）"。若要提高对词义的准确掌握，最好的方法就是多侧重词的英文定义，在日常学习中，注意词在语境中的使用，这样才能全面提高语言措辞能力。

二、句法、语篇、逻辑类错误

1. 词义重复、措辞冗长

汉语和英语的对等与不对等是辩证的，由于汉语的作者试图从完全对等思维方式去表达英文，于是会出现大量的冗词重复现象。

例一：Retrospective analysis of adverse reactions of antibiotics from document reviewing.

抗生素不良反应的文献资料回顾分析。

【析】句中 retrospective 和 document reviewing 形成了语义上的重复，retrospective、document、reviewing 均表示对过去的资料回顾分析，此句可改为 "Retrospective analysis of adverse reactions of antibiotics" 或 "Adverse reactions of antibiotics from document."。

例二：Each group was further randomly subdivided into 4 groups of 5 animals for the hormonal studies.

每个小组再随机分为 4 个小组，每组 5 只动物，用于激素研究。

【析】句子中 further 和 subdivided 形成了重复，subdivide 本身已经包含了 "to divide a part or parts of into smaller parts"（再分）之意。此句应修改为 "Each group was randomly subdivided into 4 groups of 5 animals for the hormonal studies."。

例三：Chloride channel blockers display certain protective effects against neuronal injury induced by NO.

氯通道阻滞剂对 NO 诱导的神经元损伤有保护作用。

【析】原句语义冗长，修改后："Chloride channel blockers can protect against neuronal injury induced by NO."。

例四：As for axons, the non-linear accelerated-decelerated movement, caused by rotation along coronal plane, would induce shearing force.

冠状平面突然旋转引发的非线性加速-减速运动导致剪切力变化，从而损害轴突。

【析】原句语义冗长，松散，且缺乏逻辑。修改后："It is likely that the non-linear accelerated-decelerated motion, caused by sudden rotaton in the coronal plane, induced shearing force that damages axons."。

2. 单复数误用

英语和汉语语言之间在名词的"数"方面差异有着很重要的意义。汉语句法结构中，无论是表示离散还是集合，均可用具有复数意义的名词"们"，不仅如此，也无谓语动词一致性要求。例如，"他是医生"，"他们是医生"。而英语却不一样，因为名词的数决定了与之连用的动词的数。以名词的形式来分类，英语中名词分为可数与不可数，可数与不可数是英语名词的最基本类别。凡表示可以计数的事物的名词，称可数名词，反之，凡表示不可以计数的事物的名词，称不可数名词。但问题是，英语中表示抽象概念的不可数名词通常可以用于个体名词，这一转变，不仅导致谓语动词数的变化，更重要的是名词本身的意义也会随之发生变化。例如："The **death** resulted from an infectious disease；

The infectious diseases resulted in 1000 **deaths**.”前者指“死亡”,属抽象概念,后者表示“死亡人数”,属具体概念。另外, 由于英语名词屈折变化的结果, 某些保留了-ics 结尾的名词使用时就较为复杂。一般情况下, 如果以-ics 结尾的名词表示“学科”概念时, 通常当单数, 除此之外, 当复数看待。

例一：Pharmacokinetics of luteinizing hormone-releasing hormone **in rat.**
　　　LHRH 药代动力学试验。
　　　【析】表示动物的名词一般都是可数名词, 使用时有两种情况, 一是加表示复数概念的词尾-s；另一种是加定冠词 the 表示泛指。此句可修改为：“Pharmacokinetics of luteinizing hormone-releasing hormone **in rats**” 或 “Pharmacokinetics of luteinizing hormone-releasing hormone **in the rat**”。

例二：Statistics **are** an important means to sum the number.
　　　统计学是统计数字的重要手段。
　　　【析】句中 statistics 表示学科,谓语动词应用单数。此句应改写为：Statistics is an important means to sum the number.

例三：**Risks** score for predicting death, myocardial infarction, and stroke in patients with stable angina, based on a large randonlised trial cohort of patients.
　　　基于一个大型随机试验预测稳定型心绞痛队列患者死亡、心肌梗死和卒中的危险评分。
　　　【析】“名词+名词”构成的名词词组, 前面部分的名词要用单数, 这类错误在国内医学期刊中甚为常见。此句应改写为“Risk score for predicting death …”。

例四：Uncomplicated lower respiratory tract infection is most often seen between the **age** of 2 and 10 years.
　　　单纯急性下呼吸道感染最常见于2~10 岁儿童。
　　　【析】句中 age 应用 ages, 因为本句语境提示, 这是聚散性的复数, 即由个体集中而来, 故应改写为 “Uncomplicated lower respiratory tract infection is most often seen between the **ages** of 2 and 10 years.”。

名词的单、复数问题不仅涉及其自身概念表达, 而且还影响语义理解、主谓一致性及代词的使用。在句法结构中, 代词, 包括其具有限定性质的形式, 在篇章指向上必须保持一致。例如：“Where vaginal hysterectomy is not possible, laparoscopic hysterectomy is preferable to abdominal hysterectomy, although **it** brings a higher chance of bladder or ureter injury.” 中的 “it”（it 指 laparoscopic hysterectomy）；“In HIV infected patients it remains a major pathogen in those who are unaware of **their** HIV serostatus.” 中的 “their”（their 限定前文的代词 those）。

3. 名词修饰语问题

名词作为名词的修饰语时, 实际上没有了数的概念而起着形容词的作用, 因此, 通常用单数形式。例如，不能表达为 "humans gene"，而应表达为 " human gene"。除此之外，在表示某种事物的类别，而非其性质时，名词的修饰语只能是名词，不可用形容词。例如：不能表达为 "pregnant rate" 而应表达为 "pregnancy rate"。例如：

　　例：To determine whether data on proteinuria are useful for refining estimates of risk based on kidney function alone,and whether the results of **kidneys function tests** can be a useful adjunct to data on proteinuria.

　　　　确定蛋白尿的数据是否有助于完善仅依据肾功能进行风险评估,肾功能检测结果是否是对蛋白尿数据的有力补充。

　　　　【析】从理论上说，人类有双肾，貌似应用复数。但是，肾功能检测指特定的检测项目，因而只能用单数形式作名词修饰语。原句应改为 "…kidney function tests…"。

尽管在现代英语中有复数名词作修饰语的现象，如 "dressings trolley"。但这类名词基本上都是由抽象名词或物质名词派生出来的具体名词。又如：

"At embryonic 4 weeks"（在胚胎 4 周时）应改为 "At embryonic week 4"。

4. 动词时态、语态类错误

动词的时态错误主要表现在同一结构中出现两种不同的动词形式，而语态错误则以误用那些无被动式的动词或短语动词及在同一结构中随意改变语态。

　　例一：**It indicated that** ultrasound **has** no mutating effect on reproductive cells and somatic cells within a certain scope.

　　　　超声辐照在一定剂量范围内对体细胞和生殖细胞没有致突变作用。

　　　　【析】主干结构中的动词用了过去式 indicated，而从句中却用了一般式 has。因此，主句、从句动词形式不一致。应改为 "**It indicated that** ultrasound **had** no…"。

一般情况下，从属结构中的谓语动词形式必须与主干句保持一致，但有例外。例如：

　　例二：This result **suggests** that HspA **might** be an effective protein vaccine for prevention and treatment of the infection of *H.pylori.*

　　　　结果表明，HspA 有可能作为一种有效的蛋白质疫苗用于幽门螺杆菌感染的预防和治疗。

　　　　【析】此类情况是出于措辞的考虑，如果作者认为其研究结果值得进一步探讨，完全可以借助某些功能词来表达作者的思想。另一种情况是，如果从属结构中陈述的为恒久性状态或行为，从属结构中的谓语动词不受主干结构的动词形式制约。例如下例。

　　例三：This findings **suggested** that hepatitis A **is** an infectious disease.

　　　　研究发现，甲型肝炎是传染性疾病。

例四：**We found** the whole blood cell scan was abnormal in 12 of the total 24 cases and a good clinical correlation **was obtained** in 11 of the 13.

24 例患者中，我们发现了 12 例患者全血细胞扫描异常，其中 13 例中的 11 例有良好的临床相关性。

【析】由于 and 在句中起并列关系作用，因此，前后分句必须保持结构上一致。显然，本句随意改变了语态，导致结构不平行。本句可以修改为："We found the whole blood cell scan was abnormal in 12 of the total 24 cases and obtained a good clinical correlation in 11 of the 13. "，或略去冗词，简化为："The whole blood cell scan was abnormal in 12 of the total 24 cases and a good clinical correlation was obtained in 11 of the 13. "。

除了上述问题外，还要注意英文中某些动词或动词短语的特殊结构和表达。例如：

例五：The neutralizing antibody level in children of 7-12 months **was proved** to be the lowest.

中和抗体含量在 7 至 12 个月的婴儿组最低。

【析】prove 一般无被动式，可以直接用主动式表示被动意义。所以原句宜改为 "The neutralizing antibody level in children of 7-12 months **proved** to be the lowest. "。

例六：The control group **was consisted of** 8 healthy subjects.

控制组有 8 位健康者组成。

【析】短语动词 "consist of"（包括，由……组成），不能用被动式。它有别于 "be composed of"（包括，由……组成）。该句应改为 "Eight healthy subjects consisted of the control group."。此外，不能用作被动关系的词有 "belong to、happen to、cost、lack、fail" 等。

例七：This paper **was** a brief summary based on 20 cases.

本文综述了 20 个病例。

【析】该句谓语 was 应改为 is。表示论文 "报道、介绍、综述、推荐" 等的动词时态，如 "本文报道（介绍，综述等）……" 是文摘中使用频率较高的一种句式，通常用一般现在时，偶尔用现在完成时。

例八：We **are failed to** find any infection in follow-up.

随访未发现感染情况。

【析】本句正确的说法是 "We failed to find any infection in follow-up."。英语中某些表示状态的及物动词，如 "have、own、possess、suffice、cost、lack、want、fit、resemble、fail、last" 等作谓语时通常不用被动语态。

5. 非谓语动词类逻辑错误

在上一章我们介绍的非谓语动词的用法，由于非谓语动词本身仍然保留了动词的某些特性，尤其是分词作状语时，要特别注意其逻辑主语是否与句中谓语动词的主语相一致，否则分词必须带有自己的主语，分词逻辑主语可以是分词动作的执行者，也可以是分词动作的承受者。

例一：**As applying random amplified polymorphic DNA (RAPD) technique to detecting genetic polymorphism, location of different genes, identification of races, etc,** its reliability has been generally suspected owing to poor repeatability and homology of co-migrating bands in the experiment.

　　　　随着随机扩展多态性 DNA 技术（RAPD）应用于遗传多样性检测、基因定位、品系鉴定等领域，由于发现其重复性较差，共迁移的 RAPD 标记间有时无同源性等问题，其可靠性逐渐受到怀疑。

　　　　【析】句子中 "As applying…identification of races, etc" 为现在分词与介词 as 构成的时间状语，分词的逻辑主语应为 some people，这与主句中的主语"its reliability"不一致，因此，应改写为 "As applying random amplified polymorphic DNA (RAPD) technique to detecting genetic polymorphism, location of different genes, identification of races, etc, some people have generally suspected its reliability owing to poor repeatability and homology of co-migrating bands in the experiments."。

例二：**Comparing with the control group,** the lead content in the rats' whole blood, faeces and urine of the poisoning group was significantly higher.

　　　　与对照组相比，铅中毒组大鼠全血、粪便和尿液中铅含量均显著升高。

　　　　【析】句子中分词短语 "comparing with" 与名词词组 "control group" 为动宾关系，即 "control group" 为动作承受者，显然因逻辑错误导致分词使用不当，该句应改写为 "Compared with the control group, the lead content in the rats' whole blood, faeces and urine of the poisoning group was significantly higher."。

例三：**Taken into consideration,** polio eradication program should have started simultaneously in all regions in the world.

　　　　考虑所有因素，消灭脊髓灰质炎运动应该在全世界各个国家和地区同时进行。

　　　　【析】从逻辑关系分析，分词短语的逻辑主语与主句不一致，主句的主语也非分词短语 "taken into consideration" 的逻辑主语，分词短语和主句分别表示不同的概念。为了让分词短语和主句达到逻辑上的关联，分词短语必须增加其独立的主语，根据句意，可以改写为 "Everything（being）taken into consideration, polio eradication program should have started simultaneously in all regions in the world."。当使用这类分词结构时需要特别谨慎，否则会导致语篇模糊而难以完成交际任务。

例四：**Investigating of us showed that,** out of ninety babies, 21 babies (23.34%) had seizures associated with hypoglycemia .

　　　　我们的调查结果表明，90 名婴儿中，21 名（23.34%）癫痫发作与血糖过低有关。

【析】从全句看，这是动名词的所有格用法错误。动名词是一种抽象名词，为了表示动名词的动作执行者是谁，可以在动名词之前增加一个所有格名词或代词，构成逻辑上的主谓关系。据此，本句应是"Our investigating showed that, out of ninety babies, 21 babies (23.34%) had seizures associated with hypoglycemia."。

6. 比较（级）关系错误

摘要写作中涉及对事物之间的比较，突出某种事物、现象或结果时，需要借助比较关系结构。对两种事物进行比较，除了常见的动词短语"compare with/to"等之外，更为常见的是借助形容词或副词的比较等级，如等同比较（"as…as"结构）、拉丁比较（某些来自拉丁语的外来词本身就提示比较关系，如"superior/inferior to"）及等差比较（采用…than…结构）。采用等同比较和拉丁比较时一般不会出现较大失误，失误较多的是描述等差比较关系，通常因结构错误而导致比较对象缺乏对应。

例一：For patients with reduced EF, moderate or severe diastolic dysfunction was more common than **that** when EF was preserved.

与 EF 正常的患者相比，EF 降低的患者合并中、重度舒张功能不全的比例较高。

【析】EF, ejection fraction, 射血分数。本句中比较的对象是 EF 处于两种不同的状态下所产生的结果，因而，对应关系是两个状语分句（"reduced EF" 和 "preserved EF"）。句子中增加了不必要的代词 that，造成比较关系混乱，that 要省略。

例二：The patients treated with ceftriaxone had **a slightly shorter time to defervescence than those treated with ofloxacin.**

用头孢曲松治疗的患者退热速度要比氧氟沙星快。

【析】从表面上看，似乎不太容易发现本句中存在的问题，如果仔细分析，本句比较的中心是动作关系，即 treat。因此，than 在此句中的词性为连词，故此句应改写为："The patients treated with ceftriaxone had a slightly shorter time to defervescence than **did** those treated with ofloxacin."。

例三：To evaluate patient clinical characteristics associated with receiving more intensive treatment; and to assess whether AMI patients residing in regions with more intensive invasive treatment and management strategies have better long-term survival **than that** residing in regions with more intensive medical management strategies.

评价接受积极治疗患者的相关临床特征；评估居住于积极采取介入治疗策略地区的 AMI 患者与居住于积极采取药物治疗策略地区的患者相比，是否具有更好的远期生存率。

【析】本句比较的对象为 patients，因此，代词应用对应的复数形式，所以，应改成"To evaluate patient clinical characteristics associated with receiving more intensive treatment; and to assess whether AMI patients residing in regions with more intensive invasive treatment and management strategies have better long-term survival **than those** residing in regions with more intensive medical management strategies."。

上述错误在写作中较具普遍性，要避免这类错误的发生，首先要充分熟悉英语基本句型结构，其次，表达时要仔细斟酌比较的对象是什么。

例四： Prior randomized trials suggested that revascularization of diabetic patients by coronary artery bypass grafting (CABG) **produced more superior results than** balloon angioplasty.

以往的随机研究建议糖尿病患者采取冠状动脉搭桥手术（CABG）进行血运重建，其效果优于球囊扩张血管成形术。

【析】superior（高级的），为外来词。该词在使用中有其特定的结构，即"…superior to…"。此外，英语中类似的词还有 inferior（低级的）、perfect（完美的）、unique（唯一的，独特的）、prior（优先的，在前的）、anterior（较早的）、junior（年少的，下级的）、senior（年长的，高级的）。这类词没有最高级，但可用于比较关系，后接介词 to。据此，原句改为"Prior randomized trials suggested that revascularization of diabetic patients by coronary artery bypass grafting (CABG) **produced results superior to** balloon angioplasty."。

例五： The **levels** of sIL-2R (soluble IL-2 receptor), sICAM-1(soluble intercellular adhesion molecule-1) and sVCAM-1 (soluble vascular cell adhesion molecule 1) were significantly higher in patients than **the controls**.

患者的可溶性白细胞介素，可溶性细胞间黏着分子 1 和可溶性血管细胞黏着分子 1 明显高于控制组。

【析】本例中，levels 比较的对象应该是"levels in the controls"，而不是"the controls"。据此，该句应改为"The **levels** of sIL-2R（soluble IL-2 receptor），sICAM-1（soluble intercellular adhesion molecule-1）and sVCAM-1（soluble vascular cell adhesion molecule 1）were significantly higher in patients than the **levels**（**or: those**）of the controls."。这类错误属于比较对象不一致，也是写作中常见的错误，主要原因是忽略了语篇中的逻辑关系所致。如果从话语结构上仔细分析，弄清比较对象，这类错误基本可以避免。

例六： The results showed that this new surgical technique is **more perfect than** the conventional one.

研究结果显示，新的手术方法比传统方式更完善。

【析】英语中某些具有绝对概念的形容词（副词），如 perfect、unique、

supreme、superior（inferior）、right 等，没有比较级形式，也无最高级形式。因此，"more perfect" 为误用。正确表达为 "The results showed that this new surgical technique is superior to the conventional one 或 The results showed that this new surgical technique is perfect."（借助含蓄比较方式）。

7. 副词的位置对语义的影响

按词汇意义划分，副词可以分为时间副词（如 before、ago、immediately 等）、位置空间副词（如 above、across、under 等）、程度副词（如 nearly、almost 等）、频度副词（如 always、often、seldom 等）。副词作为修饰语，在英语句中总体上可以有 3 个位置，即句首、句中、句末。对于这些副词的意义及使用，基本上没有什么大障碍，如果有什么疑问，查阅语法参考书或查阅词典即可解决。然而，我们可能忽略的是某些副词在句子中的特殊位置或与某些词，如 not 连用时语法意义的差异。试比较：

例一：1）**Almost** 80% of cases and deaths are in Asia.
　　　　　差不多 80%的病例和死亡均在亚洲。
　　　2）80% of cases and deaths are **almost** in Asia.
　　　　　80%的病例和死亡几乎在亚洲。

【析】以上两例中副词 almost 因位置改变，所表示的意义是不一样的。第 1 句的话语中心在强调百分比，第 2 句则重点说明地点。

例二：1）The patient lost **nearly** 1000 ml of blood during the operation.
　　　　　手术中患者失血量大约为 1000 ml。
　　　2）The patient **nearly** lost 1000 ml of blood during the operation.
　　　　　手术中患者差不多失去了 1000 ml 的血。

【析】以上两个句子所表达的意思的主要差别在于：第 1 句提示的信息是患者失血量为 1000 ml 左右，传递的是真实信息；第 2 句所传递的信息是一种夸张，事实并非如此。

8. 否定（词）的问题

"否定"是对"肯定"而言，凡是肯定的东西都有其相反的否定的对应。"否定"是语言的一个逻辑范畴。从表达的内容来说，"否定"可分为一般否定和特殊否定。根据否定的意思来分，又有完全否定、基本否定、部分否定等。对于作者来说，需要小心谨慎的是否定词的位置变化及否定词和某些特殊词（如不定代词中的 all、every 用作形容词时，everything 等）连用时所产生的意义变化。

例一：1）**Every** blood vessel is **not** visible.
　　　　　所有的血管都看不见。
　　　2）**Not every** blood vessel is visible.
　　　　　并非所有的血管都看不见。

【析】上述两个句子因否定词位置不同，所传递的信息不同。第 1 句表示全部否定，无一例外；第 2 句为部分否定，提示有例外情况。

例二：1）These adverse reactions are **not** incorporated into drug reference sources in a systematic manner.

这些药物的毒副反应没有系统地写入药物信息参考。

2）**Not** these adverse reactions are incorporated into drug reference sources in a systematic manner.

这些药物的毒副反应没有全部系统地写入药物信息参考。

英语否定中除了使用否定词之外，另一种手段是借助具有否定意义的副词、名词、形容词及动词等来达到否定的目的。由于这类词本身具有否定含义，因此，译词时切莫画蛇添足，造成信息传递错误。

例三：Mesothelioma is an **umcommon** tumor.

间皮瘤是一种罕见的肿瘤。

【析】如果将本句中加上否定词 not，改写成"Mesothelioma is **not an uncommon** tumor."，其意思就变成了"间皮瘤是一种常见的肿瘤"。这就与原义大相径庭。

例四：Lipid-lowering agents are widely prescribed in the United States. Reliable estimates of rhabdomyolysis risk with various lipid-lowering agents are **hardly** available.

在美国降脂药物已获广泛应用。但是对各种降脂药物发生肌溶解症的危险性目前尚缺乏可靠的估计。

【析】同上句一样，该句中 hardly 本身提示否定意义，如若再加上否定词 not，变为" Lipid-lowering agents are widely prescribed in the United States. Reliable estimates of rhabdomyolysis risk with various lipid-lowering agents are **not hardly** available. "，其意思就变成了肯定。

9. 逻辑修辞错误

英文摘要写作，国内绝大多数作者基本采用的是翻译手段，即对照中文摘要用英文表达。长期以来我们的外语学习者受到双重困扰，一是外环境，包括学校的教学手段和外语测试手段；二是内环境，包括学习者对外语学习的价值取向，如被动应试，急功近利地"考证"等。这些消极因素导致我们的外语学习者缺乏全面而系统的语言训练，更不用说对语言学基本常识的了解，如语义、语用等。以至于英文摘要写作"中式化"，语篇缺乏连贯。例如，句子与段落之间缺乏同一性，句子与句子、段落之间缺乏连贯性，语言表达缺乏简明性。

例一：This animal model, (which was) used for selection of kinds of regulatory mutants with high efficiency, was based on definite selectors and moderators.

该动物模型基于一定的选择剂和调节剂，可高效选择某些调控突变体。

【析】按全句逻辑关系分析，主句"this animal model was based on..."的提示，短语"used for selection of..."只起到附加说明的作用。该句为摘要中的一句，按整个摘要的语篇分析，应改写为"This animal model, based on definite selectors and moderators, was used for selection of kinds of regulatory mutants with high efficiency."。

简单而言，一个句子只允许叙述一个中心思想。如果用一个句子表达两个思想内容时，总是把主要思想或内容放在主句中表达，将次要内容用从句或短语表达，从而体现主次关系。该句显然违背了这一原则，造成主从颠倒。

例二： The division frequency of protoplasts was lower in the liquid medium than that embedded in the medium containing agarose.

原生质体在液体培养基中的分裂频率低于包埋在含有琼脂糖的培养基中的分裂频率。

【析】对照该句的汉语，用 that 替代"the division frequency of protoplasts"，在语法上不存在什么问题，但从修辞方面考虑，that 替代的主体 frequency 不能被埋在含有琼脂糖的培养基中，被埋的只能是 protoplasts，故英语句中缺少了替代 protoplasts 的 those，导致句子意思不完整。句意残缺主要表现在各种句子成分之间的关系不协调，如成分残缺、结构混乱、主题表达不充分、不具体导致意思不明确等。据此，该句应改写为"The division frequency of protoplasts was lower in the liquid medium than that of those embedded in the medium containing agarose."。

例三： If we attempt to employ meta-analysis of published and unpublished tabular data from randomised trials, several difficulties are encountered.

如果我们试图对已发表和未发表随机试验的表格资料进行荟萃分析，会存在一些困难。

【析】状语从句中的主语、语态与主句中的主语和语态不一致。这是英文写作中常见的语态随意改变现象。从连贯性角度考虑，语态的随意改变、叙事主体对象的突然改变、缺乏必要的过渡性连接词均可能破坏句子内部平衡。根据连贯性原则，该句应改写为"If we attempt to employ meta-analysis of published and unpublished tabular data from randomised trials, we'll encounter several difficulties."。又如下例，缺少必要的过渡性连词。

例四： Where vaginal hysterectomy is not possible, laparoscopic hysterectomy is preferable to abdominal hysterectomy, it brings a higher chance of bladder or ureter injury.

在不可能行阴式子宫切除术时，腹腔镜子宫切除术优于经腹手术，尽管前者损伤膀胱或输尿管的机会有所增加。

【析】从本句所提示的语境意义来看，由于句子之间缺乏必要的连接词衔接，导致句子意义显得松散。为了达到连贯一致，本句必须增加适当的连词，将其改写为"Where vaginal hysterectomy is not possible, laparoscopic hysterectomy is preferable to abdominal hysterectomy, **although** it brings a higher chance of bladder or ureter injury."。

例五： ERBD is an effective treatment for MOJ with the advantages of a smaller cut, safety and less complications. It is possible to help the patients to remain their lifetime longer and to improve the life quality.

经内镜置放胆道支架是治疗恶性梗阻性黄疸的有效方法，其优点是创伤小、安全性好、并发症少，并能提高患者生活质量及延长生存时间。

【析】 本句在表达上试图完全对等汉语，是典型的"中式"表达。不仅用词重复，更是舍近求远，不够简明。可改写成"ERBD is effective in treatment of MOJ with less invasion and complication. What's more, it can improve the quality of the patients' life and even prolong their life span."。

三、关键词列举不当

关键词列举不当也是作者常犯的错误。主要问题如下所述。

1. 关键词遗漏

研究论文所选关键词应突出反映研究主题内容，任何遗漏都会导致文献检索被漏检。例如：①标题为"Relationship between infection of *Helicobacter pylori* and activity of chronic gastritis and peptic ulcer"（幽门螺杆菌感染与慢性胃炎和消化性溃疡活动期的关系）。原摘要后标注的关键词有"*Helicobacter pylori*, superficial gastritis, atrophic gastritis"，而漏标了"peptic ulcer"；②标题为"Analysis on the risk factors related to hyperuricemia in population in northern Anhui province"，原摘要后标注的关键词："physical examination, blood uric acid, risk factors"，但漏标了"Metabolic diseases, cardiovascular diseases"。

2. 错误概念标识

医学写作概念或术语表达应准确无误，不可出现任何差池，否则会导致信息传递错误，不仅如此，也反映出作者的专业水平。如将"*Bacillus tetani*"（破伤风杆菌）标成"tetanus"破伤风（Tetanus is a serious illness caused by *Clostridium* bacteria）；"schistosome"（血吸虫）标成"schistosomiasis"（血吸虫病）；"digitalis"（洋地黄）标成"digitalization"（洋地黄化）等。

3. 重复标注

重复标注关键词，不仅导致关键词过多列举，同样，也反映出作者的专业水平。例如：标题为"Analysis of mycoplasma infection and drug resistance in genitourinary tract"（泌

尿生殖道支原体感染和耐药性分析）一文，其摘要后罗列的关键词是 Mycoplasma（支原体）；*Ureaplasma urealyticum*（解脲脲原体）；*Mycoplasma hominis*（人型支原体）；Drug sensitivity test（药物敏感试验）"。显然，*Ureaplasma urealyticum* 和 *Mycoplasma hominis* 都属于 *Mycoplasma*；又如，某个作者在其文摘后将关键词这样标注："Trace elements、iron、zinc、copper、calcium、magnesium"（微量元素；铁；锌；铜；钙；镁），显然不当，因为 "iron、zinc、copper、calcium、magnesium" 都属于 "trace elements"。

4. 关键词标引顺序不当

有时，作者仅考虑关键词标注的完整性，而忽略了关键词标注的顺序问题。其实，这个问题表面看，似乎无伤大雅，但恰恰违背了一定的逻辑关系。众所周知，文章标题是全文的高度浓缩体，摘要是正文浓缩出来的小短文，这是由大到小的蕴含关系。同理，关键词标注时，也应遵循这一准则，通过位置关系，体现出主次顺序。例如："Clinical classification and microsurgical procedures of gliomas of the limbic system"（边缘系统胶质瘤的临床分型及显微手术治疗）一文，作者给出的关键词顺序是 "limbic system；glioma；microsurgery"（边缘系统；胶质瘤；显微手术），正确顺序应改为 "glioma；limbic system；microsurgery" 才妥当。又如："Effect of antipsychotics on serum total bile acid levels in patietns with schizophrenia"（抗精神病药物对精神分裂症患者血清总胆汁酸的影响），原标关键词的顺序是 "antipsychotic drugs；schizophrenia；total bile acid"（抗精神病药物；精神分裂症；总胆汁酸），而正确的位置应该是首先标注 "schizophrenia"。

5. 其他不当标注

除了上述常见错误之外，还有一些不当标注方式，如 "Staphylococcal pneumonia"（葡萄球菌性肺炎），应该采用概念交叉组配方式标注为 "*Staphylococcus aureus*，pneumonia"；同样，"Pediatric neuroblastoma"（小儿神经母细胞瘤）应改标为 "neuroblastoma，pediatrics"；"simultaneous kidney-pancreas transplant"（胰肾联合移植）应采用并列概念词组配后再标注为 "kidney tranplantaiton, pancreas transplantation"；"anus temperature"（肛温）应组配为 "rectum, body temperature"；"acute intestinal obstruction"（急性肠梗阻）借助限定概念组配标注为 "intestinal obstruction，acute disease"。此外，还应避免使用动词或形容词作为关键词使用，如 "obstructive" 应改写为 "obstructive disease"。

6. 使用淘汰的医学概念

今天的医学科学发展日新月异，随着研究的不断深入，一些科学理论不断更新，因此，医学概念术语表达也随之赋予新的定义。例如：Adolescent psychology（旧）→psychology，adolescent（新）；aldosterone synthase（旧）→Cytochrome P-450 CYP11B2（新）；neuronal migration disorders（旧）→malformations of cortical development，group Ⅱ（新）；receptor，erB-2（旧）→receptor，ErB-2（新）；Eeiter disease（旧）→Reiter syndrome（新）；replication factor A（旧）→replication protein A（新）；spectrum analysis，mass（旧）→ mass spectrometry

（新）等。这些概念术语变化，对医学写作及关键词标引都会产生极大影响。这些影响包括论文质量评估、检索文献效率、文献被检索引用率等。

7. 英美英语差异问题

中国作者在用英文写作时，通常还会忽视医学概念术语在欧美国家及其他方面的差异，这种差异主要有：①单词拼写差异，如 "diarrhea（美），diarrhea（英）；leukemia（美），leukaemia（英）"。②药品通用名称的差异。导致这种差异的原因受到 British Approved Name（英国药典委员会批准的非专利药品名称，BAN）和 recommended International Non-Proprietary Name（国际非专有药名，INN）的影响。虽然 BAN 和 INN 有大量共同表达，但仍然存在一些差异，如 "grusemid（BAN），furosemide（INN）；amethocaine（BAN），tetracaine（INN）；amoxycillin（BAN），amoxicillin（INN）；cephalexin（BAN），cefalexin（INN）；dicyclomine（BAN），dicycloverine（INN）" 等。

总之，医学英文摘要写作中所表现出的种种问题不胜枚举。对于作者来说，要想有效地避免不合乎英文规范的表达，作者（学习者）应注意做到下述几点。

（1）多读一些以英语为母语作者写就的英文著作以体会地道的英语。

（2）了解一些应用语言学的有关知识，如语义、语用以提高措辞能力。

（3）积累一点英语国家的相关文化背景常识，从而避免"中式"思维干扰。

有道是："拳不离手，曲不离口"，对于英语学习也是如此。要持之以恒，不要为了发表论文而写作。语言学习需要长期积累，没有捷径可循。学习并掌握一门语言，只有一条捷径，那就是 "Practice，practice and practice"。

四、练 习

11-1 选择适当的词填空

1. There were no skeletal deformities or neurocutaneous _____(markers/indicators).

2. Complete lissencephaly is synonymous with agyria, _____(however/whereas) incomplete lissencephaly refers to brains with shallow sulci and a relatively smooth surface.

3. Classic lissencephaly (type I) is a brain malformation caused by abnormal neuronal migration _____(on/at) 9 to 13 weeks' gestation.

4. Familial inheritance should be kept in mind and to be considered in antenatal counseling. Patients with LIS detected by MRI should _____(conduct/undergo) cranial tomography to rule out intracranial calcification as these families have low risk of recurrence.

5. Disease_____(advancement/progression) was related to development of symptoms before 5 years of age, persistent atelectasis, and right lower lobe involvement.

6. A _____(retrospective/prospective) review of charts for all patients referred to the pulmonary clinic for evaluation of recurrent chest infection during the period Jan. 1993-Aug. 2005 at King Faisal specialist hospital.

7. They measured depression (SCL-20), overall functional _____(damage/impairment) and quality of life (SF-12), physical functioning (PCS-12), depression treatment, and satisfaction with care.

8. Although treatment of depression in primary care has improved, few improvements deal with the specific needs of_____(elderly/older) patients.

9. Patients were aged 60 or older and met_____(standard/criteria) for major depression or dysthymia, or both, according to the structured clinical interview for DSM-IV axis I disorders (SCID).

10. _____(Outcome/Result) variables included self-reported use of antidepressants and psychotherapy, satisfaction with care.

11. _____(Medium/Mean) age at loss of ambulation was 8.1y but at the time of the study when_____(mean/average) age was 10.1y only 63% were non-ambulatory.

12. We retrieved published case reports of suspected adverse drug reactions and _____(established/developed) whether each case report had been followed by more definitive studies.

13. Alternatively, if a validation study did not cite the original case report, we would not have found it through the citation_____(index/marker) search.

14. All the subjects were asymptomatic and long-term follow-up of pulmonary function is good despite minor radiological anomalies _____(like/such as) compensatory lobar hyperinflation.

15. Quality scores increased_____(with/by) clinical team size (measured by the whole time equivalent number of principals, non-principals, and practice nurses).

16. Practices with fewer than four _____(completed/whole) time equivalent clinicians had lower quality recorded.

17. Neutrophil counts_____(at/on) 12 hours after birth range from 7,000 to 15,000/mcL in term infants, and at times are higher in preterm neonates compared with children and adults.

18. _____(Temperature/Fever) was noted in roughly half of the patients.

19. Since one of our goals was to assess the reliability of Jones criteria and since no alternative diagnostic system has been formally proposed yet, the gold_____(criteria/standard)for ARF in this study was based on the authors' clinical judgement.

20. Apical systolic_____(sound/murmur) was by far the most common clinical cardiac sign.

21. Cystic fibrosis is initially a disease of the airways which eventually progresses to parenchymal destruction. The extent of this destructive process varies between_____(regions/district)of the lung, rather than being uniformly distributed.

22. The regulation of cell proliferation and apoptosis is linked at the level of the cell _____(period/cycle).

23. _____(Duration/Period) of residence was obtained from a questionnaire either completed at the Vitamin A Program or mailed to the subject.

24. These initial stress stimuli in the tubular compartment are known to cause cell_____(impairment/injury)and death.

25. In an _____(*in vitro/in vivo*)model of _____(trauma/wound) healing using injured alveolar epithelial cells, hydrogen peroxide has been shown to cause cell death via caspase-dependent apoptosis.

26. Immunofluorescence _____(microscope/microscopy) images of PNA-positive cells exhibited an increase in galectin-3 protein expression with acidosis.

27. Based on the results of these tests and the patient's _____(professional/ occupational) exposure to cotton inhalation, the cellulose fibres were concluded to be cotton.

28. These observations suggest a role for WNK1 gene products in the regulation of distal nephron Na$^+$ transport, but their_____(relationship/relation) to the pathogenesis of FHHt remains unclear.

29. Starting ICS at a constant moderate or low dose is equally _____(effective/ efficacious) to starting at a high dose and then stepping down.

30. A 6 year old girl was_____(admitted/hospitalized) with recurrent episodes of loss of consciousness. ECG showed prolonged QT interval and macroscopic T Wave alternans.

31. Hyperuricemia is also commonly observed in metabolic syndrome, as well as in secondary insulin resistance syndromes such as that associated with gout, diuretic_____ (usage/use), or preeclampsia.

32. Wound dehiscence near the port with an active infection, failure to thrive, catheter obstruction, or visceral-to-parietal peritoneal adhesions at laparotomy were, _____ (however/while), used as criteria for removing an animal from the study.

33. All _____(cases/subjects) gave their informed consent and the study was approved by the human research ethics committee of the University of Western Australia and the Clinical Drug Trials Committee of the Sir Charles Gairdner Hospital, Nedlands, Western Australia.

34. The potential of these results to indicate the clinical use of EGF in _____ (subjects/cases)of adult obstruction is limited by the fact that the study used neonates and that EGF treatment was initiated from the start of UUO.

35. We suggest a larger study with equal _____(doses/dosages) of two vaccines with estimation of antibodies to pre-S antigens to confirm our findings.

11-2 找出句中的错误并改正

1. It is important to consider LIS in the diagnosis of developmental delay as many patients may be diagnosed than cerebral palsy. It may have familial occurrence and can occur in sibs of same family often leading to a diagnostic problem.

2. To authors knowledge there is no case reports or care series reported in Indian subcontinent except for a recent report from India.

3. One-year-old boy, presented to Pediatric Neurology Clinic of a tertiary care hospital with myoclonic seizures from 4 month of age,

4. His birth weight were 3.25 kg and there was history of consistent weight gain.

5. Magnetic resonance imaging of brain revealed thickening agyric cortex with diminished thickness of white matter suggestive of lissencephaly.

6. They were probably belonged to pure isolated variety of LIS, which contributes to about 15%-20% of patients.

7. Published reports from some developing countries suggest that childhood bronchiectasis may not be disappearing, and that it represents a more common problem than that in developed countries.

8. The present report agrees other reports of early start of symptoms before 5 years of age in 83% of our population.

9. Published case reports of suspected adverse reactions are of limited value as suspicions seldom are subjected to confirmatory investigation.

10. To determine whether individual case reports fulfilled their role as early warnings signals that stimulated more detailed studies we used two methods to establish whether such additional validation studies had been carried out.

11. This may have been because for the lack of data confirming the link between the drug and the adverse event.

12. They are consisted of pulmonary sequestration (PS), cystic adenomatoid malformation (CCAM), congenital lobar emphysema (CLE), and bronchogenic cyst (BC).

13. Plain X-ray along side chest CT scans were chosen as diagnostic modalities for all of patients, which revealed involvement of right upper lobe in two cases, right middle lobe was involved in 1 case, right lower lobe in 1 and left lower lobe in 2 cases.

14. In two patients left-upper lobe were impacted and one subject had bilobar involvement of upper and middle lobes of left side.

15. Linear regression analysis used, we estimated the univariate associations between possible determinants of quality and the quality score.

16. Subjects were included in the study if: a) their age ranged from 5 to 15 years; b) they had a clinical diagnosis of a first episode of ARF agreed by at least 2 board-certified rheumatologists; and c) this diagnosis was sustained for 6 months and 2 or more visits.

17. Carditis, in the form of valvulitis, usually occur in more than three-quarters of patients with ARF.

18. Although any layer of the heart can be affected, mitral valve insufficiency was present in more than 90% of patients who performed echo-Doppler, as has been reported by other authors

19. Necrotizing enterocolitis are the most common gastrointestinal emergency of the neonate, affecting 5%-10% of infants, yet the pathogenesis remains unclear.

20. The rate of deaths or suicidal ideation are consistent with older primary care veterans reported by Oslin and colleagues

21. Adult female Wistar rats were injected daily for 7 days with 2 g of BSA or an equivalent volume of sterile normal saline everyday.

22. Our studies were approved by our Institutional Animal Care and Use Committee and were performed in accordance to the Guide for the Care and Use of Laboratory Animals of the National Institutes of Health.

23. Immunohistochemical analysis was performed, as previously described, on tissue sections fixed in 10% neutral buffered formalin and embedded them in paraffin.

24. Glomerular disease may incur the chemical alteration of albumin before their filtration into the urinary space.

25. In addition to having appreciable inhibitory effects on amastigote multiplication within macrophages (IC50, 4.6 μg/ml), complete elimination of liver and spleen parasite burden was achieved by18-glycyrrhetinic acid (GRA) at a dosage of 50 mg/(kg·d), given three times, 5 days apart, in a 45-day mice model of visceral leishmaniasis (利什曼病).

26. Each 15 days after infection up to 45 days, single-cell suspensions were prepared using splenocytes from infected mice as described previously.

附录1　致谢（Acknowledgement）

根据国际惯例及刊物的投稿要求，对于那些在研究过程中提供过各种帮助但又不符合作者资格的人，作者应在研究论文之后，参考文献之前一一表示感谢。致谢范围包括研究设计方案的指导、技术支持、对整个研究的审核、研究设施设备的提供、研究对象的参与配合度及研究经费的资助等。

例一：感谢提供研究设施。

The authors are grateful to the Tamilnadu Veterinary and animal Science University, Chennai for the facilities provided during the course of study.

引自：*Vet World*, 2012, 5(5): 284

例二：感谢对本研究思路的指导、审核。

We acknowledge the major intellectual contribution, comments, criticisms and advice of Drs. Cristinane S. Carvalho, Michel Rabinovitch, and Genevieve Milon. We would like to thank the *Plate-form Imagerie Dynamique* staff, Institute Pasteur, France, for technical support and advice, especially Dr. Spencer Shorte, Emmanuelle Perret, and Christophe Machu. We also acknowledge Drs. Eric Prina, Rogerio Amino, Erico Carmo, and Thierry Lang for their most generous support and exciting discussion. This manuscript has been proofread and edited by native English speakers with related backgrounds from BioMed Proofreading, LLC.

引自：*PLoS Neglected Tropical Diseases*, 2012,6(2): e1518

例三：感谢帮助处理数据及数据资料收集。

We thank the Statistics and Data Department at the Malawi-Liverpool-Wellcome Trust Clinical Research Program, the data management team of the Blantyre Malaria Project, and John Cashman for their contribution to the data abstraction. We also extend special thanks to the patients at QECH, the medical and nursing staff of the QECH medical and pediatric wards, and the Malawi-Liverpool-Wellcome Trust Clinical Research Ward for their contribution to this work.

引自：*Emerging Infectious Diseases*, 2012, 18(2): 272

例四： 感谢资金支持。

Sources of funding: this work was supported by operating grants from the Canadian Institute of Health Research and GlaxoSmithKline, Canada.

引自：*Disease Models & Mechanisms*, 2009, 2: 282

例五： 感谢技术及研究思路审核。

We than Adrian Dixon, Sri Aitken, and the radiography staff at addenbrooke's Hospital for their assistance with imaging studies; Fiona Tulloch and Keith Bruling, who performed the biochemical assays, and David Moller for helpful discussions; the patients and volunteers for their participation; and the physicians involved in the Genetics of Obesity Study.

引自：*N Engl J Med*, 2009, 360: 52

【致谢常用句型】

(1) to thank…for…

(2) to be thankful to…for…

(3) to be grateful to…for….

(4) to be indebted to…for…

(5) to acknowledge…; To be acknowledged

(6) to express…thanks to…for…

(7) to appreciate

(8) to express…appreciation to…for…

附录 2 投稿信（Cover letter）

　　研究论文投稿时一般均要求附有 Cover letter，中文的意思是指随文稿一起提交的投稿信或声明信，简言之，就是作者学术道德的自律声明。尽管各刊物一般会在其投稿说明中有相应要求，但 Cover letter 总体格式和内容无外乎涉及说明本研究的主题意义、主要价值、论文文题、投稿刊物的名称、作者对稿件的处理有无特殊要求、伦理学要求符合度、通信作者的姓名、联系地址和联系方式等。写作时无须长篇大论，能将重要问题说明清楚即可，字数一般在 80～200 字左右为宜。

　　备注：下列例证结合网络素材，经作者加工改写。

例一：

(Address of Author)

Marie Taylor

324 Maple Street

Newmarket, MA 02357

(Date)

September 20, 2012

Dear Editor,

We are sending you the manuscript entitled *"Vertebroplasty and kyphoplasty for the treatment of vertebral compression fractures: an evidenced-based review of the liberature"* for consideration for publication in your journal, ***The Spine Journal***.

This study has not been duplicate publication or submission elsewhere. The authors received no financial support for the research and/or authorship of this article. The authors declare that they have no conflict of interest to the publication of this article. The Local Ethics Committee approval was obtained.

I look forward to hearing from you at your earliest convenience.

Thanks for your evaluation.

Best Regards,

(Signature)

Marie Taylor

(Name of Corresponding author)

Matthew J. McGirt. 600N. Wolfe Street, Meyer 8-161, Baltimore, MD 21287, USA. Tel: (410)292-7026. E-mail: mmcgirt1@jhmi.edu

例二：

(Address of Author)

Instituto Superiore di Sanita,

Viale Regina Elena 299, 00161 Rome, Italy

(Date)

February 24, 2003

Dear Sir,

I attach herewith a manuscript entitled "*Case report: An unusual late relapse of Plasmodium vivax malaria*" for your kind consideration for publication in your journal, *Am. J. Trop. Med. Hyg.,*.

The manuscript is the first case report about relapse of "*Plasmodium vivax malaria*" in "*Intaly*". This report also supports our previous relapse case report of "*Plasmodium vivax malaria*" with "*Carlo Severini and Michela Menegon*".

I declare that all authors have agreed on the submission of this article and it is not currently under any consideration for publication anywhere.

You may communicate with me in all aspects of the publication.

Thank you for your cooperation in anticipation.

Sincerely,

Signature (Name of Corresponding author)

Ciancarlo Majori

例三：

(Address of Author)

Department of Surgery,

Kouseiren Takaoka Hospital 5-10,

Eiraku-cho, Takaoka, 933-8555, Japan

(Date)

August 7, 2006

Dear Editor,

May we submit the manuscript "*Asymptomatic spontaneous pneumoperitoneum complicating duodenal diverticulum*" for publication as a "Case Report" in "*Indian J Surg*".

The manuscript has not been published and is not simultaneously being submitted elsewhere. There is no financial support or other benefits from commercial sources for the work reported in the manuscript, or any other financial interest of the authors, which could create a potential conflict of interest.

We are looking forward to receiving your response.

With kind regards

(Signature of corresponding author)
Yasumitsu Hirano

例四：

(Address of Author)
Departmento de Parasitologia,
Escuela Nacional de Cinecias Biologicas-IPN,
Mexico DF, 11340
Mexico

(Date)
April 8, 2009

Dear The Editor,

I am enclosing a manuscript entitled: "*Mixed Hymenolepis species infection in two members: two-case report from an urban area of Chilpancingo, Guerrero, Mexico*" by Name of first author, et al. to be considered for publication in your journal, *Tropical Gastroenterology*.

The significance of the paper to the readers of the *Tropical Gastroenterology* is:

1. This is the first report of the infection with mixed hymenolepis species infection in the man. The two cases presented in this manuscript show hymenolepiasis has a high prevalence in populations in tropical and subtropical climates characterized by poor hygiene and poverty.

2. It is of interest that the doses of **praziquantel** used was not able to eliminate the infection, so the use of **Niclosamide** is recommended as an alternative treatment.

3. Our sanitary and health authorities should put more attention to the information that is published in worldwide international journals, as is the case of the *Tropical Gastroenterology*, so it will be more feasible to implement support to the communities with poor sanitation indicated in this article.

I hereby certify that this is an original paper which has not been published elsewhere, that it is not under consideration for publication elsewhere, that its publication is approved by all authors and tacitly or explicitly by the responsible authorities where the work was carried out, and that, if accepted, it will not be published elsewhere including electronically in the same form, in English or in any other language, without the written consent of the copyright-holder. We have not any relationships or support which might be perceived as constituting a conflict of interest. All authors have participated in the study and concur with the submission and subsequent revisions submitted by the corresponding author.

(Signature of Corresponding author)
Dr. Benjamín Nogueda-Torres
Email: bnogueda@hotmail.com

附录3 研究论文文后参考文献书写

参考文献是研究论文必不可少的组成部分。我国有 GB/T 7714—2015 标准，国际上也有相应准则。有关详细要求，作者可参考具体规定或投稿说明等。为读者写作参考方便，特将该部分内容写作要点、难点综合如下。

1. 相关基本术语

（1）主要责任者（primary responsibility）：对文献的知识内容负主要责任的个人或团体。主要责任者包括著者、编者、学位论文撰写者、专利申请者或所有者、报告撰写者、标准提出者、析出文献的作者等。

（2）专著（monographs）：以单行本形式或多卷册形式，在限定的期限内出版的非连续性出版物。它包括以各种载体形式出版的普通图书、学位论文、技术报告、会议文集、汇编、多卷书、丛书等。

（3）连续出版物（serials）：一种载有卷期号或年月顺序号、计划无限期地连续出版发行的出版物。它包括以各种载体形式出版的期刊、报纸等。

（4）析出文献（contribution）：从整本文献中析出的具有独立篇名的文献。

（5）电子文献（electronic documents）：以数字方式将图、文、声、像等信息存储在磁、光、电介质上，通过计算机、网络或相关设备使用的记录有知识内容的文献信息资源，包括电子书刊、数据库、电子公告等。

2. 文献类型及载体类型标识

根据 GB 3469—83 规定，各种参考文献类型以大写英文字母标识，即专著[M]、论文集[C]、报纸文章[N]、期刊文章[J]、学位论文[D]、报告[R]、标准[S]、专利[P]、数据库[DB]、计算机程序[CP]、电子公告[EB]、著和论文集中的析出文献[A]、磁盘[DK]、光盘[CD]、联机网络[OL]。

3. 参考文献常用格式模板及举例

1）连续出版物
[序号]主要责任者. 文献题名[J]. 刊名，出版年份，卷号（期号）：起止页码.

例如：［1］Schuetz P, Christ crain M, Muller B. Biomarkers to improve diagnostic and prognostic accuracy in systemic infections［J］. Curr Opin Crit Care, 2007,13(2): 578-585.

2）专著

［序号］主要责任者. 文献题名［M］. 出版地：出版者，出版年：起止页码.

例如：［2］Burton J Bogitsh, Thomas C. Cheng. Human Parasitology［M］.USA: Academic Press, 1998：79-108.

3）论文集

［序号］主要责任者. 文献题名［C］//主编. 论文集名. 出版地：出版者，出版年：起止页码.

例如：［3］王咪咪. 中国急性传染病学［C］. 时逸人医学论文集//二十世纪初中医名家医学文集丛编. 北京：学苑出版社，2011：233-257.

4）学位论文

［序号］主要责任者. 文献题名［D］. 保存地：保存单位，年份.

例如：［4］唐秀云. 淮南地区粉螨群落结构和多样性的初步研究［D］. 淮南：安徽理工大学，2009.

5）报告

［序号］主要责任者. 文献题名［R］. 报告地：报告会主办单位，年份.

例如：［5］PEPFAR Male Circumcision Technical Working Group. The President's Emergency Plan for AIDS Relief［R］. USA:National Press Club, 2009.

6）专利文献

［序号］专利所有者. 专利题名［P］. 专利国别：专利号，发布日期.

例如：［6］姜锡洲. 一种温热外敷药制备方案［P］. 中国专利:881056078,1983-08-12.

7）国际、国家标准

［序号］标准代号，标准名称［S］. 出版地：出版者，出版年.

例如：［7］GB 3101—93，有关量、单位和符号的一般原则［S］. 北京：中国标准出版社，1994.

8）报纸文章

［序号］主要责任者. 文献题名［N］. 报纸名，出版日期（版次）.

例如：［8］Jennifer Huget. Loneliness linked to older people's death, disability［N］. The Washington Post, 2012-06-21.

9）电子文献

［序号］主要责任者. 电子文献题名［文献类型/载体类型］.出版物名称，发表或更新的日期/引用日期（任选）. 电子文献的出版或可获得地址.

例如：［9］Christine M. Plant Physiology: Plant biology in the Genome Era［J/OL］. Science, 1998, 281:331-332. http://www.sciencemag. Org/cgi/collection/anatmorp.

10）专著中析出的文献

［序号］析出责任者. 析出题名［A］//专著责任者. 书名［M］. 出版地:出版者,出版年:起止页码.

　　例如：[10] Nancy F, Krebs. Normal Childhood Nutrition & Its Disorders[A]//William W. Hay, Jr., Anthony R. Hayward, Myron J. Levin, Judith M. Sondheimer. Current Pediatric Diagnosis & Treatment[M]. New York, USA:The McGraw-Hill Companies, 2000:43-67.

附录 4　典型摘要例证 25 篇

　　本部分所附摘要例证，表面看来，似画蛇添足，但我们认为这些例证对于读者来说还是大有裨益的。写作的成功之路在于效仿，若要达到意到笔随之功，必须得博取众家之长。为了让广大读者感受真实性（authentic）的语料，该部分所选例证除少数几篇来源于国内期刊外，其余均取材于国外出版物。这些文摘的作者均以英语为其母语或第二语言，所选摘要的版式，包括字体、格式完全按原版排样。鉴于篇幅的限制，实难覆盖所有出版物，当然，也无此必要。此外，由于我们重点讨论的是结构式摘要写作，为了弥补其他类型，如报道性摘要、指示性摘要、报道-指示性摘要例证不足的缺憾，所选文摘不完全拘泥于结构式摘要，目的是为广大读者提供一个全方位的视角。在这些文摘中，有些虽出自同一期刊，却在结构式上有着迥然不同的子项，所以，这类文摘在以下例证中我们采用了复选方式。

摘　要　实　例

Passage 1

Abstract

Importance: The pandemic of coronavirus disease 2019 (COVID-19) caused by the novel severe acute respiratory syndrome coronavirus 2 (SARS-CoV-2) presents an unprecedented challenge to identify effective drugs for prevention and treatment. Given the rapid pace of scientific discovery and clinical data generated by the large number of people rapidly infected by SARS-CoV-2, clinicians need accurate evidence regarding effective medical treatments for this infection.

Observations: No proven effective therapies for this virus currently exist. The rapidly expanding knowledge regarding SARS-CoV-2 virology provides a significant number of potential drug targets. The most promising therapy is remdesivir. Remdesivir has potent *in vitro* activity against SARS-CoV-2, but it is not US Food and Drug Administration approved and currently is being tested in ongoing randomized trials. Oseltamivir has not been shown to have efficacy, and corticosteroids are currently not recommended. Current clinical evidence does not support stopping angiotensin-converting enzyme inhibitors or angiotensin receptor blockers in patients with COVID-19.

Conclusions and Relevance: The COVID-19 pandemic represents the greatest global public health crisis of this generation and, potentially, since the pandemic influenza outbreak of 1918. The speed and volume of clinical trials launched to investigate potential therapies for COVID-19 highlight both the need and capability to produce high-quality evidence even in the middle of a pandemic. No therapies have been shown effective to date.

引自: JAMA, 2020, 323(18): 1824-1836

Passage 2

Abstract

Importance: Given the shortage of donor hearts and improvement in outcomes with left ventricular assist device (LVAD) therapy, a relevant but, to date, unanswered question is whether select patients with advanced heart failure should receive LVAD destination therapy as an alternative to heart transplant.

Objective: To determine whether a strategy of LVAD destination therapy is associated with similar survival benefit as wait-listing for heart transplant with or without LVAD therapy among patients with advanced heart failure.

Design, Setting, and Participants: This retrospective propensity-matched cohort analysis used data on heart transplants from the United Network for Organ Sharing registry and LVAD implants from the Interagency Registry for Mechanically Assisted Circulatory Support from January 1, 2010, to December 31, 2014. The matched LVAD destination therapy cohort included 3411 patients. Data analysis for this study was conducted from December 22, 2017, to May 24, 2019.

Main Outcomes and Measures: Survival at 5 years was analyzed using Cox proportional hazards models.

Results: In total, 8281 patients had albumin level, creatinine level, and BMI data recorded and were included in the analysis. Despite propensity score matching, the 3411 patients receiving LVAD destination therapy still tended to be slightly older than the 3411 patients wait-listed for heart transplant (64.0 years [interquartile range, 55.0-70.0 years] *vs.* 60.0 [interquartile range, 54.0-65.0 years]; $P<0.001$), but there was no significant difference in sex (2701 men [79.2%] *vs.* 2648 men [77.6%]; $P=0.13$). After propensity score matching for age, sex, body mass index, renal function, and albumin level, 3411 patients were wait-listed for heart transplant. This included 1607 patients with bridge to transplant LVAD therapy and 1804 patients without LVAD. The strategy of wait-listing for heart transplant was associated with better 5-year survival than LVAD destination therapy (risk ratio, 0.42; 95% CI, 0.38-0.46) after matching and adjusting for key clinical factors. This survival advantage was associated with heart transplant (adjusted risk ratio for time-dependent transplant status, 0.27; 95% CI, 0.24-0.32).

Conclusions and Relevance: The present analysis suggests that heart transplant with or without bridge to transplant LVAD therapy was associated with superior 5-year survival compared with LVAD destination therapy among patients matched on several relevant clinical factors. Continued improvement in LVAD technology, along with prospective comparative research, appears to be needed to amend this strategy.

引自: *JAMA Cardiol*, 2020, 5(6): 652-659

Passage 3

Abstract

Importance: Pityriasis rubra pilaris is a rare and disabling cutaneous disease that is frequently recalcitrant to conventional therapies and appears to involve interleukin (IL)-17 overexpression.

Objective: To investigate the clinical response and safety of ixekizumab in treating pityriasis rubra pilaris.

Design, Setting, and Participants: Single-arm, investigator-initiated trial conducted in adult patients with moderate to severe pityriasis rubra pilaris at a single-center academic university from June 2018 to January 2020. A total of 41 patients were screened, 12 were enrolled, and 11 completed the full duration of therapy. A referred, consecutive sample was used during participant selection. The treatment period and primary outcome occurred over 24 weeks with additional patient follow-up through 36 weeks.

Intervention: Subcutaneous administration of ixekizumab, a humanized IgG4 antibody that binds IL-17A, at the US Food and Drug Administration-approved dosing schedule for treatment of psoriasis for 24 weeks.

Main Outcomes and Measures: The primary outcome was the mean change in Psoriasis Area and Severity Index at 24 weeks. Secondary outcome included change in affected body surface area, quality of life, induction of sustained remission, and association of improvement with *CARD14* genetic variations and cutaneous cytokine expression.

Results: A total of 12 white patients (mean [SD] age, 49.8 [15.1] years; 8 male [67%]) were enrolled between June 2018 and April 2019, with 11 completing the full course of intervention. The mean (SEM) improvements in Psoriasis Area and Severity Index, affected body surface area, and Dermatology Life Quality Index were 15.2 (2.1) ($P < 0.0001$), 29.8% (9.3%) ($P = 0.009$), and 9.5 (2.5) ($P = 0.004$), respectively. The 4 participants with the most improvement in Psoriasis Area and Severity Index at week 24 stayed in remission at week 36 (defined as lack of increase in Psoriasis Area and Severity Index from week 24 through week 36), off therapy. Relative dermal IL-17A expression decreased by a 1.9 log-fold change. No participants had known pathogenic *CARD14* variations. There were no serious adverse events.

Conclusions and Relevance: In this single-armed trial, ixekizumab was associated with reduced clinical signs and symptoms of pityriasis rubra pilaris in a subset of patients, including those in whom other systemic therapies have failed.

引自: *JAMA Dermatol*, 2020, 156(6): 668-675

Passage 4

Abstract

Background: It is recommended that patients with acute upper gastrointestinal bleeding undergo endoscopy within 24 hours after gastroenterologic consultation. The role of endoscopy performed within time frames shorter than 24 hours has not been adequately defined.

Methods: To evaluate whether urgent endoscopy improves outcomes in patients predicted to be at high risk for further bleeding or death, we randomly assigned patients with overt signs of acute upper gastrointestinal bleeding and a Glasgow-Blatchford score of 12 or higher (scores range from 0 to 23, with higher scores indicating a higher risk of further bleeding or death) to undergo endoscopy within 6 hours (urgent-endoscopy group) or between 6 and 24 hours (early-endoscopy group) after gastroenterologic consultation. The primary end point was death from any cause within 30 days after randomization.

Results: A total of 516 patients were enrolled. The 30-day mortality was 8.9% (23 of 258 patients) in the urgent-endoscopy group and 6.6%(17 of 258) in the early-endoscopy group (difference, 2.3 percentage points; 95% confidence interval [CI], −2.3 to 6.9). Further bleeding within 30 days occurred in 28 patients(10.9%) in the urgent-endoscopy group and in 20(7.8%) in the early-endoscopy group (difference, 3.1 percentage points; 95% CI, −1.9 to 8.1). Ulcers with active bleeding or visible vessels were found on initial endoscopy in 105 of the 158 patients (66.4%) with peptic ulcers in the urgent-endoscopy group and in 76 of 159 (47.8%) in the early-endoscopy group. Endoscopic hemostatic treatment was administered at initial endoscopy for 155 patients (60.1%) in the urgent-endoscopy group and for 125 (48.4%) in the early-endoscopy group.

Conclusions: In patients with acute upper gastrointestinal bleeding who were at high risk for further bleeding or death, endoscopy performed within 6 hours after gastroenterologic consultation was not associated with lower 30-day mortality than endoscopy performed between 6 and 24 hours after consultation.

引自: *N Engl J Med*, 2020, 382: 1299-1308

Passage 5

Abstract

Background: Multidrug-resistant (MDR) bacteria that are commonly associated with health care cause a substantial health burden. Updated national estimates for this group of pathogens are needed to inform public health action.

Methods: Using data from patients hospitalized in a cohort of 890 U.S. hospitals during the period 2012-2017, we generated national case counts for both hospital-onset and community-onset infections caused by methicillin-resistant *Staphylococcus aureus* (MRSA), vancomycin-resistant enterococcus (VRE), extended-spectrum cephalosporin resistance in Enterobacteriaceae suggestive of extended-spectrum beta-lactamase (ESBL) production, carbapenem-resistant Enterobacteriaceae, carbapenem-resistant acinetobacter species, and MDR

Pseudomonas aeruginosa.

Results: The hospital cohort in the study accounted for 41.6 million hospitalizations (>20% of U.S. hospitalizations annually). The overall rate of clinical cultures was 292 cultures per 1000 patient-days and was stable throughout the time period. In 2017, these pathogens caused an estimated 622,390 infections (95% confidence interval [CI], 579,125 to 665,655) among hospitalized patients. Of these infections, 517,818 (83%) had their onset in the community, and 104,572 (17%) had their onset in the hospital. MRSA and ESBL infections accounted for the majority of the infections (52% and 32%, respectively). Between 2012 and 2017, the incidence decreased for MRSA infection (from 114.18 to 93.68 cases per 10,000 hospitalizations), VRE infection (from 24.15 to 15.76 per 10,000), carbapenem-resistant acinetobacter species infection (from 3.33 to 2.47 per 10,000), and MDR *P. aeruginosa* infection (from 13.10 to 9.43 per 10,000), with decreases ranging from −20.5% to −39.2%. The incidence of carbapenem-resistant Enterobacteriaceae infection did not change significantly (from 3.36 to 3.79 cases per 10,000 hospitalizations). The incidence of ESBL infection increased by 53.3% (from 37.55 to 57.12 cases per 10,000 hospitalizations), a change driven by an increase in community-onset cases.

Conclusions: Health care-associated antimicrobial resistance places a substantial burden on patients in the United States. Further work is needed to identify improved interventions for both the inpatient and outpatient settings.

引自: *N Engl J Med*, 2020, 382: 1309-1319

Passage 6

Abstract

Acute kidney disease (AKD), or renal dysfunction persisting >7 days after an initiating event of acute kidney injury, is a rising concern. This study aimed to elucidate the clinical course of AKD after cardiac surgery with data on post-cardiac surgery patients admitted to intensive care units (ICU) at 18 Japanese hospitals during 2012-2014. Using multivariable logistic models, we evaluated the association of AKD with 90-day mortality and the 50% eGFR decline during 2-year follow-up compared to eGFR at 90 days. AKD was defined as an elevation in serum creatinine to at least 1.5-fold from baseline in >7 days after ICU admission. Of the 3,605 eligible patients undergoing cardiac surgery, 403 patients (11.2%) had AKD. Multivariable analysis revealed that the adjusted odds ratio (OR) of AKD for 90-day mortality was 63.0 (95% confidence interval [CI], 27.9-180.6). In addition, the adjusted OR of AKD for 50% eGFR decline was 3.56 (95% CI, 2.24-5.57) among hospital survivors. In conclusion, AKD after cardiac surgery was associated with higher 90-day mortality and renal function decline after hospital discharge.

引自: *Nature*, 2020, 6490

Passage 7

Abstract

Introduction: Primary aldosteronism (PA) contributed to the cardiovascular disease and metabolic alterations independent of the blood pressure level. Evidence exists that aldosterone excess also affects calcium and mineral homeostasis. PA subjects have been shown to have greater prevalence of vitamin D deficiency. However, the impact of vitamin D treatment in this population has never been assessed.

Objective: This study aimed to evaluate the effect of vitamin D treatment on clinical and biochemical outcomes of PA patients.

Methods: Two hundred forty hypertensive subjects were screened, 31 had positive ARR, and 17 patients with newly confirmed PA following positive confirmatory test that has not been subjected for definitive treatment were enrolled. Clinical parameter (blood pressure) and biochemical parameters (renal profile, plasma aldosterone concentration, plasma renin activity, serum calcium, vitamin D, intact parathyroid hormone, 24-hour urinary calcium) were measured at baseline and 3 months of treatment with Bio-D3 capsule. Primary outcomes were the changes in the blood pressure and biochemical parameters.

Results: About 70% of our PA subjects have low vitamin D levels at baseline. Three months following treatment, there were significant: (a) improvement in 25(OH)D levels; (b) reduction in systolic blood pressure and plasma aldosterone concentration; and (c) improvement in the eGFR. The vitamin D deficient subgroup has the greatest magnitude of the systolic blood pressure reduction following treatment.

Conclusions: This study demonstrated significant proportion of PA patients has vitamin D insufficiency. Vitamin D treatment improves these interrelated parameters possibly suggesting interplay between vitamin D, aldosterone, renal function and the blood pressure.

引自: *Clin Endocrinol(Oxf)*, 2020, 92(6): 509-517

Passage 8

Summary

The recent emergence of the novel, pathogenic SARS-coronavirus 2 (SARS-CoV-2) in China and its rapid national and international spread pose a global health emergency. Cell entry of coronaviruses depends on binding of the viral spike (S) proteins to cellular receptors and on S protein priming by host cell proteases. Unravelling which cellular factors are used by SARS-CoV-2 for entry might provide insights into viral transmission and reveal therapeutic targets. Here, we demonstrate that SARS-CoV-2 uses the SARS-CoV receptor ACE2 for entry and the serine protease TMPRSS2 for S protein priming. A TMPRSS2 inhibitor approved for clinical use blocked entry and might constitute a treatment option. Finally, we show that the sera from convalescent SARS patients cross-neutralized SARS-2-S-driven entry. Our results reveal important commonalities between SARS-CoV-2 and SARS-CoV infection and identify a potential target for antiviral intervention.

引自: *Cell*, 2020, 181(2): 271-280. e8

Passage 9

Abstract

Background: The association of milk intake with cardiovascular disease(CVD) and cause-specific mortality remained controversial and evidence among the Chinese population was limited. We aimed to study the relationship between milk intake and CVDs among general Chinese adults.

Methods: A total of 104,957 participants received questionnaire survey. Results of physical examination such as anthropometric measurements and biochemical tests during 2007 to 2008, demographic data and their information on milk intake were collected through standardized questionnaires. Cox proportional hazard regression models were used to calculate hazard ratios (HRs) and their corresponding 95% confidence intervals (CIs) of CVD incidence, cause-specific mortality andall-cause mortality related to milk intake. Restricted cubic splines (RCSs) were applied to examine dose-response associations.

Results: Among the 91,757 participants with a median follow-up period of 5.8 years, we documented 3877 CVD cases and 4091 all-cause deaths. Compared with participants who never consumed milk, the multivariate-adjusted HRs (95% CIs) of CVD incidence for 1 to 150 g/day, 151 to 299 g/day, and ≥300 g/day were 0.94 (0.86-1.03) (P >0.05), 0.77 (0.66-0.89) (P<0.05), and 0.59 (0.40-0.89) (P<0.05), respectively; each 100 g increase of daily milk intake was associated with 11% lower risk of CVD incidence (HR, 0.89; 95% CI: 0.85-0.94; P<0.001), and 11% lower risk of CVD mortality (HR, 0.89; 95% CI: 0.82-0.97; P= 0.008) after adjustment for age, sex, residential area, geographic region, education level, family history of CVD, smoking, alcohol drinking, physical activity level, body mass index, and healthy diet status (ideal or not). RCS analyses also showed a linear dose-response relationship with CVD (P for overall significance of the curve <0.001; P for non-linearity = 0.979; P for linearity <0.001) and stroke (P for overall significance of the curve = 0.010; P for non-linearity = 0.998; P for linearity = 0.002)incidence, and CVD mortality (P for overall significance of the curve=0.045; P for non-linearity =0.768; P for linearity= 0.014) within the current range of daily milk intake.

Conclusions: Daily milk intake was associated with lower risk of CVD incidence and mortality in a linear inverse relationship. The findings provide new evidence for dietary recommendations in CVD prevention among Chinese adults and people with similar dietary pattern in other countries.

引自：*Chin Med J*, 2020, 133(10): 1144-1154

Passage 10

Abstract

Antiphospholipid syndrome (APS) is a thromboinflammatory disease with a variety of clinical phenotypes. Primary thrombosis prophylaxis should take an individualized risk stratification approach. Moderate-intensity vitamin K antagonist such as warfarin remains the primary strategy for secondary thrombosis prophylaxis among APS patients, especially for patients with predominantly venous disease. For now, direct oral anti-coagulants should be avoided in most APS patients, especially those with history of arterial manifestations. Obstetric APS management should be tailored based on an individual patient's antiphospholipid antibody profile, and obstetric and thrombotic history. Pharmacological agents beyond anticoagulants may be considered for the management of microthrombotic and nonthrombotic manifestations of APS, although more data are needed. A relatively recent discovery in the area of APS pathogenesis is the implication of neutrophil extracellular traps in thrombin generation and initiation of inflammatory cascades. APS is a complex thromboinflammatory disease with a broad clinical spectrum. Personalized therapy according to an individual's unique thrombosis and obstetric risk should be advocated.

引自: *Chin Med J*, 2020, 133(8): 929-940

Passage 11

Abstract

Background: Food insecurity affects 1 in 8 households in Canada, with serious health consequences. We investigated the association between household food insecurity and all-cause and cause-specific mortality.

Methods: We assessed the food insecurity status of Canadian adults using the Canadian Community Health Survey 2005-2017 and identified premature deaths among the survey respondents using the Canadian Vital Statistics Database 2005-2017. Applying Cox survival analyses to the linked data sets, we compared adults' all-cause and cause-specific mortality hazard by their household food insecurity status.

Results: Of the 510 010 adults sampled (3 390 500 person-years), 25 460 died prematurely by 2017. Death rates of food-secure adults and their counterparts experiencing marginal, moderate and severe food insecurity were 736, 752, 834 and 1124 per 100 000 person-years, respectively. The adjusted hazard ratios (HRs) of all-cause premature mortality for marginal, moderate and severe food insecurity were 1.10 (95% confidence interval [CI] 1.03-1.18), 1.11 (95% CI 1.05-1.18) and 1.37 (95% CI 1.27-1.47), respectively. Among adults who died prematurely, those experiencing severe food insecurity died on average 9 years earlier than their food-secure counterparts (age 59.5 v. 68.9 yr). Severe food insecurity was consistently associated with higher mortality across all causes of death except cancers; the association was particularly pronounced for infectious-parasitic diseases (adjusted HR 2.24, 95%CI 1.42-3.55), unintentional injuries (adjusted HR 2.69, 95%CI 2.04-3.56) and suicides (adjusted HR 2.21, 95% CI 1.50-3.24).

Interpretation: Canadian adults from food-insecure households were more likely to die prematurely than their food-secure counterparts. Efforts to reduce premature mortality should consider food insecurity as a relevant social determinant.

引自: *CMAJ*, 2020, 192(3): E53-E60

Passage 12

Summary

Background: Catheter-based renal denervation has significantly reduced blood pressure in previous studies. Following a positive pilot trial, the SPYRAL HTN-OFF MED (SPYRAL Pivotal) trial was designed to assess the efficacy of renal denervation in the absence of antihypertensive medications.

Methods: In this international, prospective, single-blinded, sham-controlled trial, done at 44 study sites in Australia, Austria, Canada, Germany, Greece, Ireland, Japan, the UK, and the USA, hypertensive patients with office systolic blood pressure of 150 mm Hg to less than 180 mm Hg were randomly assigned 1:1 to either a renal denervation or sham procedure. The primary efficacy endpoint was baseline-adjusted change in 24-h systolic blood pressure and the secondary efficacy endpoint was baseline-adjusted change in office systolic blood pressure from baseline to 3 months after the procedure. We used a Bayesian design with an informative prior, so the primary analysis combines evidence from the pilot and Pivotal trials. The primary efficacy and safety analyses were done in the intention-to-treat population.

Findings: From June 25, 2015, to Oct 15, 2019, 331 patients were randomly assigned to either renal denervation (n=166) or a sham procedure (n=165). The primary and secondary efficacy endpoints were met, with posterior probability of superiority more than 0.999 for both. The treatment difference between the two groups for 24-h systolic blood pressure was −3.9 mmHg (Bayesian 95% credible interval −6.2 to −1.6) and for office systolic blood pressure the difference was −6.5 mmHg (−9.6 to −3.5). No major device-related or procedural-related safety events occurred up to 3 months.

Interpretation: SPYRAL Pivotal showed the superiority of catheter-based renal denervation compared with a sham procedure to safely lower blood pressure in the absence of antihypertensive medications.

引自: *The Lancet*, 2020, 395(10234): 1444-1451

Passage 13

Abstract

Objectives: To compare standard high flow oxygen treatment with titrated oxygen treatment for patients with an acute exacerbation of chronic obstructive pulmonary disease in the prehospital setting.

Design: Cluster randomised controlled parallel group trial.

Setting: Ambulance service in Hobart, Tasmania, Australia.

Participants: 405 patients with a presumed acute exacerbation of chronic obstructive pulmonary disease who were treated by paramedics, transported, and admitted to the Royal Hobart Hospital during the trial period; 214 had a diagnosis of chronic obstructive pulmonary disease confirmed by lung function tests in the previous five years.

Interventions: High flow oxygen treatment compared with titrated oxygen treatment in the prehospital (ambulance/paramedic) setting.

Main outcome measure: Prehospital or in-hospital mortality.

Results: In an intention to treat analysis, the risk of death was significantly lower in the titrated oxygen arm compared with the high flow oxygen arm for all patients (high flow oxygen n=226; titrated oxygen n=179) and for the subgroup of patients with confirmed chronic obstructive pulmonary disease (high flow n=117; titrated n=97). Overall mortality was 9% (21 deaths) in the high flow oxygen arm compared with 4% (7 deaths) in the titrated oxygen arm; mortality in the subgroup with confirmed chronic obstructive pulmonary disease was 9% (11 deaths) in the high flow arm compared with 2% (2 deaths) in the titrated oxygen arm. Titrated oxygen treatment reduced mortality compared with high flow oxygen by 58% for all patients (relative risk 0.42, 95% confidence interval 0.20 to 0.89; P=0.02) and by 78% for the patients with confirmed chronic obstructive pulmonary disease (0.22, 0.05 to 0.91; P=0.04). Patients with chronic obstructive pulmonary disease who received titrated oxygen according to the protocol were significantly less likely to have respiratory acidosis (mean difference in pH 0.12 (SE 0.05); P=0.01; n=28) or hypercapnia (mean difference in arterial carbon dioxide pressure −33.6 (16.3) mm Hg; P=0.02; n=29) than were patients who received high flow oxygen.

Conclusions: Titrated oxygen treatment significantly reduced mortality, hypercapnia, and respiratory acidosis compared with high flow oxygen in acute exacerbations of chronic obstructive pulmonary disease. These results provide strong evidence to recommend the routine use of titrated oxygen treatment in patients with breathlessness and a history or clinical likelihood of chronic obstructive pulmonary disease in the prehospital setting.

引自：*BMJ*, 2010, 341: c5462

Passage 14

Abstract

To investigate the effect of GRACE scores on prediction of 30-day cardiovascular adverse events in acute chest pain patients. A prospective, observational analysis was conducted in the patients with acute chest pain in Emergency Department (ED) from January 1, 2016 through January 1, 2017. Data including characteristics and GRACE scores were collected. All causes leading to MACE were followed up at 30th day after the onset of acute chest pain. Among a total of 600 patients presenting with acute chest pain enrolled in this study, 302 were male (50.3%) and 298 were female (49.7%). The range of age was 20-80 years old. During follow-up period, 102 patients had MACE, 498 patients had no MACE. When compared with non-MACE group, factors including number of Smoker, Hypercholesterolemia, Diabetes, Hypercholesterolemia and patients admitted in CCU as well as GRACE scores, were significantly higher in MACE group (P<0.05). The predictive ROC curve area of GRACE scores in 30-day MACE was 0.739 (0.687 to 0.791). The probability of 30-day cardiovascular adverse events in various GRACE score risk stratification was 2.0% (low-risk), 5.33% (medium-risk), and 9.67% (high-risk), respectively. The GRACE score was a useful predictor to the occurrence of 30-day cardiovascular adverse events in acute chest pain patients. Patients with low GRACE score risk stratification have a low risk of 30-dayMACE, which may be able to convey risk quickly and efficiently.

引自: *Clin Exp Med*, 2020, 8(1): 1-5

Passage 15

Abstract

Objectives: We describe results of programmed death ligand 1 (PD-L1) immunohistochemical assessment in methotrexate (MTX)-associated lymphoproliferative disorders (LPDs) and highlight the characteristics of classic Hodgkin lymphoma (CHL) type MTX-LPD.

Methods: Fifty cases of MTX-LPD, including CHL type (n=9), diffuse large B-cell lymphoma type (n=15), and polymorphic B-cell LPD (n=21), were investigated.

Results: Staining with anti-PD-L1 clone SP142 was exclusively found in CHL type (89%) but not in the others. Cases of CHL type MTX-LPD involved nodal disease and were associated with Epstein-Barr virus. They were histopathologically characterized by a vaguely nodular pattern, predominance of mononuclear cells, and strong expression of at least one pan-B-cell marker. Their clinical course was variable, with spontaneous regression in 5 patients, relapse in 2, and a fatal course in 1.

Conclusions: The PD-L1 (clone SP142) workup aids the diagnostic approach to patients with MTX-LPD. CHL type MTX-LPD appears to represent a unique morphologic variant of CHL.

引自: *AJCP*, 2020, 153(5): 571-582

Passage 16

Abstract

Objectives: Biomarkers are widely used for rapid diagnosis of sepsis. This study evaluated the diagnostic accuracy of presepsin, procalcitonin (PCT), and C-reactive protein (CRP) in differentiating sepsis severity as well as their association with Sepsis-related Organ Failure Assessment (SOFA) score.

Methods: One hundred septic patients from two university clinical centers were enrolled in the study during two time periods. New Sepsis-3 definitions were used for sepsis stratification. Biomarkers and SOFA score were evaluated four times during the illness. A sandwich ELISA kit was used for presepsin measurement. Generalized linear mixed effects model was used to test the changes in biomarkers concentrations and SOFA score values during the illness and to estimate the differences between severity groups. Multivariate analysis was used to test the association of biomarkers with SOFA score.

Results: Presepsin concentrations were significantly higher on admission in patients with septic shock (n=34) compared to patients with sepsis (n= 66), mean ± SD: 128.5 ± 47.6 ng/mL *vs*. 88.6 ± 65.6 ng/mL, respectively (P < 0.001). The same was not observed for PCT and CRP;

their concentrations did not differ significantly between severity groups. A strong correlation of presepsin with SOFA score was also found ($P < 0.0001$).

Conclusions: Presepsin had a good diagnostic ability to differentiate septic shock from sepsis in the study groups. PCT and CRP failed in differentiating sepsis severity.

引自: *Int J Infect Dis*, 2020, 95: 1-7

Passage 17

Abstract

Owing to the breakdown of health systems, mass population displacements, and resettlement of vulnerable refugees in camps or locations prone to vector breeding, malaria is often a major health problem during war and the aftermath of war. During the initial acute phase of the emergency, before health services become properly established, mortality rates may rise to alarming levels. Establishing good case management and effective malaria prevention are important priorities for international agencies responsible for emergency health services. The operational strategies and control methods used in peacetime must be adapted to emergency conditions, and should be regularly re-assessed as social, political and epidemiological conditions evolve. During the last decade, research on malaria in refugee camps on the Pakistan-Afghanistan and Thailand-Burma borders has led to new methods and strategies for malaria prevention and case management, and these are now being taken up by international health agencies. This experience has shown that integration of research within control programmes is an efficient and dynamic mode of working that can lead to innovation and hopefully sustainable malaria control. United Nations' humanitarian and non-governmental agencies can play a significant part in resolving the outstanding research issues in malaria control.

引自: *Ann Trop Med Parasitol*, 2001, 95(8): 741-754

Passage 18

Abstract

The list of pharmacological agents that can modify the gut microbiome or be modified by it continues to grow at a high rate. The greatest amount of attention on drug-gut microbiome interactions has been directed primarily at pharmaceuticals used to treat infection, diabetes, cardiovascular conditions and cancer. By comparison, drugs of abuse and addiction, which can powerfully and chronically worsen human health, have received relatively little attention in this regard. Therefore, the main objective of this study was to characterize how selected synthetic psychoactive cathinones (aka "Bath Salts") and amphetamine stimulants modify the gut microbiome. Mice were treated with mephedrone (40 mg/kg), methcathinone (80 mg/kg), methamphetamine (5 mg/kg) or 4-methyl-methamphetamine (40 mg/kg), following a binge regimen consisting of 4 injections at 2 h intervals. These drugs were selected for study because they are structural analogs that contain a β-keto substituent (methcathinone), a 4-methyl group (4-methyl-methamphetamine), both substituents (mephedrone) or neither (methamphetamine).

Mice were sacrificed 1, 2 or 7 days after treatment and DNA from caecum contents was subjected to 16S rRNA sequencing. We found that all drugs caused significant time- and structure-dependent alterations in the diversity and taxonomic structure of the gut microbiome. The two phyla most changed by drug treatments were Firmicutes (methcathinone, 4-methyl-methamphetamine) and Bacteriodetes (methcathinone, 4-methyl-methamphetamine, methamphetamine, mephedrone). Across time, broad microbiome changes from the phylum to genus levels were characteristic of all drugs. The present results signify that these selected psychoactive drugs, which are thought to exert their primary effects within the CNS, can have profound effects on the gut microbiome. They also suggest new avenues of investigation into the possibility that gut-derived signals could modulate drug abuse and addiction via altered communication along the gut-brain axis.

引自: *PLoS One*, 2020,15(1): e0227774

Passage 19

Abstract

Background: Aging may detrimentally affect cognitive and motor function. However, age is also associated with experience, and how these factors interplay and affect outcomes following surgery is unclear. We sought to evaluate the effect of surgeon age on postoperative outcomes in patients undergoing common surgical procedures.

Methods: We performed a retrospective cohort study of patients undergoing 1 of 25 common surgical procedures in Ontario, Canada, from 2007 to 2015. We evaluated the association between surgeon age and a composite outcome of death, readmission and complications. We used generalized estimating equations for analysis, accounting for relevant patient-, procedure-, surgeon- and hospital-level factors.

Results: We found 1 159 676 eligible patients who were treated by 3314 surgeons and ranged in age from 27 to 81 years. Modelled as a continuous variable, a 10-year increase in surgeon age was associated with a 5% relative decreased odds of the composite outcome (adjusted odds ratio [OR] 0.95, 95% confidence interval [CI] 0.92 to 0.98, $P=0.002$). Considered dichotomously, patients receiving treatment from surgeons who were older than 65 years of age had a 7% lower odds of adverse outcomes (adjusted OR 0.93, 95% CI 0.88-0.97, $P=0.03$; crude absolute difference = 3.1%).

Interpretation: We found that increasing surgeon age was associated with decreasing rates of postoperative death, readmission and complications in a nearly linear fashion after accounting for patient-, procedure-, surgeon- and hospital-level factors. Further evaluation of the mechanisms underlying these findings may help to improve patient safety and outcomes, and inform policy about maintenance of certification and retirement age for surgeons.

引自: *CMAJ*, 2020, 192 (15): E385-E392

Passage 20

Abstract

Background: FLU-v is a broad-spectrum influenza vaccine that induces antibodies and cell-mediated immunity.

Objective: To compare the safety, immunogenicity, and exploratory efficacy of different formulations and dosing regimens of FLU-v versus placebo.

Design: Randomized, double-blind, placebo-controlled, single-center phase 2b clinical trial. (ClinicalTrials. gov: NCT02962908; EudraCT: 2015-001932-38)

Setting: The Netherlands.

Participants: 175 healthy adults aged 18 to 60 years.

Intervention: 0.5-mL subcutaneous injection of 500 μg of adjuvanted (1 dose) or nonadjuvanted (2 doses) FLU-v (A-FLU-v or NA-FLU-v) or adjuvanted or nonadjuvanted placebo (A-placebo or NA-placebo) (2:2:1:1 ratio).

Measurements: Vaccine-specific cellular responses at days 0, 42, and 180 were assessed via flow cytometry and enzyme-linked immunosorbent assay. Solicited information on adverse events (AEs) was collected for 21 days after vaccination. Unsolicited information on AEs was collected throughout the study.

Results: The AEs with the highest incidence were mild to moderate injection site reactions. The difference between A-FLU-v and A-placebo in the median fold increase in secreted interferon-γ (IFN-γ) was 38.2-fold (95% CI, 4.7- to 69.7-fold; $P= 0.001$) at day 42 and 25.0-fold (CI, 5.7- to 50.9-fold; $P < 0.001$) at day 180. The differences between A-FLU-v and A-placebo in median fold increase at day 42 were 4.5-fold (CI, 2.3- to 9.8-fold; $P < 0.001$) for IFN-γ-producing CD4$^+$T cells, 4.9-fold (CI, 1.3- to 40.0-fold; $P < 0.001$) for tumor necrosis factor-α (TNF-α), 7.0-fold (CI, 3.5- to 18.0-fold; $P < 0.001$) for interleukin-2 (IL-2), and 1.7-fold (CI, 0.1- to 4.0-fold; $P= 0.004$) for CD107a. At day 180, differences were 2.1-fold (CI, 0.0- to 6.0-fold; $P= 0.030$) for IFN-γ and 5.7-fold (CI, 2.0- to 15.0-fold; $P < 0.001$) for IL-2, with no difference for TNF-α or CD107a. No differences were seen between NA-FLU-v and NA-placebo.

Limitation: The study was not powered to evaluate vaccine efficacy against influenza infection.

Conclusion: Adjuvanted FLU-v is immunogenic and merits phase 3 development to explore efficacy.

引自: *Ann Intern Med*, 2020, 172(7): 453-462

Passage 21

Abstract

Our understanding of Alzheimer's disease (AD) pathophysiology remains incomplete. Here we used quantitative mass spectrometry and coexpression network analysis to conduct the largest proteomic study thus far on AD. A protein network module linked to sugar metabolism emerged as one of the modules most significantly associated with AD pathology and cognitive impairment. This module was enriched in AD genetic risk factors and in microglia and astrocyte protein markers associated with an anti-inflammatory state, suggesting that the biological functions it represents serve a protective role in AD. Proteins from this module were elevated in cerebrospinal fluid in early stages of the disease. In this study of>2,000 brains and nearly 400 cerebrospinal fluid samples by quantitative proteomics, we identify proteins and biological processes in AD brains that may serve as therapeutic targets and fluid biomarkers for the disease.

引自: *Nat Med*, 2020, 26(5): 769-780

Passage 22

Abstract

Among the most urgent public health threats is the worldwide emergence of carbapenem-resistant Enterobacteriaceae[1,2,3,4], which are resistant to the antibiotic class of 'last resort'. In the United States and Europe, carbapenem-resistant strains of the *Klebsiella pneumoniae* ST258 (ref.[5]) sequence type are dominant, endemic[6,7,8] and associated with high mortality[6,9,10]. We report the global evolution of pathogenicity in carbapenem-resistant *K. pneumoniae*, resulting in the repeated convergence of virulence and carbapenem resistance in the United States and Europe, dating back to as early as 2009. We demonstrate that *K. pneumoniae* can enhance its pathogenicity by adopting two opposing infection programs through easily acquired gain- and loss-of-function mutations. Single-nucleotide polymorphisms in the capsule biosynthesis gene *wzc* lead to hypercapsule production, which confers phagocytosis resistance, enhanced dissemination and increased mortality in animal models. In contrast, mutations disrupting capsule biosynthesis genes impair capsule production, which enhances epithelial cell invasion, *in vitro* biofilm formation and persistence in urinary tract infections. These two types of capsule mutants have emerged repeatedly and independently in Europe and the United States, with hypercapsule mutants associated with bloodstream infections and capsule-deficient mutants associated with urinary tract infections. In the latter case, drug-tolerant *K. pneumoniae* can persist to yield potentially untreatable, persistent infection.

引自: *Nat Med*, 2020, 26(5): 705-711

Passage 23

Abstract

Purpose: To evaluate the performance of machine-learning-based computed tomography (CT) radiomic analysis to differentiate high-risk thymic epithelial tumours (TETs) from low-risk TETs according to the WHO classification.

Method: This retrospective study included 155 patients with a histologic diagnosis of high-risk TET (*n*= 72) and low-risk TET (*n*=83) who underwent unenhanced CT (UECT) and contrast-enhanced CT (CECT). The radiomic features were extracted from the UECT and CECT of each patient at the largest cross-section of the lesion. The classification performance was evaluated with a nested leave-one-out cross-validation approach combining the least absolute shrinkage and selection operator feature selection and four classifiers: generalised linear model (GLM), k-nearest neighbor (KNN), support vector machine (SVM) and random forest (RF). The receiver-operating characteristic curve (ROC) and the area under the curve (AUC) were used to evaluate the performance of the classifiers.

Results: The combination of UECT and CECT radiomic features demonstrated the best performance to differentiate high-risk TETs from low-risk TETs for all four classifiers. Among these classifiers, the RF had the highest AUC of 0.87, followed by GLM (AUC=0.86), KNN (AUC=0.86) and SVM (AUC=0.84).

Conclusions: Machine learning-based CT radiomic analysis allows for the differentiation of high-risk TETs and low-risk TETs with excellent performance, representing a promising tool to assist clinical decision making in patients with TETs.

引自: *Int J Stroke*, 2018, 13(6): 612-632

Passage 24

Abstract

Aim: Real-world data inform the outcome comparisons and help the development of new therapeutic strategies. To this end, we aimed to describe the full characteristics and outcomes in the Epidemiological Strategy and Medical Economics (ESME) cohort, a large national contemporary observational database of patients with metastatic breast cancer (MBC).

Methods: Women aged $\geqslant 18$ years with newly diagnosed MBC and who initiated MBC treatment between January 2008 and December 2016 in one of the 18 French Comprehensive Cancer Centers (N=22,109) were included. We assessed the full patients' characteristics, first-line treatments, overall survival (OS) and first-line progression-free survival, as well as updated prognostic factors in the whole cohort and among the 3 major subtypes: hormone receptor positive and HER2-negative (HR+/HER2−, n=13,656), HER2-positive (HER2+, n=4017) and triple-negative (n=2963) tumours.

Results: The median OS of the whole cohort was 39.5 months (95% confidence interval [CI], 38.7-40.3). Five-year OS was 33.8%. OS differed significantly between the 3 subtypes (p<0.0001) with a median OS of 43.3 (95% CI, 42.5-44.5) in HR+/HER2−; 50.1 (95% CI, 47.6-53.1) in HER2+; and 14.8 months (95% CI, 14.1-15.5) in triple-negative subgroups, respectively. Beyond performance status, the following variables had a constant significant negative prognostic impact on OS in the whole cohort and among subtypes: older age at diagnosis of metastases (except for the triple-negative subtype), metastasis-free interval between 6 and 24 months, presence of visceral metastases and number of metastatic sites$\geqslant 3$.

Conclusions: The ESME program represents a unique large-scale real-life cohort on MBC. This study highlights important situations of high medical need within MBC patients.

引自: *Eur J Cancer*, 2020,129: 60-70

Passage 25

Abstract

Introduction: The number of occupational therapy degree programs in Australia has increased substantially over the last decade. During this time, Australian academics have produced a significant amount of scholarship focussed on entry-level education; however, the landscape of this scholarship has not been examined. The aim of this study was to review the literature on the scholarship of entry-level Australian occupational therapy education programs, specifically the topics explored and methods employed.

Methods: An extensive search of nine databases produced 1,002 papers related to occupational therapy education. Two researchers screened each paper using inclusion and exclusion criteria. Seventy‐six articles, published between 2000 and September 2019, were included. Data were extracted using a coding tool, and entered into NVivo, where data were analysed using queries and tallies of the characteristics of the articles.

Results: Sixty‐eight articles were research and eight were other peer reviewed literature. Articles primarily focussed on student characteristics and perceptions. Quantitative research designs were predominant with surveys the most frequently used method. There were few articles that addressed the topic of teaching methods and approaches, and of these none addressed occupation-centred teaching. No articles addressed the learning environment. Four articles reported on an educational intervention that targeted participation, and attitudes/perceptions or knowledge/skills of students and/or academics. These findings inform understanding about what has been completed so far in the scholarship; and what topic focus and research designs could address gaps in existing knowledge.

Conclusions: This review elucidated topics that have been well researched (student focus), as well as gaps in the scholarship (teaching methods and approaches including occupation-centred teaching, and the learning environment). It showed that quantitative designs were predominant, with qualitative approaches less frequently adopted. The results of this review could assist academics and researchers to focus their scholarship on topics that require further investigation and diversify research methods.

引自: *Aust Occup Ther J,* 2020, 67(4): 373-395

练习参考答案

主要参考文献

陈浩元, 1998. 科技期刊标准化 18 讲. 北京: 北京师范大学出版社

陈续跃, 2002. 医学论文中英语摘要写作典型用词错误分析. 遵义医学院学报, 25(3): 291-294

崔正勤, 1992. 现代英语句式转换. 济南: 山东教育出版社

范华泉, 冷怀明, 郭建秀, 2004. 我国医学期刊论文英文摘要典型错误分析. 中国科技期刊研究. 15(1): 104-106

范华泉, 罗明奎, 余党会, 等, 2004. 中英美科技期刊论文题目特征的比较分析. 中国科技期刊研究, 15(5): 542-544

范晓晖, 2005. 论医学论文英文摘要中被动语态的滥用. 中国科技翻译, 18(4): 11-14

国林祥, 2002. 医学英语写作与翻译. 北京: 高等教育出版社

李朝品, 王先寅, 王健, 2009. 医学论文英文摘要写作. 北京: 人民卫生出版社

李传英, 2005. 医学论文英文摘要写作中的语法修辞手段. 武汉大学学报(医学版), 26(6): 808-810

李传英, 潘承礼, 2015. 医学英语写作与翻译. 武汉: 武汉大学出版社

李慎安, 李寿星, 1997. 计量单位实用指南. 北京: 中国计量出版社. 319-540

李照国, 2008. 中医常用语句英译探析(一). 中西医结合学报, 6(1):107-110

陆刚, 2003. 论文章标题英译的功能对等. 中国科技翻译, 16(4): 28-30

钱尔凡, 王先寅, 2010. 科技论文中英文摘要的人称与语态问题. 编辑学报, 22(4):319-321

钱寿初, 2002. 医学英语写作技巧和词语辨析. 北京: 人民军医出版社

钱寿初, 2001. 作者署名和作者的贡献. 中国科技期刊研究, 12(1): 1-3

任胜利, 2014. 英语科技论文撰写与投稿. 2 版. 北京: 科学出版社

单其昌, 1990. 汉英翻译技巧. 北京: 外语教学与研究出版社

腾真如, 2004. 采用第一人称撰写科技论文摘要的探讨. 中国科技期刊研究, 15(4):492-493

汪佳明, 汪颖, 何玲, 2002. 科技论文英文摘要写作中的一些问题. 中国科技期刊研究, 2002, 13(4): 360-362

王桂梅, 2016. 中国知网与万方中文医学期刊数据库比较研究. 图书情报导刊, 1(9): 123-126

王健, 周玉梅, 2005. 医学英语的语用翻译. 中国科技翻译, 18(3): 17-19

王先寅, 钱尔凡, 2012. 医学论文英文摘要写作常见问题分析. 皖南医学院学报.31(6):511-515

王征爱, 宋建武, 2002. 医学科技论文英文摘要的时态、语态和人称. 第一军医大学学报, 22(6): 574-576

王征爱, 宋建武, 2002. 英文医学科技论文写作中词的选择与搭配. 第一军医大学学报, 22(9): 862-865

王征爱, 许瑾, 宋建武, 2002. 医学科技论文几个高频词的用法. 第一军医大学学报, 22(11): 1053-1056

王征爱, 许瑾, 张丽莉, 2003. 英语医学科技论文中冠词的使用. 第一军医大学学报, 23(5): 512-514

新闻出版署图书管理司, 1998a. 科学技术报告、学位论文和学术论文的编写格式: GB 7713—87. 北京: 中国标准出版社, 264-271

新闻出版署图书管理司, 1998b. 文摘编写规则: GB 6447—86. 北京: 中国标准出版社, 259-263

于双成, 张云秋, 李正红, 2004. 向国外医学期刊投稿要注意关键词的标引. 中国科技期刊研究, 15(1): 116-117

张鹏, 2005. 论对等翻译的限度. 天津外国语学院学报, 12(2): 25-27

张宗美, 1992. 科技汉英翻译技巧. 北京: 宇航出版社

章恒珍, 2004. 医学英文摘要写作. 广州: 暨南大学出版社

章振邦, 1997. 新编英语语法(第三版). 上海: 上海外语教育出版社

赵萱, 郑仰成, 2006. 科技英语翻译. 北京: 外语教学与研究出版社

照日格图, 2006. 关于医学论文英文摘要的撰写要求(二). 中华口腔医学杂志, 41(5): 316-318

照日格图, 2006. 关于医学论文英文摘要的撰写要求(六). 中华口腔医学杂志, 41(9): 570-571

照日格图, 2006. 关于医学论文英文摘要的撰写要求(三). 中华口腔医学杂志, 41(6): 383-384

照日格图, 2006. 关于医学论文英文摘要的撰写要求(四). 中华口腔医学杂志, 41(7): 443-445

中华人民共和国国家质量监督检验检疫总局, 中国国家标准化管理委员会, 2012. 汉语拼音正词法基本规则: GB/T 16159—2012.https://www.doc88.com/p-1106692088129.html[2015-11-05]

周英智, 孙瑶, 2007. 国内医学论文英文题名问题调查与分析. 中国科技期刊研究, 18(3): 524-526

Advice to contributors. http://bmj.bmjjournals.com/advice

Haynes RB, Mulrow CD, Huth EJ, et al, 1990. More informative abstracts revised. Ann Intern Med, 113(1): 69-76

Joseph H. Greenberg, 1984. Some Universals of Grammar with Particular Reference to the Order of Meaningful Elements: Joseph H. Greenberg(ed.) University of Language. London: MIT Press, 73:113

Nation P, 2000. Learning Vocabulary in Another Language. Cambridge England: CUP

Uniform Requirements for Manuscripts Submitted to Biomedical Journals: Writing and Editing for Biomedical Publication. www.icmje.org (Updated April 2010)